Post-Traumatic Arthritis

Savyasachi C. Thakkar
Erik A. Hasenboehler

Editors

Post-Traumatic Arthritis

Diagnosis, Management and Outcomes

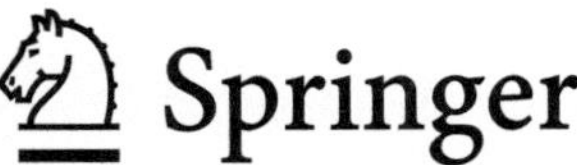 Springer

Editors
Savyasachi C. Thakkar
Hip & Knee Reconstruction Surgery
Johns Hopkins
Department of Orthopaedic Surgery
Columbia, MD
USA

Erik A. Hasenboehler
Department of Orthopaedic Surgery
Adult Trauma Service
The Johns Hopkins Medical Institution
Baltimore, MD
USA

ISBN 978-3-030-50415-1   ISBN 978-3-030-50413-7   (eBook)
https://doi.org/10.1007/978-3-030-50413-7

This Springer imprint is published by the registered company Springer Nature Switzerland AG
The registered company address is: Gewerbestrasse 11, 6330 Cham, Switzerland

I would like to dedicate this book to my parents Mrs. Heena C. Thakkar and Dr. C.J. Thakkar for their dedicated upbringing and commitment towards excellence in life. I would also like to dedicate the book to my wife Dr. Rashmi S. Thakkar and my children Sahuri and Shaarav who have provided me with untiring support, love and patience. Without these individuals, I would not be where I am today!

Savyasachi C. Thakkar, MD

This book is dedicated to my beloved father Dr. Giorgio Hasenboehler, who passed years ago of cancer, and to my mother Elfriede Hasenboehler, whom have always supported me and have fostered my passion for medicine and the surgical specialty. I also would like to acknowledge my love Ana Torregrosa for her infinite support, and last my dearest children Nikolas and Lukas to whom this book shall be an example of commitment to teaching, learning and dedication to a fulfilling profession.

Erik A. Hasenboehler, MD

Preface

The incidence and prevalence of post-traumatic arthritis is increasing globally due to longevity of life, increased activity and injuries. Orthopaedic surgeons are skilled at treating traumatic injuries to the extremities and joints. Early anatomic stabilization is required when it comes to traumatic joint reconstructions. Unfortunately, post-traumatic osteoarthritis (PTOA) of a joint is an unpredictable consequence that can occur at any time, in different presentations, severity and complexity after an injury. Delayed post-traumatic complications require a thorough understanding of anatomic principles, meticulous planning and symphonic surgical execution. Timing of treatment and subsequent care of PTOA are the most essential aspects to achieve excellent outcomes in this challenging group of patients.

The book is broadly divided into two parts – upper extremity and lower extremity – to encompass the breadth of the subject while delving into the unique challenges of each joint. Additional parts of the book will also cover the basic science of cartilage degeneration in response to trauma, dedicated imaging modalities that optimize visualization and surgical planning of the arthritic joint and the economic impact of post-traumatic osteoarthritis.

It is our hope that the readers of this book will receive a comprehensive framework to base their clinical decisions and learn about the latest techniques in managing these challenging injuries. The book is geared towards general orthopaedic surgeons and sub-specialty trained orthopaedic surgeons with equal measure. The book has also been written for orthopaedic surgeons in training who require a broad overview of this subject to complement their education.

This book would not have been possible without the tremendous synergy between basic science experts, radiologists and orthopaedic surgeons with a passion for teaching by example. On behalf of the editors and the authors, we hope that you enjoy reading this book and apply the principles of managing post-traumatic osteoarthritis for the benefit of your patients.

Columbia, MD, USA
Baltimore, MD, USA

Savyasachi C. Thakkar
Erik A. Hasenboehler

Acknowledgments

The creation of this book has been a collective effort of several professionals. First, we would like to thank the authors who have provided us their invaluable time and energy to assemble various surgical cases that highlight the sentinel principles of post-traumatic arthritis. Second, we would like to acknowledge Ms. Meera V. Shanbhag who has devoted her talents as a pre-medical student at Vanderbilt University in reviewing manuscripts and collating the contents of this book.

Third, this book would not have been possible without the oversight and planning provided by Mr. Kristopher Spring and Ms. Abha Krishnan. Both of them have provided us with tremendous resources to make this book a reality.

Finally, we would like to thank our families for providing us with incredible support and motivation to devote time to projects such as this.

Contents

Part I   Background and Assessment of Post-traumatic Arthritis

1   The Role of TGF-β in Post-traumatic Osteoarthritis   3
Gehua Zhen and Xu Cao

2   Imaging Modalities for Post-traumatic Arthritis.   15
Filippo Del Grande, Luca Deabate, and Christian Candrian

**3   Economic Implications of Post-traumatic Arthritis of the Hip and
Knee**   25
Richard Iorio, Kelvin Y. Kim, Afshin A. Anoushiravani, and
William J. Long

Part II   Post-traumatic Arthritis of the Upper Extremity

4   Post-traumatic Glenohumeral Arthritis   45
Uma Srikumaran and Eric Huish

5   Post-traumatic Arthritis of the Elbow.   59
Kevin O'Malley, Ryan Churchill, Curtis M. Henn, and Michael
W. Kessler

6   Post-traumatic Arthritis of the Wrist   73
Sophia A. Strike and Philip E. Blazar

7   Post-traumatic Arthritis of the Hand   97
Andrew P. Harris, Thomas J. Kim, and Christopher Got

Part III   Post-traumatic Arthritis of the Lower Extremity

8   Post-traumatic Arthritis of the Acetabulum.   111
Savyasachi C. Thakkar, Erik A. Hasenboehler, and Chandrashekhar
J. Thakkar

9   Post-traumatic Arthritis of the Proximal Femur   135
Raj M. Amin, Erik A. Hasenboehler, and Babar Shafiq

10   Post-traumatic Arthritis of the Distal Femur   153
Karthikeyan Ponnusamy and Ajit Deshmukh

11   Post-traumatic Arthritis of the Proximal Tibia   167
Stefanie Hirsiger, Lukas Clerc, and Hermes H. Miozzari

12   Post-traumatic Arthritis of the Ankle   185
Nigel N. Hsu and Lew Schon

13   Post-traumatic Arthritis of the Foot   199
Ram K. Alluri and Eric W. Tan

Index   219

Contributors

Ram K. Alluri, MD Department of Orthopaedic Surgery, Keck School of Medicine of USC, Los Angeles, CA, USA

Raj M. Amin, MD Department of Orthopaedic Surgery, The Johns Hopkins Medical Institutions, Baltimore, MD, USA

Afshin A. Anoushiravani, MD Department of Orthopaedic Surgery, Albany Medical Center, Albany, NY, USA

Philip E. Blazar, MD Brigham and Women's Hospital, Boston, MA, USA

Christian Candrian, MD Servizio di ortopedia, Ospedale Regionale di Lugano, Ticino, Switzerland

Xu Cao, PhD Department of Orthopaedic Surgery, The Johns Hopkins University, Baltimore, MD, USA

Ryan Churchill, MD Medstar Georgetown University Hospital, Department of Orthopaedics, Washington, DC, USA

Lukas Clerc, MD Division of Orthopaedic and Traumatology, Department of Surgery, Geneva University Hospitals, Faculty of Medicine, University of Geneva, Geneva, Switzerland

Luca Deabate, MD Servizio di ortopedia, Ospedale Regionale di Lugano, Ticino, Switzerland

Filippo Del Grande, MD Clinica di Radiologia EOC, Istituto di Imaging della Svizzera Italiana, Ente Ospedaliero Cantonale, Ticino, Switzerland

Ajit Deshmukh, MD Department of Orthopaedic Surgery, New York University, New York, NY, USA

Christopher Got, MD Brown University, Warren Alpert Medical School, Providence, RI, USA

Andrew P. Harris, MD Warren Alpert Medical School of Brown University, Providence, RI, USA

Erik A. Hasenboehler, MD Department of Orthopaedic Surgery, Adult Trauma Service, The Johns Hopkins Medical Institution, Baltimore, MD, USA

Curtis M. Henn, MD Medstar Georgetown University Hospital, Department of Orthopaedics, Washington, DC, USA

Stefanie Hirsiger, MD Division of Orthopaedic and Traumatology, Department of Surgery, Geneva University Hospitals, Faculty of Medicine, University of Geneva, Geneva, Switzerland

Nigel N. Hsu, MD Department of Orthopaedic Surgery, Johns Hopkins University, Baltimore, MD, USA

Eric Huish, DO Stanislaus Orthopaedics & Sports Medicine Clinic, Modesto, CA, USA

Richard Iorio, MD Brigham and Women's Hospital, Member of the Faculty, Harvard Medical School, Boston, MA, USA

Michael W. Kessler, MD Medstar Georgetown University Hospital, Department of Orthopaedics, Washington, DC, USA

Kelvin Y. Kim, MD Department of Orthopaedic Surgery, UNLV School of Medicine, Las Vegas, NV, USA

Thomas J. Kim, MD Brown University, Warren Alpert Medical School, Providence, RI, USA

William J. Long, MD, FRCSC ISK Institute, Department of Orthopaedic Surgery, NYU Langone Medical Center, Hospital for Joint Diseases, New York, NY, USA

Hermes H. Miozzari, MD Division of Orthopaedic and Traumatology, Department of Surgery, Geneva University Hospitals, Faculty of Medicine, University of Geneva, Geneva, Switzerland

Kevin O'Malley, MD Medstar Georgetown University Hospital, Department of Orthopaedics, Washington, DC, USA

Karthikeyan Ponnusamy, MD Pinnacle Orthopaedics, Canton, GA, USA

Lew Schon, MD Department of Orthopaedic Surgery, Mercy Medical Center, Baltimore, MD, USA

Babar Shafiq, MD Department of Orthopaedic Surgery, The Johns Hopkins Medical Institutions, Baltimore, MD, USA

Uma Srikumaran, MD, MBA The Johns Hopkins University, Division of Shoulder and Elbow Surgery, Columbia, MD, USA

Sophia A. Strike, MD Johns Hopkins University School of Medicine, Baltimore, MD, USA

Eric W. Tan, MD Department of Orthopaedic Surgery, Keck School of Medicine of USC, Los Angeles, CA, USA

Chandrashekhar J. Thakkar, MS (Ortho) Joints Masters Institute, Mumbai, Maharashtra, India

Breach Candy Hospital, Mumbai, Maharashtra, India

Lilavati Hospital, Mumbai, Maharashtra, India

Hinduja Hospital, Mumbai, Maharashtra, India

Savyasachi C. Thakkar, MD Hip & Knee Reconstruction Surgery, Johns Hopkins Department of Orthopaedic Surgery, Columbia, MD, USA

Gehua Zhen, MD Department of Orthopaedic Surgery, The Johns Hopkins University, Baltimore, MD, USA

Part I
Background and Assessment of Post-traumatic Arthritis

Chapter 1
The Role of TGF-β in Post-traumatic Osteoarthritis

Gehua Zhen and Xu Cao

Key Points
- Osteoarthritis is a disease that affects the whole joint. Biochemical and biomechanical interactions among different components within the joint actively participate in and contribute to the development and progression of the disease.
- TGF-β plays an important role in the pathogenesis of osteoarthritis. Temporal and spatial regulation of TGF-β activity is critical for maintenance of homeostasis of joint tissues.
- The effects of TGF-β differ according to tissue type within the joint and may vary at different time points. Various tissue-specific treatments targeting TGF-β signaling may produce optimal therapeutic effects.

Introduction

Osteoarthritis is the most common degenerative joint disease. Although osteoarthritis develops in joints naturally over time, it progresses rapidly after traumatic injury. Extreme physical demands or injuries to bones, ligaments, menisci, or articular cartilage predispose patients to post-traumatic osteoarthritis (PTOA) [1]. Despite surgical reconstruction of the joint components, osteoarthritis still develops at a high rate after joint injuries. PTOA accounts for an estimated 12% of all cases of osteoarthritis, with approximately 5.6 million people in the United States living with PTOA [2]. The symptoms of PTOA, including joint pain, swelling, stiffness, and

G. Zhen · X. Cao (✉)
Department of Orthopaedic Surgery, The Johns Hopkins University, Baltimore, MD, USA
e-mail: gzhen1@jhmi.edu; xcao11@jhmi.edu

© Springer Nature Switzerland AG 2021
S. C. Thakkar, E. A. Hasenboehler (eds.), *Post-Traumatic Arthritis*,
https://doi.org/10.1007/978-3-030-50413-7_1

limited movement, are similar to symptoms of other types of osteoarthritis. The pathological characteristics of PTOA include articular cartilage degeneration, abnormal bone formation, and aberrant angiogenesis in subchondral bone.

The risk of developing PTOA can be minimized by preventing injuries to the joint. According to osteoarthritis management guidelines, treatment of PTOA often starts with lifestyle modifications, including weight loss, low-impact exercise, and strengthening of the muscles surrounding the joint [2]. Analgesics and anti-inflammatory medications are the primary nonsurgical approach to control symptoms. However, these medications can cause gastrointestinal complications and their efficacy quickly becomes blunted. To date, there is no approved pharmacologic agent, biologic therapy, or procedure to prevent progressive destruction of the osteoarthritic joint. Many agents have been developed and tested to treat osteoarthritis-related abnormalities. Glucosamine sulfate, chondroitin sulfate, sodium hyaluronan, and matrix metalloproteinase (MMP) inhibitors have been tested in various clinical trials [3]. Unfortunately, the ability of these medications to stop or reverse osteoarthritis progression is still limited. In end-stage PTOA, when medications are no longer effective to control symptoms, surgical treatment such as arthroscopic debridement, reconstruction, or joint replacement is usually necessary.

A new treatment paradigm relies heavily on novel findings in pathogenesis studies. Progress in exploring new biologic and pharmaceutical interventions has been impeded because the pathomechanical cause of PTOA is still poorly understood. Currently, most patients in the United States receive appropriate surgery and/or physical therapy immediately after an acute joint injury. However, PTOA develops eventually in a considerable proportion of these patients. Surgical reconstruction may not fully restore normal joint kinematics, causing an altered mechanical environment that may lead to secondary cartilage degeneration and joint abnormalities [4]. Osteoarthritis risk factors such as obesity, aging, and joint malalignment accelerate decline of joint function. These factors directly or indirectly change the mechanical environment of the joint after traumatic injury. This evidence collectively indicates that chronic alteration of mechanical stress could be the one of the primary triggers of PTOA onset and progression. Because osteoarthritis affects the whole joint, changes in biochemical and/or biomechanical properties of one tissue may influence the homeostasis and integrity of other parts of the joint.

The Functional Unit of Articular Cartilage and Subchondral Bone

Recently, patient-specific finite element stress analysis has been used to measure cartilage stress from residual surface incongruity after traumatic joint injury. However, factors that trigger stress alterations in cartilage are not limited to cartilage itself. As a functional unit, the joint involves constant interaction between various tissues [5]. Because of the physical contact between cartilage and bone, the mechanical influence of the subchondral bone on articular cartilage is critical to the maintenance of cartilage homeostasis. Articular cartilage buffers loading force and prevents mechanical damage to subchondral bone, while subchondral bone provides structural support for the overlying articular cartilage. Thus, the homeostasis and integrity of these two tissues rely on the biochemical and biomechanical interplay between them [5]. A finite element simulation study indicated that slight expansion of subchondral bone volume or elevation of subchondral bone stiffness dramatically increases the mechanical stress in the overlying articular cartilage [6]. Subchondral bone responds rapidly to changes in the mechanical environment, and its structural changes can be detected during the early stages of osteoarthritis. When the ability of subchondral bone to provide stable mechanical support is impaired, one would expect the stress distribution in articular cartilage to alter accordingly. The mechanical impact of subchondral bone on articular cartilage is translated into biochemical signals that influence cartilage homeostasis [7]. Therefore, exploring how subchondral bone responds to an abnormal environment and how it subsequently affects cartilage homeostasis is critical to understanding the pathogenesis of PTOA.

To maintain proper levels of calcium and phosphorus in circulation and reshape the micro-damage that occurs during normal activities, adult bone is constantly resorbed and formed in a process called bone remodeling. To provide stable support to the overlying cartilage, normal subchondral bone maintains the turnover rate at a very low level compared with that of the long bone trabeculae. However, the bone turnover rate increases dramatically in osteoarthritic subchondral bone [8]. The sequence of events that occurs in normal bone remodeling is disrupted, and the discordant behavior of osteoblast and osteoclast lineage cells results in abnormal bone formation with hypo-mineralization. The de novo bone formation in the osteoarthritic subchondral bone suggests that the new bone does not form in the resorption pit of the bone surface but rather in the bone marrow cavity, without appropriate connections to the original trabeculae. Understanding the mechanism that underlies the uncoupled bone resorption and formation is imperative for developing effective measures to mitigate subchondral bone abnormality and consequent cartilage degeneration. In the osteoarthritic environment, particularly during adaptation to the new mechanical environment, subchondral bone is destroyed by highly activated osteoclasts. Consequently, high levels of active transforming growth factor-β (TGF-β) are released from the sequestration of bone matrix, triggering sequential pathological events at the onset and during the progression of osteoarthritis [6].

TGF-β

TGF-β is a cytokine that belongs to the TGF-® superfamily, members of which have been highly conserved through evolution and are involved in a broad range of biological processes [9]. TGF-β is one of four major subfamilies of this superfamily. There are three TGF-β isoforms: TGF-β1, TGF-β2, and TGF-β3. These isoforms have distinct tissue-specific expression profiles but use the same receptor-signaling systems [10]. On secretion, the homodimers of mature TGF-β peptide link nonco-valently to latency-associated peptide (LAP), with LAP masking its receptor-binding domains and rendering it inactive [11]. The small latent complex formed by LAP and TGF-β further interacts with latent TGF-β binding protein in the extracel-lular matrix and forms the large latent complex. Although TGF-β synthesis is wide-spread, activation is localized to sites where TGF-β is released from latency. Temporal-spatial regulation of TGF-® activation is crucial for appropriate function of this cytokine, and the abundant latent TGF-®s that are deposited in the extracel-lular matrix ensure that sufficient TGF-β can be activated when necessary. The TGF-β activation mechanism is tissue-specific and cellular context-dependent [12]. For example, enzyme-mediated proteolytic cleavage has been reported to be the dominant pathway for TGF-β to be activated in tumors or metastasis, whereas pul-monary fibrosis is induced by integrin-mediated excessive TGF-β activation. Multiple mechanisms of TGF-β activation may be used or switched from one to another depending on the cellular context or environmental stimuli [11].

TGF-βs signal via the heteromeric complexes of two related transmembrane ser-ine/threonine kinase receptors, TGF-β type I and type II receptors (TβR-I and TβR-II). TβR-I is also termed activin receptor-like kinase (ALK). The dimeric ligand of TGF-β binds to the extracellular domains of TβR-I and TβR-II, inducing close proximity of the receptors. Unlike TβR-II, which is unique to its ligand, dis-tinctive TβR-Is can be phosphorylated by TβR-II, which determines the specificity of the downstream signaling pathway [13]. Smad2 and Smad3 are substrates of ALK5, whereas ALK1 phosphorylates Smad1, Smad5, and Smad8. After phosphor-ylation by the receptor, the phosphorylated receptor-regulated Smad forms a com-plex with the common mediator Smad4 and translocates to the nucleus where they interact with other transcription factors (cofactors) to regulate transcriptional responses. In addition to the Smad-dependent canonical pathway, TGF-β also sig-nals through the Smad-independent or noncanonical pathways. The tumor necrosis factor receptor-associated factor 4 (TRAF4), TRAF6, p38 mitogen-activated pro-tein kinase (p38 MAPK), TGF-β-activated kinase 1 (TAK1; also known as MAP3K7), Ras homolog gene family, phosphoinositide 3-kinase (PI3K), protein kinase B, extracellular signal-regulated kinase (ERK), JUN N-terminal kinase (JNK), and nuclear factor-κB (NF-κB) have all been reported to mediate the TGF-β signaling pathway [14].

The Role of TGF-β in Osteoarthritic Subchondral Bone

Temporal-spatial regulation of the TGF-β activation process is the prerequisite for TGF-β to function appropriately. Additionally, the effect of TGF-β is influenced by the expression levels and activity of TGF-β receptors, as well as downstream fac-tors. When TGF-β signaling is up- or downregulated, tissue homeostasis fails in the affected organs. Abnormal TGF-β signaling has been observed in various immune diseases, cancer, heart disease, diabetes, Camurati-Engelmann disease, Marfan syn-drome, Loeys-Dietz syndrome, Parkinson disease, and acquired immune deficiency syndrome [15]. Premature activation of TGF-βs and the consequent pathological events in subchondral bone were found to contribute to the development and progression of osteoarthritis. In physiological conditions, TGF-βs in the matrix are activated and released into the interstitial space or lumens during tissue injury or remodeling. Stem cells or progenitor cells harbored in the nearby tissue are then recruited to the remodeling site with the highest TGF-β concentration [16]. In conjunction with other signals, TGF-βs further regulate whether the stem cells differentiate or self-renew. In this way, TGF-β acts as the key coupling factor during bone remodeling that directs the migration of mesenchymal stem cells (MSCs) in normal conditions [17].

Intra-articular injury alters the mechanical environment of the joint dramatically. Osteoclastic bone resorption is substantially elevated in adaptation to the new mechanical environment, which results in the release of a large quantity of active TGF-βs in the relatively confined space of subchondral bone. The normal pattern of TGF-β gradients from the bone resorption site to the bone marrow cavity is then disrupted because of the excessive liberation of TGF-β. As a result, MSCs or osteoprogenitors cluster in the bone marrow cavity or randomly deposit on bone surfaces. De novo bone formation at inappropriate times and/or locations ensues [6].

TGF-β also regulates stem cell behavior through its direct or indirect effects in modulating the bone marrow microenvironment. For example, bone formation always couples with angiogenesis and vascularization, which creates an environment rich in MSCs. TGF-β can promote angiogenesis, which provides an environment favorable to bone formation and therefore contributes to the abnormal bone formation in osteoarthritic subchondral bone. TGF-β signaling plays an important role in epithelial-mesenchymal and endothelial-mesenchymal transitions [18]. In the context of different morphogenetic events, epithelial or endothelial cells transdifferentiate into stromal lineage cells, which are involved in many pathological conditions such as fibrosis [19]. Therefore, aberrant elevated active TGF-β could be associated with formation of poorly mineralized bone and increased marrow perfusion and fibrosis in osteoarthritic subchondral bone. When active TGF-β1 is released prematurely by osteoblastic cells in the transgenic mouse, early onset of osteoarthritic-like changes in knee joints is common [6]. In these mice, the abnormally elevated TGF-β levels in subchondral bone induce abnormal bone formation and structure alteration and consequently contribute to articular cartilage degeneration [6]. The linkage of gain of function of Smad3 mutations with the early onset of hip and knee osteoarthritis in humans also supports this notion [20]. Indeed, osteoarthritis progression can be attenuated substantially in the mouse PTOA model when the TGF-β signaling pathway in MSCs is blocked genetically [6].

The Role of TGF-β in Osteoarthritic Articular Cartilage

Cartilage degeneration is another major concern in osteoarthritis. Articular cartilage has limited self-repair capability, and cartilage lesions rarely heal if the damage is larger than 3 mm in diameter [21]. The role of TGF-β in cartilage is different than its role in subchondral bone. For example, genetically deleting TβR-II or Smad3 in chondrocytes resulted in early onset of osteoarthritis in animal models, as evidenced by the hypocellularity and decreased matrix protein synthesis of chondrocytes [22]. The effects of TGF-β in stimulating chondrogenic condensation, proliferating chondroprogenitors, and inhibiting terminal differentiation of chondrocytes have been evidenced in multiple in vitro studies. These findings suggest that TGF-β is critical to maintaining articular cartilage's functional and structural integrity [23]. The abundant latent TGF-β storage (~300 ng/mL) in the extracellular matrix of cartilage provides sufficient raw material for TGF-β activation [24]. In physiological conditions, minimal amounts of active TGF-βs are needed for the maintenance of cartilage physiological function. In osteoarthritic cartilage, many mechanisms involved in the process of TGF-β activation such as MMPs or integrins are altered [25], which may lead to excessive or insufficient activation of TGF-β. Intra-articular injury likely alters the mechanical stress distribution in articular cartilage directly or indirectly through subchondral bone. Subchondral bone changes its structure constantly in response to the mechanical environment. During the period of structural fluctuation, the capacity of subchondral bone to dissipate the mechanical load is altered or impaired. Because physiological mechanical stimulation is indispensable for maintaining the function and structural integrity of articular cartilage, abnormal mechanical stress (altered intensity or frequency) can promote catabolic events and induce cartilage degeneration [26]. Although the soluble factors responsible for propagating mechanical signals into biochemical signaling are still unclear, evidence suggests an important role of TGF-β in mechanical transduction pathways in chondrocytes [27]. In addition to TGF-β activation pathways, it has been reported that shear forces can liberate active TGF-β from the sequestration of LAP in synovial fluid [28]. TβR-I-specific inhibitor eliminated the anabolic effect of shear stress in stimulating protein synthesis in the superficial zone of articular cartilage [29]. These findings indicate that abnormal biomechanical and biochemical environments alter the TGF-β activation process, and excessive or insufficient levels of TGF-β, in turn, effect the chondrocytes' survival and function.

The responsiveness of chondrocytes to TGF-β also depends on the expression levels and activity of its receptors. The canonic TGF-β signaling pathway includes the formation of the heteromeric complexes of type I and type II receptors. A sequential phosphorylation and nuclear translocation of downstream Smads ultimately triggers the expression of the target genes. Dysregulation of TGF-β signaling pathways or differential expression of TGF-β receptors in the chondrocytes has been reported in various in vivo studies, including a surgically induced PTOA animal model. TβR-II degradation and decreased TβR-I expression blunt the sensitivity of articular chondrocytes to TGF-β, contributing to cartilage degeneration [30]. The expression pattern of TβR-I in chondrocytes is markedly different in osteoarthritic cartilage. The dominant TβR-I receptor shifts from ALK5 to ALK1 [31]. TGF-β signals from these two pathways influence the metabolism of chondrocytes in an opposing fashion [32]. TGF-β acts as an anabolic factor on chondrocytes, stimulating matrix protein production when signaling through ALK5, and as a catabolic factor when ALK1 is mediating its downstream signaling [33]. In addition, there are several other factors involved in the signaling transduction pathway of TGF-β by modulating the sensitivity of receptors to the ligand or the internalization process of the receptors. For example, endoglin can facilitate the binding of TGF-β to its receptors with the preference to recruit ALK1 [34]. Therefore, elevated expression of endoglin in chondrocytes may promote the catabolic effect by making ALK1/pSmad1/5/8 the dominant signaling pathway of TGF-β. Betaglycan is a homolog of endoglin but it has distinctive functions in regulating the TGF-β pathway. Betaglycan can direct clathrin-mediated endocytosis of TβR-I and TβR-II [35] and increase the sensitivity of TβR-II to its ligands [36]. CD109 is another identified TGF-β co-receptor. It negatively regulates TGF-β signaling by promoting TGF-β receptor internalization and degradation [37]. Thus, during osteoarthritis development, the altered TGF-β signaling in articular cartilage may potentially be corrected by targeting these co-receptors or modulators.

The Role of TGF-β in the Osteoarthritic Synovial System

As avascular tissue, articular cartilage is nourished mainly by the synovial fluid that is secreted by the synovium. Therefore, articular cartilage is vulnerable to pathological changes in the synovial system. Although osteoarthritis is defined as "non-inflammatory arthritis," synovial hyperplasia, macrophage infiltration, and angiogenesis are common characteristics of osteoarthritic abnormality [38]. Histologically recognizable synovitis occurs in more than one-third of patients with symptomatic osteoarthritis. Persistent or episodic synovitis has been found to be related closely to osteoarthritic pain. The cytokines released by synovium have been recognized as being of pathological and clinical importance in the development of osteoarthritis. Notably, human and animal studies suggest that the concentration of TGF-β1 might be used as a prognostic indicator for PTOA. In a rabbit meniscectomy model, early postoperative concentrations of TGF-β1 in synovial lavage fluid were correlated positively with the severity of PTOA [39]. In patients with acute or chronic anterior cruciate ligament rupture, the levels of TGF-β in the synovial fluid were consistent with the persistence of inflammatory reactions, and their synovial fluid cytokine profiles were associated with the risk of developing PTOA [40]. TGF-β typically serves as an important immune suppressor during the process of inflammation. Knocking out TGF-β1 in mice is usually lethal because it induces severe inflammatory events. TGF-β receptors are expressed widely in immune cell types and have broad activities in immune regulation. In most immune reactions, TGF-β acts as a suppressor. Conversely, TGF-β sometimes plays a pro-inflammatory role by promoting the differentiation of TH17 lineage cells [41]. TGF-β was found to induce the differentiation from "attacking" type I macrophages toward "inflammatory molecule secreting" type II macrophages [42, 43]. This may underlie the mechanism of TGF-β in augmenting the tumor necrosis factor-α- or interleukin

(IL)-1β-induced expression of MMP3, IL-6, IL-8, and macrophage inflammation protein 1α in synoviocytes [44]. Therefore, TGF-β and its downstream signaling could potentially be therapeutic targets for osteoarthritic synovitis.

Modulation of TGF-β Activity as a Potential Therapy for Osteoarthritis

Currently, no medications have shown the disease-modifying efficacy and clinically meaningful effects needed to gain regulatory approval. In animal studies and clinical trials, controlling subchondral bone abnormality seems to mitigate the advancement of osteoarthritis. Increased osteoclast activity and bone turnover rate are known pathological characteristics of subchondral bone in osteoarthritis. For this reason, the efficacy of the common antiresorptive medicine, bisphosphonate, has been tested for treating osteoarthritis in clinical trials [45]. Though the results in humans have not been as encouraging as those in animal osteoarthritis models, some drugs within the bisphosphonate class have shown beneficial effects in human studies. It is conceivable that the level of active TGF-β released from bone matrix will decrease substantially when osteoclast bone resorption is inhibited by bisphosphonate. Aberrantly activated TGF-β signaling induces abnormal bone formation in subchondral bone and contributes to osteoarthritis progression. This at least partially explains the efficacy of bisphosphonates in treating osteoarthritis. TGF-β-neutralizing antibodies or TβR inhibitors may achieve a high specificity in suppressing TGF-β signaling in subchondral bone, and their ability to attenuate degeneration of articular cartilage was observed in anterior cruciate ligament transection osteoarthritis rodent models [6]. However, as a critical growth factor, TGF-β has a broad spectrum of functional activities such as growth inhibition, cell migration, cell invasion, epithelial-mesenchymal transition, and immune regulation. The role of TGF-β in maintaining the homeostasis of articular cartilage is different than that of subchondral bone. Thus, systemic administration of a TβR-I inhibitor might disrupt tissue homeostasis of other organs, resulting in unwanted adverse effects and chemical toxicity. Novel approaches that inhibit TGF-β signaling, specifically in subchondral bone, may reduce potential adverse effects while maintaining the therapeutic efficacy of the TβR-I inhibitor.

The function and behavior of cells are not only cell-context-dependent but are also regulated by the local microenvironment. Aberrant elevation of TGF-β is one of the primary factors in the microenvironment that drives the sequence of pathological changes in osteoarthritic subchondral bone such as clustering of osteoprogenitors, de novo bone formation, and neovascularization in marrow cavities. Many other growth factors or cytokines such as Wnts, bone morphogenetic protein (BMP), and insulin-like growth factor are also reported to be involved in the development of subchondral bone abnormality [46]. Parathyroid hormone (PTH) plays an important role in bone metabolism and calcium homeostasis. Recently, PTH was found to orchestrate the signaling of local factors and thereby improve the microenvironment in bone marrow [47]. TβR-II can form a complex with PTH type I receptor (PTH1R). The binding of PTH with PTH1R downregulates TGF-β signaling by inducing internalization of the TβR-II/PTH1R complex [47]. It is known that BMP and Wnt signaling can promote the commitment of MSCs to osteoblastic lineage cells [48]. PTH upregulates BMP and Wnt signaling and, therefore, positively regulates osteogenesis. Additionally, angiogenesis is always coupled with osteogenesis during bone formation. PTH has been shown to reduce the distance between newly formed vessels and sites of bone formation [49]. Therefore, by coordinating the effects of these osteogenic factors, PTH may alleviate abnormal bone formation while stimulating normal bone turnover at the right location. Moreover, PTH is a well-recognized anabolic factor during cartilage development and maintenance [50]. PTH may be developed as a therapeutic agent because of its potential ability to rescue pathological changes in both osteoarthritic cartilage and subchondral bone.

Summary

The diarthrodial joint works as a functional unit, and osteoarthritis affects almost all of its structural components. TGF-β is a crucial factor that regulates the physiological turnover of subchondral bone and articular cartilage. Dysregulation of TGF-β1 signaling leads to failure in maintenance of joint homeostasis during the development and progression of osteoarthritis. Because the effects of TGF-β may differ according to tissue type within the joint and may vary at different time points, differential and tissue-specific treatments targeting TGF-β signaling may produce optimal therapeutic effects.

References

1. Maffulli N, Longo UG, Gougoulias N, Caine D, Denaro V. Sport injuries: a review of outcomes. Br Med Bull. 2011;97:47–80. https://doi.org/10.1093/bmb/ldq026.
2. Riordan EA, Little C, Hunter D. Pathogenesis of post-traumatic OA with a view to intervention. Best Pract Res Clin Rheumatol. 2014;28:17–30. https://doi.org/10.1016/j.berh.2014.02.001.
3. Hunter D. Osteoarthritis. Best Pract Res Clin Rheumatol. 2011;25:801–14. https://doi.org/10.1016/j.berh.2011.11.008.
4. Dare D, Rodeo S. Mechanisms of post-traumatic osteoarthritis after ACL injury. Curr Rheumatol Rep. 2014;16:448. https://doi.org/10.1007/s11926-014-0448-1.
5. Lories RJ, Luyten FP. The bone-cartilage unit in osteoarthritis. Nat Rev Rheumatol. 2011;7:43–9. https://doi.org/10.1038/nrrheum.2010.197.
6. Zhen G, et al. Inhibition of TGF-beta signaling in mesenchymal stem cells of subchondral bone attenuates osteoarthritis. Nat Med. 2013;19:704–12. https://doi.org/10.1038/nm.3143.
7. Burr DB. The importance of subchondral bone in osteoarthrosis. Curr Opin Rheumatol. 1998;10:256–62.

8. Goldring SR. Alterations in periarticular bone and cross talk between subchondral bone and articular cartilage in osteoarthritis. Ther Adv Musculoskelet Dis. 2012;4:249–58. https://doi.org/10.1177/1759720X12437353.

9. Massague J. TGF-beta signaling in development and disease. FEBS Lett. 2012;586:1833. https://doi.org/10.1016/j.febslet.2012.05.030.

10. Cupp AS, Kim G, Skinner MK. Expression and action of transforming growth factor beta (TGFbeta1, TGFbeta2, and TGFbeta3) during embryonic rat testis development. Biol Reprod. 1999;60:1304–13.

11. Annes JP, Munger JS, Rifkin DB. Making sense of latent TGFbeta activation. J Cell Sci. 2003;116:217–24.

12. Murphy-Ullrich JE, Poczatek M. Activation of latent TGF-beta by thrombospondin-1: mechanisms and physiology. Cytokine Growth Factor Rev. 2000;11:59–69.

13. Heldin CH, Miyazono K, ten Dijke P. TGF-beta signalling from cell membrane to nucleus through SMAD proteins. Nature. 1997;390:465–71. https://doi.org/10.1038/37284.

14. Zhang YE. Non-Smad pathways in TGF-beta signaling. Cell Res. 2009;19:128–39. https://doi.org/10.1038/cr.2008.328.

15. Blobe GC, Schiemann WP, Lodish HF. Role of transforming growth factor beta in human disease. N Engl J Med. 2000;342:1350–8. https://doi.org/10.1056/NEJM200005043421807.

16. Kalinina NI, Sysoeva VY, Rubina KA, Parfenova YV, Tkachuk VA. Mesenchymal stem cells in tissue growth and repair. Acta Nat. 2011;3:30–7.

17. Tang Y, et al. TGF-beta1-induced migration of bone mesenchymal stem cells couples bone resorption with formation. Nat Med. 2009;15:757–65. https://doi.org/10.1038/nm.1979.

18. Piera-Velazquez S, Li Z, Jimenez SA. Role of endothelial-mesenchymal transition (EndoMT) in the pathogenesis of fibrotic disorders. Am J Pathol. 2011;179:1074–80. https://doi.org/10.1016/j.ajpath.2011.06.001.

19. Stone RC, et al. Epithelial-mesenchymal transition in tissue repair and fibrosis. Cell Tissue Res. 2016;365:495–506. https://doi.org/10.1007/s00441-016-2464-0.

20. Loughlin J. Genetics of osteoarthritis. Curr Opin Rheumatol. 2011;23:479–83. https://doi.org/10.1097/BOR.0b013e3283493ff0.

21. Vinatier C, et al. Cartilage tissue engineering: towards a biomaterial-assisted mesenchymal stem cell therapy. Curr Stem Cell Res Ther. 2009;4:318–29.

22. Shen J, et al. Deletion of the transforming growth factor beta receptor type II gene in articular chondrocytes leads to a progressive osteoarthritis-like phenotype in mice. Arthritis Rheum. 2013;65:3107–19. https://doi.org/10.1002/art.38122.

23. Yang X, et al. TGF-beta/Smad3 signals repress chondrocyte hypertrophic differentiation and are required for maintaining articular cartilage. J Cell Biol. 2001;153:35–46.

24. Morales TI, Joyce ME, Sobel ME, Danielpour D, Roberts AB. Transforming growth factor-beta in calf articular cartilage organ cultures: synthesis and distribution. Arch Biochem Biophys. 1991;288:397–405.

25. Maeda S, Dean DD, Gomez R, Schwartz Z, Boyan BD. The first stage of transforming growth factor beta1 activation is release of the large latent complex from the extracellular matrix of growth plate chondrocytes by matrix vesicle stromelysin-1 (MMP-3). Calcif Tissue Int. 2002;70:54–65. https://doi.org/10.1007/s002230010032.

26. Farquhar T, et al. Swelling and fibronectin accumulation in articular cartilage explants after cyclical impact. J Orthop Res. 1996;14:417–23. https://doi.org/10.1002/jor.1100140312.

27. Hinz B. The extracellular matrix and transforming growth factor-beta1: tale of a strained relationship. Matrix Biol. 2015;47:54–65. https://doi.org/10.1016/j.matbio.2015.05.006.

28. Albro MB, et al. Shearing of synovial fluid activates latent TGF-beta. Osteoarthr Cartil. 2012;20:1374–82. https://doi.org/10.1016/j.joca.2012.07.006.

29. Neu CP, Khalafi A, Komvopoulos K, Schmid TM, Reddi AH. Mechanotransduction of bovine articular cartilage superficial zone protein by transforming growth factor beta signaling. Arthritis Rheum. 2007;56:3706–14. https://doi.org/10.1002/art.23024.

30. Serra R, et al. Expression of a truncated, kinase-defective TGF-beta type II receptor in mouse skeletal tissue promotes terminal chondrocyte differentiation and osteoarthritis. J Cell Biol. 1997;139:541–52.

31. van der Kraan PM, Blaney Davidson EN, van den Berg WB. A role for age-related changes in TGFbeta signaling in aberrant chondrocyte differentiation and osteoarthritis. Arthritis Res Ther. 2010;12:201. https://doi.org/10.1186/ar2896.

32. Goumans MJ, et al. Activin receptor-like kinase (ALK)1 is an antagonistic mediator of lateral TGFbeta/ALK5 signaling. Mol Cell. 2003;12:817–28.

33. van der Kraan PM, Goumans MJ, Blaney Davidson E, ten Dijke P. Age-dependent alteration of TGF-beta signalling in osteoarthritis. Cell Tissue Res. 2012;347:257–65. https://doi.org/10.1007/s00441-011-1194-6.

34. Finnson KW, et al. Endoglin differentially regulates TGF-beta-induced Smad2/3 and Smad1/5 signalling and its expression correlates with extracellular matrix production and cellular differentiation state in human chondrocytes. Osteoarthr Cartil. 2010;18:1518–27. https://doi.org/10.1016/j.joca.2010.09.002.

35. Santander C, Brandan E. Betaglycan induces TGF-beta signaling in a ligand-independent manner, through activation of the p38 pathway. Cell Signal. 2006;18:1482–91. https://doi.org/10.1016/j.cellsig.2005.11.011.

36. Lopez-Casillas F, et al. Structure and expression of the membrane proteoglycan betaglycan, a component of the TGF-beta receptor system. Cell. 1991;67:785–95.

37. Bizet AA, et al. The TGF-beta co-receptor, CD109, promotes internalization and degradation of TGF-beta receptors. Biochim Biophys Acta. 2011;1813:742–53. https://doi.org/10.1016/j.bbamcr.2011.01.028.

38. Mathiessen A, Conaghan PG. Synovitis in osteoarthritis: current understanding with therapeutic implications. Arthritis Res Ther. 2017;19:18. https://doi.org/10.1186/s13075-017-1229-9.

39. Fahlgren A, Andersson B, Messner K. TGF-beta1 as a prognostic factor in the process of early osteoarthrosis in the rabbit knee. Osteoarthr Cartil. 2001;9:195–202. https://doi.org/10.1053/joca.2000.0376.

40. Cameron ML, Fu FH, Paessler HH, Schneider M, Evans CH. Synovial fluid cytokine concentrations as possible prognostic indicators in the ACL-deficient knee. Knee Surg Sports Traumatol Arthrosc. 1994;2:38–44.

41. Yoshimura A, Muto G. TGF-beta function in immune suppression. Curr Top Microbiol Immunol. 2011;350:127–47. https://doi.org/10.1007/82_2010_87.

42. Gong D, et al. TGFbeta signaling plays a critical role in promoting alternative macrophage activation. BMC Immunol. 2012;13:31. https://doi.org/10.1186/1471-2172-13-31.

43. Gordon S. Alternative activation of macrophages. Nat Rev Immunol. 2003;3:23–35. https://doi.org/10.1038/nri978.

44. Rosengren S, Corr M, Boyle DL. Platelet-derived growth factor and transforming growth factor beta synergistically potentiate inflammatory mediator synthesis by fibroblast-like synoviocytes. Arthritis Res Ther. 2010;12:R65. https://doi.org/10.1186/ar2981.

45. Nishii T, Tamura S, Shiomi T, Yoshikawa H, Sugano N. Alendronate treatment for hip osteoarthritis: prospective randomized 2-year trial. Clin Rheumatol. 2013;32:1759–66. https://doi.org/10.1007/s10067-013-2338-8.

46. Iannone F, Lapadula G. The pathophysiology of osteoarthritis. Aging Clin Exp Res. 2003;15:364–72.

47. Qiu T, et al. TGF-beta type II receptor phosphorylates PTH receptor to integrate bone remodelling signalling. Nat Cell Biol. 2010;12:224–34. https://doi.org/10.1038/ncb2022.

48. Lin GL, Hankenson KD. Integration of BMP, Wnt, and notch signaling pathways in osteoblast differentiation. J Cell Biochem. 2011;112:3491–501. https://doi.org/10.1002/jcb.23287.

49. Prisby R, et al. Intermittent PTH(1-84) is osteoanabolic but not osteoangiogenic and relocates bone marrow blood vessels closer to bone-forming sites. J Bone Miner Res. 2011;26:2583–96. https://doi.org/10.1002/jbmr.459.

50. Orth P, et al. Parathyroid hormone [1-34] improves articular cartilage surface architecture and integration and subchondral bone reconstitution in osteochondral defects in vivo. Osteoarthr Cartil. 2013;21:614–24. https://doi.org/10.1016/j.joca.2013.01.008.

Chapter 2
Imaging Modalities for Post-traumatic Arthritis

Filippo Del Grande, Luca Deabate, and Christian Candrian

> **Key Points**
> - Magnetic field strength increases the signal to noise ratio (SNR) and can influence cartilage detection and grading.
> - T2 mapping, dGEMERIC, T1 rho, and Sodium imaging are advanced MRI techniques that allow the biochemical evaluation of the cartilage.
> - Bone marrow edema (also called bone marrow lesions) is commonly present in patients with OA mainly in areas of mechanical loading.

Introduction

Osteoarthritis (OA) is a rapidly increasing condition in US population ranging from 21 million in 1995 to 27 million in 2007 [1]. Aging population, male gender, increasing overweight, and genetic predisposition are the main general risk factors for the disease [2]. Besides these general risk factors, other local biomechanical conditions such as post-traumatic joint instability and/or misalignment are responsible for OA [2]. It is estimated that post-traumatic etiology accounts for approximately 12% of OA of lower extremities [3].

The well-known imaging findings of primary OA such as subchondral bone sclerosis, osteophytes, joint space narrowing, and subchondral cysts are similar to

F. Del Grande (✉)
Clinica di Radiologia EOC, Istituto di Imaging della Svizzera Italiana,
Ente Ospedaliero Cantonale, Ticino, Switzerland
e-mail: Filippo.delgrande@eoc.ch

L. Deabate · C. Candrian
Servizio di ortopedia, Ospedale Regionale di Lugano, Ticino, Switzerland
e-mail: luca.deabate@eoc.ch; christian.candrian@eoc.ch

© Springer Nature Switzerland AG 2021
S. C. Thakkar, E. A. Hasenboehler (eds.), *Post-Traumatic Arthritis*,
https://doi.org/10.1007/978-3-030-50413-7_2

post-traumatic OA [3]. Conventional radiography, CT imaging, and MR imaging are currently the imaging modality available in the clinical practice to assess OA. The main difference between post-traumatic OA and idiopathic OA is the joint location. Ankle joint, shoulder joint, and elbow joint are generally atypical locations for primary OA but are involved in post-traumatic OA (Figs. 2.1 and 2.2). For instance, less than 2% of hip OA are post-traumatic, whereas approximately 80% of ankle OA are post-traumatic [3].

The purpose of our chapter is to familiarize oneself with the most common imaging modalities used in clinical practice to assess post-traumatic OA, i.e., conventional radiography and MR imaging, and to review the diagnostic performance, the reliability, and the correlation of imaging findings with pain. Owing to the scarcity of the literature on imaging in post-traumatic OA, our chapter will review the general principles of imaging of OA and will focus on post-traumatic OA when possible.

Conventional Radiography

Conventional radiography (CR) is the least expensive and most widely available imaging modality to assess OA in the clinical practice. CR allows not only to detect morphological changes of OA but also to follow the disease progression by measuring the joint space narrowing (JSN) (Fig. 2.3) [4, 5]. Slowing of the JSN progression is the official criterion approved by the Federal and Drug Administration (FDA) to demonstrate efficacy of drugs in phase III trials of OA [4, 5].

JSN is a complex process that involves several anatomical structures depending on the joint. For instance, in the knee joint, cartilage loss, meniscal degeneration, and/or meniscal extrusion are involved in the joint space narrowing process [6].

In the clinical practice, radiologists don't use scoring systems to report OA. Kellgren and Lawrence (K-L) is the best-known semiquantitative grading system to assess OA and was originally developed for anteroposterior knee radiographies [7]. The 5-point K-L scoring system stratifies OA according to four conventional radiology findings: presence of bony osteophytes, joint space narrowing, presence and degree of subchondral sclerosis, and bony deformity (Fig. 2.4) [7, 8]. K-L grade 0 indicates none OA, K-L grade 1 indicates doubtful OA, K-L grade 2 indicates minimal OA, K-L grade 3 indicates moderate OA, and K-L grade 4 indicates severe OA. Although the K-L scoring system could help to increase communication between radiologists and clinicians, it shows some important limitations that prevent its introduction in clinical practice and in research protocols. One of the major limitations of K-L grading system is the grouping of the majorities of patients in the grade of moderate OA (grade 3) [4]. Furthermore, K-L method shows high interpretation variability with poor to moderate inter-observer agreement [9]. Experience and training seems to play an important role for reliability reporting. Differences arise between readers on site and an expert centralized reader as well, which highlight the importance to use a centralized reader in the research projects [10].

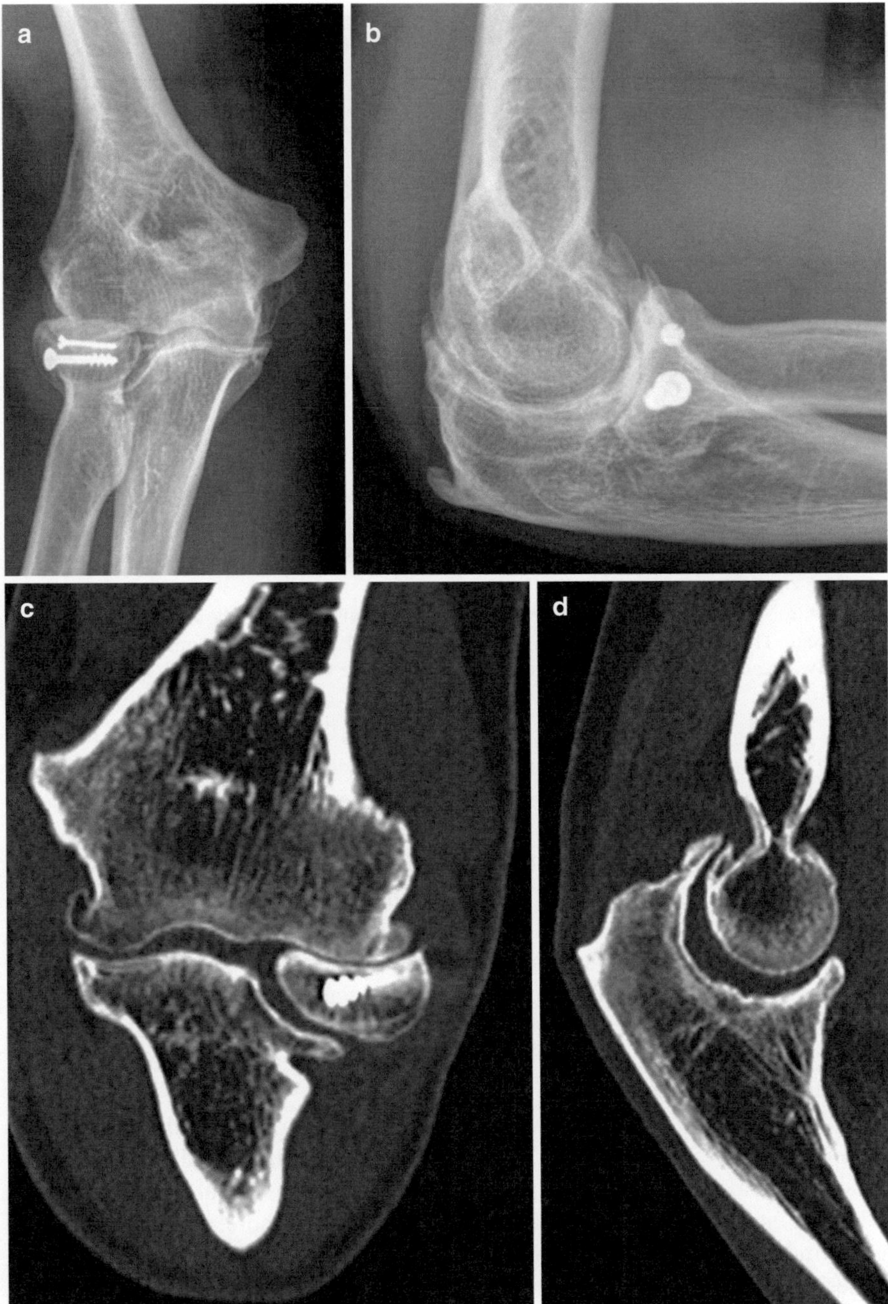

Fig. 2.1 (**a**) Anteroposterior and (**b**) lateral conventional radiographies and (**c**) coronal and (**d**) sagittal CT MPR reconstruction of the elbow of a 60-year-old patient after internal fixation of a radial head fracture. The patient developed post-traumatic OA of the elbow which is an atypical location for primary OA. Radiographs and CT show humero-ulnar and humero-radial OA. The osteophyte arising from the olecranon ulnae causes extension deficit

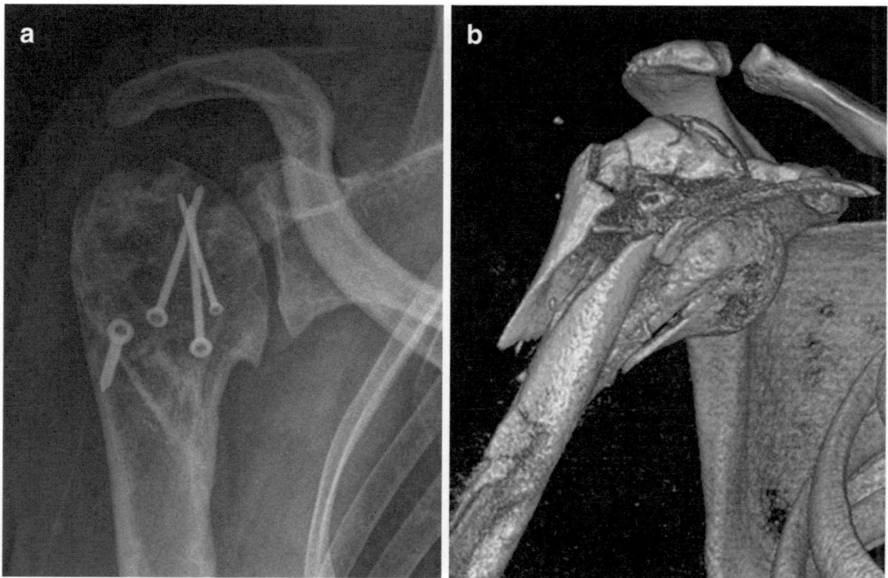

Fig. 2.2 (**a**) Anteroposterior shoulder view and (**b**) 3D reconstruction of the shoulder of a 25-year-old patient. The 3D reconstruction (**b**) shows a displaced comminuted humerus fracture after MVA. Two years later the patient developed a post-traumatic OA (**a**)

The major drawbacks of CR are lack of sensitivity [8, 11] and of reliability [9]. In clinical practice, standard anteroposterior and lateral views are generally sufficient; additional views are rarely requested. The role of additional special projection on knee MRI is debatable in the literature. In patients with arthroscopy-confirmed grade II femorotibial chondromalacia, the 45°flexion PA and the standing AP view are both insensitive to detect OA [11]. However, a more recent systematic review concluded that the 45°flexion PA view was more sensitive than the standing AP view for the detection of femorotibial OA, especially in patients suffering from advanced OA [8]. The two studies showed contradictory results, probably because of the relatively young population (average 38 years old) and the mild femorotibial OA in the first study compared to the meta-analysis.

To the best of our knowledge, to date, only two studies focus on the reliability of imaging of post-traumatic OA [12, 13]. K-L scoring system is reliable and correlates with clinical symptoms in patients with ankle OA several years after open reduction internal fixation of a malleolar fracture. Furthermore, adding the talar tilt angle (modified K-L scale) will result in even better differentiation of clinical outcomes [13].

In order to assess the reliability of grading systems for post-traumatic ankle OA, Cleassen and colleagues analyzed three different methods: the Van Dick, the Takakura, and the K-L methods. A total of 118 orthopedic surgeons and residents graded 128 ankle radiographs after bi- or trimalleolar ankle fractures. The authors

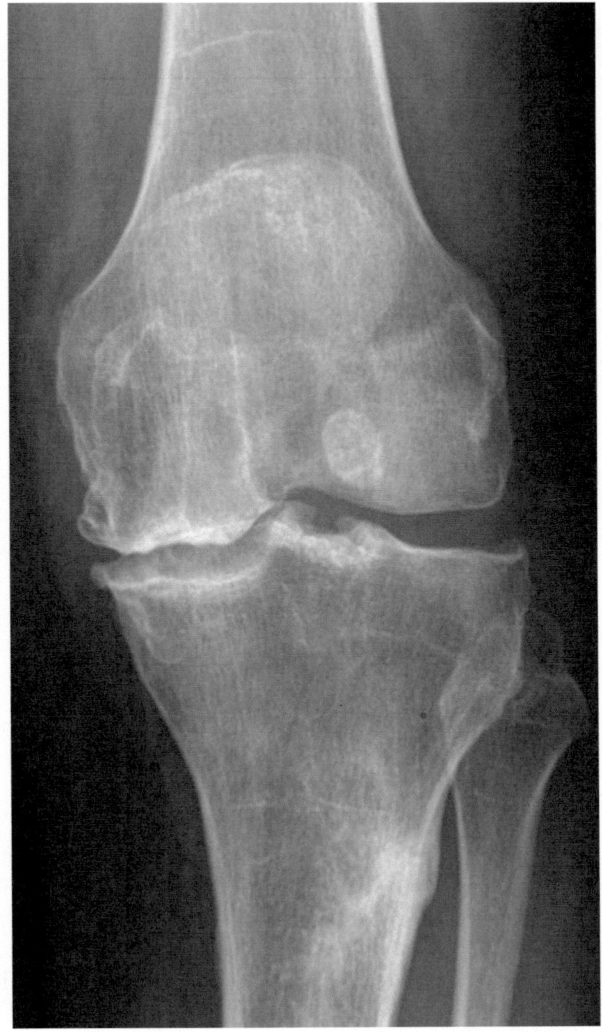

Fig. 2.3 Anteroposterior conventional radiography of medial OA of the knee with osteophytes, subchondral sclerosis, and joint space narrowing

found only fair inter-reader agreement for the Van Dick and low for the Takakura and K-L classification systems. According to the results of the study, the authors warned to use these classifications in the clinical practice [12].

MR Imaging

MRI has a high soft tissue contrast that allows to visualize the whole joint, i.e., the bone, the synovia, the ligaments, the capsule, and mainly the cartilage [5, 14, 15]. Furthermore MRIs allow to assess the morphology and the composition of the cartilage [16].

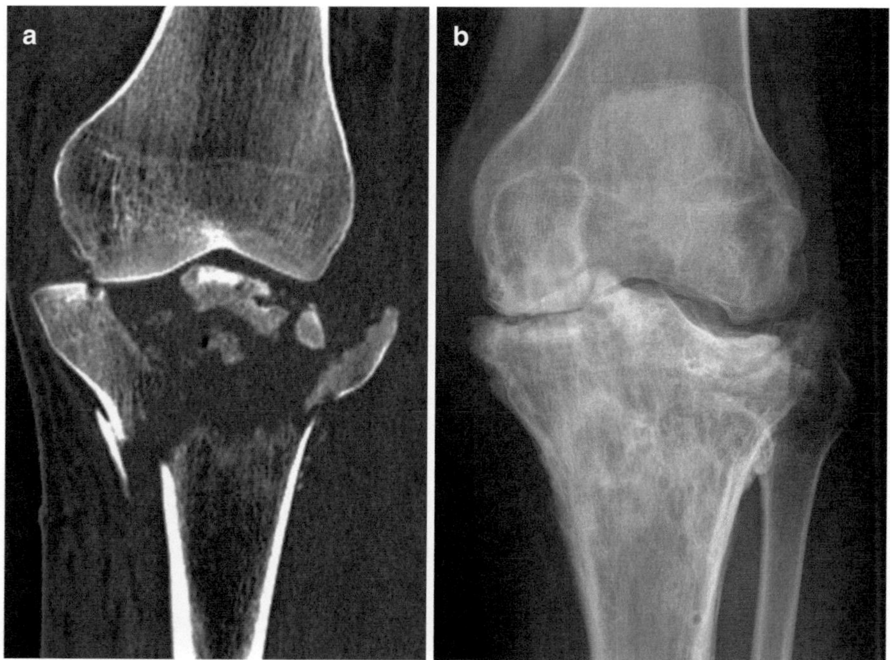

Fig. 2.4 (**a**) Coronal MPR CT reconstruction of the knee of a comminuted displaced fracture of the proximal tibia of a 36-year-old male patient after MVA. (**b**) Anteroposterior conventional radiography 6 years later shows severe medial knee OA (K-L 4)

Studies on morphological cartilage assessment show a large heterogeneity of results depending on several technical factors. A wide range of sensitivity from 0% to 86% is reported for the detection of early cartilage lesions and from 47 to 98% for the detection of more advanced cartilage lesions [17].

Among the several technical factors, higher magnetic field strength increases the signal-to-noise ratio (SNR) and can influence cartilage detection and grading. Masi and colleagues demonstrated higher accuracy in cartilage lesion detection and higher ability to grade cartilage lesions on porcine model on 3 tesla compared to 1.5 tesla MRI [18]. Kijowski et al. compared the detection of cartilage lesion of the knee on 3 tesla MRI compared to 1.5 tesla MRI with arthroscopy in two different study populations. The authors concluded that 3 tesla MRIs show higher specificity and higher accuracy but not higher sensitivity compared to 1.5 tesla MRI [19]. Wong et al. found a modest but significant increase in sensitivity and accuracy of diagnostic lesions on 3 tesla MRI compared to 1.5 tesla MRI. Additionally the authors found a higher grading and higher confidence in grading cartilage lesions [20].

T2 mapping, dGEMRIC, T1 rho, and sodium imaging are advanced MRI techniques that allow the biochemical evaluation of the cartilage [16]. A detailed description of compositional MRI techniques for cartilage evaluation will go far beyond the scope of this chapter. It is only worthy to mention that these compositional techniques are rarely used in clinical practice mainly because of long acquisition time and the need to use special pulse sequences and/or dedicated hardware [16].

Association Between Pain and Imaging Findings of OA

Association between pain and imaging findings in OA is one of the greatest challenges for researchers, radiologists, and referring physicians. Hyaline cartilage is avascular and aneural and as such cannot be the source of pain [21]. Pain transmission is probably the result of more complex and indirect mechanisms involving other articular structures [21]. It is speculated that pain could be secondary to the exposure of nociceptors of the subchondral bone, to the increased intraosseous pressure secondary to vascular congestion, and/or to cartilage damage that can lead to synovitis [21].

Prevalence studies on hip OA show only low correlation between imaging findings and pain. In the Framingham OA study, a community-based prevalence study in which symptomatic and asymptomatic subjects underwent hip radiographies, nearly one out of five subjects shows CR features of hip OA, but less than 5% were symptomatic [22].

Another population-based observational study emphasizes the low sensitivity of CR for OA and the low correlation of MRI findings of OA with pain [23]. In the study, a cohort of 710 patients without evidence of knee OA (K-L grade 0) underwent MRI of the knee. The authors assessed the prevalence of MRI finding suggestive for OA such as osteophytes, cartilage damage, bone marrow lesions, synovitis, subchondral cysts, meniscal lesions, and bone attrition. Some interesting clinical considerations came out from the study. First, 89% of subjects showed MRI features compatible with OA. Second, a high prevalence of symptomatic (97%) and asymptomatic (88%) subjects showed at least one MRI feature of OA. According to the study, MRI features of OA are so common in asymptomatic subjects that should not be used as a diagnostic tool for OA. The role of MRI will be rather to rule out other pathologies that can mimic OA such as subchondral bone fractures, osteonecrosis, and insufficiency fractures [23].

Although the correlation between pain and imaging finding is low, some imaging findings such as bone marrow edema, synovitis/effusion, and bone attrition are predictive of pain in patients with OA.

Bone marrow edema (also called bone marrow lesions) is commonly present in patients with OA mainly in areas of mechanical loading (Fig. 2.5) [24]. Bone marrow edema is considered a strong pain generator in patients with OA [25–27] and predictive for OA progression [24]. Interestingly, the fluctuation of bone marrow edema on MRI correlates with pain fluctuation [28]. Histologically, bone marrow edema in patients with OA is a mixture of fibrosis, hemorrhage, trabecular fractures,

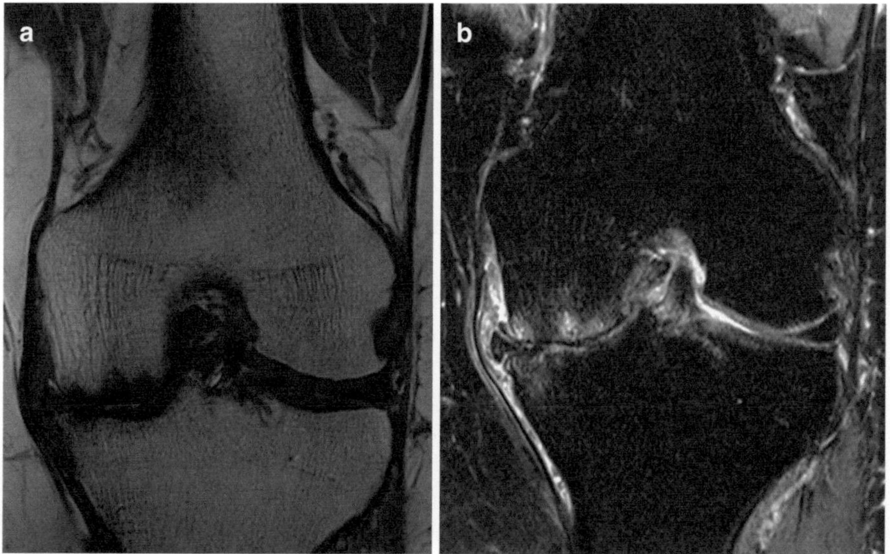

Fig. 2.5 (**a**) Coronal T1-weighted sequences and (**b**) T2-weighted sequences of a 71-year-old female patient with painful OA. Note the osteophytes arising from the medial compartment of the knee, the meniscus subluxation, and diffuse cartilage loss. T2-weighted sequences show the bone marrow edema of medial condyle and the medial tibial plateau

and only a minor component of edema [29, 30]. Bone attrition is a common bony feature in OA and plays an important role in association with bone marrow edema to generate pain [27]. Lastly, several studies emphasize the association of synovitis/joint effusion with knee pain [26, 27, 31, 32].

References

1. Lawrence RC, Felson DT, Helmick CG, Arnold LM, Choi H, Deyo RA, et al. Estimates of the prevalence of arthritis and other rheumatic conditions in the United States. Part II. Arthritis Rheum. 2008;58(1):26–35.
2. Suri P, Morgenroth DC, Hunter DJ. Epidemiology of osteoarthritis and associated comorbidities. PM R. 2012;4(5 Suppl):S10–9.
3. Brown TD, Johnston RC, Saltzman CL, Marsh JL, Buckwalter JA. Posttraumatic osteoarthritis: a first estimate of incidence, prevalence, and burden of disease. J Orthop Trauma. 2006;20(10):739–44.
4. Guermazi A, Hayashi D, Eckstein F, Hunter DJ, Duryea J, Roemer FW. Imaging of osteoarthritis. Rheum Dis Clin N Am. 2013;39(1):67–105.
5. Roemer FW, Eckstein F, Hayashi D, Guermazi A. The role of imaging in osteoarthritis. Best Pract Res Clin Rheumatol. 2014;28(1):31–60.
6. Hunter DJ, Zhang YQ, Tu X, Lavalley M, Niu JB, Amin S, et al. Change in joint space width: hyaline articular cartilage loss or alteration in meniscus? Arthritis Rheum. 2006;54(8):2488–95.
7. Kellgren JH, Lawrence JS. Radiological assessment of osteo-arthrosis. Ann Rheum Dis. 1957;16(4):494–502.

8. Duncan ST, Khazzam MS, Burnham JM, Spindler KP, Dunn WR, Wright RW. Sensitivity of standing radiographs to detect knee arthritis: a systematic review of Level I studies. Arthroscopy. 2015;31(2):321–8.

9. Vilalta C, Nunez M, Segur JM, Domingo A, Carbonell JA, Macule F. Knee osteoarthritis: interpretation variability of radiological signs. Clin Rheumatol. 2004;23(6):501–4.

10. Guermazi A, Hunter DJ, Li L, Benichou O, Eckstein F, Kwoh CK, et al. Different thresholds for detecting osteophytes and joint space narrowing exist between the site investigators and the centralized reader in a multicenter knee osteoarthritis study–data from the osteoarthritis initiative. Skelet Radiol. 2012;41(2):179–86.

11. Wright RW, Boyce RH, Michener T, Shyr Y, McCarty EC, Spindler KP. Radiographs are not useful in detecting arthroscopically confirmed mild chondral damage. Clin Orthop Relat Res. 2006;442:245–51.

12. Claessen FM, Meijer DT, van den Bekerom MP, Gevers Deynoot BD, Mallee WH, Doornberg JN, et al. Reliability of classification for post-traumatic ankle osteoarthritis. Knee Surg Sports Traumatol Arthrosc. 2016;24(4):1332–7.

13. Holzer N, Salvo D, Marijnissen AC, Vincken KL, Ahmad AC, Serra E, et al. Radiographic evaluation of posttraumatic osteoarthritis of the ankle: the Kellgren-Lawrence scale is reliable and correlates with clinical symptoms. Osteoarthr Cartil. 2015;23(3):363–9.

14. Hayashi D, Guermazi A, Crema MD, Roemer FW. Imaging in osteoarthritis: what have we learned and where are we going? Minerva Med. 2011;102(1):15–32.

15. Wenham CY, Grainger AJ, Conaghan PG. The role of imaging modalities in the diagnosis, differential diagnosis and clinical assessment of peripheral joint osteoarthritis. Osteoarthr Cartil. 2014;22(10):1692–702.

16. Crema MD, Roemer FW, Marra MD, Burstein D, Gold GE, Eckstein F, et al. Articular cartilage in the knee: current MR imaging techniques and applications in clinical practice and research. Radiographics. 2011;31(1):37–61.

17. Quatman CE, Hettrich CM, Schmitt LC, Spindler KP. The clinical utility and diagnostic performance of magnetic resonance imaging for identification of early and advanced knee osteoarthritis: a systematic review. Am J Sports Med. 2011;39(7):1557–68.

18. Masi JN, Sell CA, Phan C, Han E, Newitt D, Steinbach L, et al. Cartilage MR imaging at 3.0 versus that at 1.5 T: preliminary results in a porcine model. Radiology. 2005;236(1):140–50.

19. Kijowski R, Blankenbaker DG, Davis KW, Shinki K, Kaplan LD, De Smet AA. Comparison of 1.5- and 3.0-T MR imaging for evaluating the articular cartilage of the knee joint. Radiology. 2009;250(3):839–48.

20. Wong S, Steinbach L, Zhao J, Stehling C, Ma CB, Link TM. Comparative study of imaging at 3.0 T versus 1.5 T of the knee. Skelet Radiol. 2009;38(8):761–9.

21. Hunter DJ, Guermazi A, Roemer F, Zhang Y, Neogi T. Structural correlates of pain in joints with osteoarthritis. Osteoarthr Cartil. 2013;21(9):1170–8.

22. Kim C, Linsenmeyer KD, Vlad SC, Guermazi A, Clancy MM, Niu J, et al. Prevalence of radiographic and symptomatic hip osteoarthritis in an urban United States community: the Framingham osteoarthritis study. Arthritis Rheum (Hoboken, NJ). 2014;66(11):3013–7.

23. Guermazi A, Niu J, Hayashi D, Roemer FW, Englund M, Neogi T, et al. Prevalence of abnormalities in knees detected by MRI in adults without knee osteoarthritis: population based observational study (Framingham Osteoarthritis Study). BMJ (Clinical Research ed). 2012;345:e5339.

24. Felson DT, McLaughlin S, Goggins J, LaValley MP, Gale ME, Totterman S, et al. Bone marrow edema and its relation to progression of knee osteoarthritis. Ann Intern Med. 2003;139(5 Pt 1):330–6.

25. Felson DT, Chaisson CE, Hill CL, Totterman SM, Gale ME, Skinner KM, et al. The association of bone marrow lesions with pain in knee osteoarthritis. Ann Intern Med. 2001;134(7):541–9.

26. Lo GH, McAlindon TE, Niu J, Zhang Y, Beals C, Dabrowski C, et al. Bone marrow lesions and joint effusion are strongly and independently associated with weight-bearing pain in knee osteoarthritis: data from the osteoarthritis initiative. Osteoarthr Cartil. 2009;17(12):1562–9.

27. Torres L, Dunlop DD, Peterfy C, Guermazi A, Prasad P, Hayes KW, et al. The relationship between specific tissue lesions and pain severity in persons with knee osteoarthritis. Osteoarthr Cartil. 2006;14(10):1033–40.
28. Zhang Y, Nevitt M, Niu J, Lewis C, Torner J, Guermazi A, et al. Fluctuation of knee pain and changes in bone marrow lesions, effusions, and synovitis on magnetic resonance imaging. Arthritis Rheum. 2011;63(3):691–9.
29. Bergman AG, Willen HK, Lindstrand AL, Pettersson HT. Osteoarthritis of the knee: correlation of subchondral MR signal abnormalities with histopathologic and radiographic features. Skelet Radiol. 1994;23(6):445–8.
30. Zanetti M, Bruder E, Romero J, Hodler J. Bone marrow edema pattern in osteoarthritic knees: correlation between MR imaging and histologic findings. Radiology. 2000;215(3):835–40.
31. Baker K, Grainger A, Niu J, Clancy M, Guermazi A, Crema M, et al. Relation of synovitis to knee pain using contrast-enhanced MRIs. Ann Rheum Dis. 2010;69(10):1779–83.
32. Hill CL, Gale DG, Chaisson CE, Skinner K, Kazis L, Gale ME, et al. Knee effusions, popliteal cysts, and synovial thickening: association with knee pain in osteoarthritis. J Rheumatol. 2001;28(6):1330–7.

Chapter 3
Economic Implications of Post-traumatic Arthritis of the Hip and Knee

Richard Iorio, Kelvin Y. Kim, Afshin A. Anoushiravani, and William J. Long

> **Key Points**
> - To understand how patient demographics, injury patterns, and the management of hip and knee PTOA contribute to the disease burden
> - To assess the direct and indirect economic burden associated with PTOA of the hip and knee

Introduction

There are 27 million [1] people in the United States who have been diagnosed with degenerative joint disease (DJD). Patients with osteoarthritis (OA) frequently present with joint stiffness, pain, or instability due to degeneration of the articular surface. In the event OA develops after an acute injury, this subcategory of OA is referred to as post-traumatic osteoarthritis (PTOA). Posttraumatic osteoarthritis of

R. Iorio (✉)
Brigham and Women's Hospital, Member of the Faculty, Harvard Medical School,
Boston, MA, USA
e-mail: riorio@bwh.harvard.edu

K. Y. Kim
Department of Orthopaedic Surgery, UNLV School of Medicine, Las Vegas, NV, USA

A. A. Anoushiravani
Department of Orthopaedic Surgery, Albany Medical Center, Albany, NY, USA

W. J. Long
ISK Institute, Department of Orthopaedic Surgery, NYU Langone Medical Center,
Hospital for Joint Diseases, New York, NY, USA

© Springer Nature Switzerland AG 2021
S. C. Thakkar, E. A. Hasenboehler (eds.), *Post-Traumatic Arthritis*,
https://doi.org/10.1007/978-3-030-50413-7_3

the lower extremity comprises about 12% of OA overall, of which PTOA of the hip and knee account for 0.5% and 6.3%, respectively [2].

Following the initial injury, there are two mechanisms by which OA may ultimately develop. One pathway is through damage to the articular surface of the joint at the time of injury followed by subsequent, chronic degeneration of the joint secondary to a continuous inflammatory response [3]. Another pathway is through chronic inflammation to the articular surface caused by joint instability or incongruity following an inadequately treated joint injury. The pathophysiologic mechanism in PTOA and primary OA is similar; however, PTOA is initiated by an acute traumatic episode [4].

Given the association between PTOA and acute injury, the patient population that typically develops PTOA is younger and more active than patients diagnosed with primary OA [5]. Patients with a history of lower-extremity joint trauma will on average develop OA 10 years sooner than those without a history of trauma [6]. Despite extensive research aimed at better managing PTOA, over 40% of patients with significant soft tissue injuries to the knee will develop symptomatic OA [3].

An abundant amount of resources have been dedicated to understanding the management of OA. The Agency for Healthcare Research and Quality (AHRQ) ranked OA as one of the top 5 most costly conditions in the United States [7]. Yet, there is a paucity of literature evaluating the economic effects of secondary causes of OA including PTOA. This is particularly concerning as recent studies have demonstrated that the direct costs associated with managing PTOA are substantially greater than those diagnosed with primary OA [8]. Additionally, as a growing number of individuals participate in high-risk activities, the incidence of PTOA is expected to increase. Given this growing trend, PTOA poses a substantial financial burden on the healthcare system. Thus, the aim of this review is to shed light on the clinical and economic implications of PTOA. Emphasis will be placed on the direct, indirect, and long-term costs associated with PTOA. Finally, we will present potential solutions which may improve the delivery of care and reduce the financial burden on all stakeholders.

Post-traumatic Osteoarthritis of the Knee

Post-traumatic osteoarthritis of the knee is responsible for 6.3% of the overall prevalence of OA [2]. Patients diagnosed with PTOA are on average 10 years younger, and more active than those with primary OA [2], and have a five times greater likelihood of developing PTOA with a past history significant for knee injury [9]. Specifically, the incidence of ligamentous and meniscal injury is associated with a 50% incidence of knee PTOA within 10–20 years [10]. Given the rapidly progressive nature of PTOA and the young active population often affected by this disease process, it is not uncommon to see debilitating manifestations of the disease within the third and fourth decades of life.

Types of Injuries Associated with PTOA of the Knee

Anterior Cruciate Ligament Injuries

Anterior cruciate ligament (ACL) pathology is commonly associated with PTOA and is responsible for a quarter of knee injuries subsequently resulting in degenerative changes of the knee [11]. Investigators have reported that 13% to 39% of patients with isolated ACL injuries and 21% to 48% of individuals with complex ligamentous injuries will develop symptomatic PTOA within 10 years of injury [12, 13]. Based on the severity of the injury, cartilage damage after ACL and meniscus injuries can develop into PTOA regardless of whether the ligaments or meniscus is repaired. Even in those who have their ACL reconstructed, about 50% of patients go on to develop OA within 14 years (Fig. 3.1) [14].

Meniscus Injuries

Meniscal injuries are another common cause of degenerative knee changes and are responsible for 23% of patients with PTOA [11]. Swenson et al. [15] observed that following meniscal injury, the first signs of OA were identified 10 years after injury

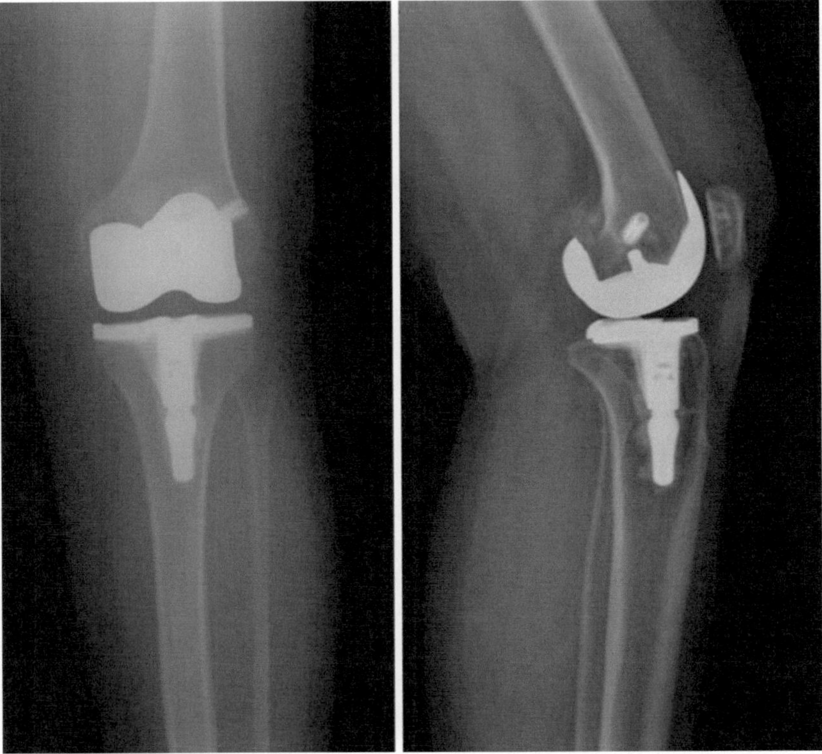

Fig. 3.1 Patient with ACL reconstruction that went on to total knee arthroplasty

at an average age of 50 years. The investigators also reported that the age of the patient at the time of the injury played a role in the timing of the onset of OA as patients who had an isolated meniscal injury between the ages of 17 and 30 developed radiologic OA after 15 years, whereas patients over the age of 30 years developed degenerative changes within 5 years [15]. A study by Badlani et al. [16] compared the characteristics of meniscal injury in those who did and did not develop PTOA within 2 years of injury. The authors reported that complex tears, extrusion of the meniscus, tears greater than one-third of the radial width of the meniscus, and injuries longer than one-third of the longitudinal length of the meniscus occurred more frequently in those who developed PTOA.

Intra-articular Fractures

Patients with fractures of the articular surface are at increased risk for developing PTOA (Fig. 3.3). Studies have demonstrated that up to 31% of these patients will develop PTOA of the knee depending on the location of the fracture [17]. In a study by Honkone [18], 44% of patients with a previous history of tibial plateau fractures developed arthritis within 7.6 years of surgery. Although Honkone and colleagues demonstrated the high prevalence of arthritis within patients with history of tibial plateau fractures, the mechanism and severity of injury is often the best prognostic indicator of PTOA. Higher load injuries are more likely to be associated with immediate damage to the surrounding cartilaginous structures, whereas joints may be more forgiving to less severe injuries [19, 20].

Management of Post-traumatic Osteoarthritis of the Knee

Primary Prevention

Primary prevention strategies are implemented in order to prevent the initial injury from occurring and are considered to be the most effective management tool for prevention of PTOA. Specifically for ACL rupture prevention, neuromuscular training, aerobic conditioning, resistance training, and plyometrics have all been shown to strengthen soft tissue around the knee, reducing the incidence of ligamentous injury [21]. Recent literature has reported a 70% risk reduction in ACL ruptures when proper exercise regimens are practiced [22]. The costs associated with primary prevention of PTOA are not unreasonable. Exercise programs using these preventative therapies have been estimated to cost between $50 and 400 USD per session and may require a 3-hour commitment per week. Given the high costs associated with ACL reconstruction ($38,121 to $88,538 USD) [23], primary prevention is particularly worthwhile among high-risk patients.

Secondary Prevention

Secondary preventative measures are indicated in individuals who have already sustained a joint injury. The goal of secondary prevention is to prevent worsening of a joint injury. Although surgical techniques and knowledge surrounding the restoration of joint stability and articular surface congruity have improved over the past 25 years, up to 50% of individuals sustaining a serious joint injury warranting surgical intervention will go on to develop OA [24]. While in the majority of patients, arthroscopic repair of soft tissue, ACL reconstruction, and partial meniscectomy are the current standard of care, the literature has not demonstrated a reduced incidence of PTOA with these interventions (Fig. 3.1) [25].

Similarly, the benefits are unclear in patients undergoing autologous chondrocyte implantation (ACI), microfracture, and chondroplasty. Knutsen et al. assessed 5-[26] and 15-year [27] outcomes following ACI and microfracture repair in symptomatic patients with cartilage defects and reported a failure rate as high as 43% and 33% for the respective procedures. In addition, the study also demonstrated that OA develops in 33% of patients undergoing ACI and microfracture repair at 5 years and greater than 50% of patients at 15 years. Given the similar long-term outlook, it is important for providers and patients to be aware of the direct and indirect costs associated with the various treatment modalities as there may be substantial differences between them.

Tertiary Prevention

When primary and secondary prevention measures have failed and PTOA has developed, alternative treatment modalities may be implemented to slow the progression of OA. In younger, more active individuals, the clinician is left with the difficult task of developing a treatment strategy aimed at minimizing pain, improving function, and delaying TKA. Such an approach requires a host of patient-centered strategies focusing on tiered interventions. The least invasive therapies should always be implemented first regardless of the patient's age. These interventions include weight loss, orthotics, knee bracing, and physical therapy. Physical exercise has been shown to provide pain relief, particularly when combined with strengthening and aerobic activities. Various pharmacological treatments commonly used in combination with first-line therapies include oral analgesic agents and intra-articular hyaluronic acid or corticosteroid injections. Although nonsurgical interventions have been shown to provide temporary relief, they do not have any impact on the reversal of the underlying joint disease.

If nonsurgical management is unsuccessful, there are multiple surgical alternatives available. Total knee arthroplasty (TKA) has been shown to alleviate knee pain and improve knee function (Fig. 3.1). Although very effective, TKA in patients with PTOA may be challenging due to anatomic malalignment, bony deficiency, joint instability, contractures, compromised soft tissue, and retained hardware [28, 29]. These obstacles contribute to high complication rates, increased length of hospital stay, readmissions, and worse functional outcomes than patients preoperatively diagnosed with primary OA [8, 30].

Another method of surgical management particularly among younger patients with significant deformities are osteotomies. These procedures are typically done in younger (<50 years) more active patients with obvious bony malalignment. Although an osteotomy has been shown to be associated with delaying the need for TKA and improved pain and function scores [31], the benefits of surgery gradually deteriorate as the disease progresses. Long-term studies have demonstrated 10-year failure rates of 24.6% [32].

For patients with localized cartilaginous defects, osteochondral grafts may be indicated. The procedure is almost exclusively conducted in younger patients and has been associated with variable outcomes. A systematic review after a mean follow-up of 58 months demonstrated an overall failure rate of 18%, while 65% of patients had little to no radiographic change in knee arthritis on follow-up [33].

In order to deliver the highest quality of care, healthcare providers must emphasize primary and secondary prevention. Tertiary prevention will frequently require costly surgical procedures which may resolve the underlying joint pathology but often with suboptimal outcomes. Thus, healthcare providers should continue to investigate the pathophysiological association between mechanical injury and the subsequent degenerative changes observed in the joint. Moreover, structured treatment protocols are needed for the management of PTOA as these patients frequently require multiple surgical interventions during their lifetime, each associated with an independent list of complications and expenditures.

Post-traumatic Osteoarthritis of the Hip

Although PTOA of the hip is substantially less common than PTOA of the knee [2], its clinical and economic implications must also be considered. Unlike in the knee, time between injury and the development of PTOA of the hip is slightly lengthier, and the population that is affected is generally older. One population-based study demonstrated that in patients who developed hip PTOA following a traumatic event to the hip, the median age at which symptoms occurred was 66 years, approximately 13 years following the injury [34]. Furthermore, the study reported that injuries to the hip have been associated with a 4.3-fold increase in the risk of hip osteoarthritis. Although there are numerous mechanisms leading to PTOA of the hip, common causes include articular incongruity and disruption of the articular surface most frequently due to fractures or hip dislocations.

Types of Injuries Associated with PTOA of the Hip

Hip/Acetabular Fractures

Hip fractures may predispose patients to secondary arthritis of the hip, mainly as a result of failed subcapital hip fixation, and to a lesser extent intertrochanteric and subtrochanteric fractures. The specific mechanisms that lead to PTOA include high-energy fracture patterns, injury to the articular surface, and nonunions following injury. In addition, avascular necrosis resulting from traumatic devascularization or hardware placement following fracture fixation may subsequently cause PTOA of the hip (Fig. 3.2) [35].

Although acetabular fractures of the hip are rare compared to other types of fractures in the hip region, up to a quarter of these patients will go on to develop PTOA [36]. Acetabular fractures have a bimodal distribution occurring in the elderly and young males. The mechanism of injury in these two populations varies significantly. Elderly patients are more likely to sustain acetabular fractures following low-energy falls, whereas younger individuals typically sustain a high-energy injury [37]. Unfortunately, acetabular fractures predominantly occur in the elderly population, and their incidence has increased substantially in the past quarter century as the geriatric population continues to be the fastest growing subgroup in the United States [38] (Fig. 3.3).

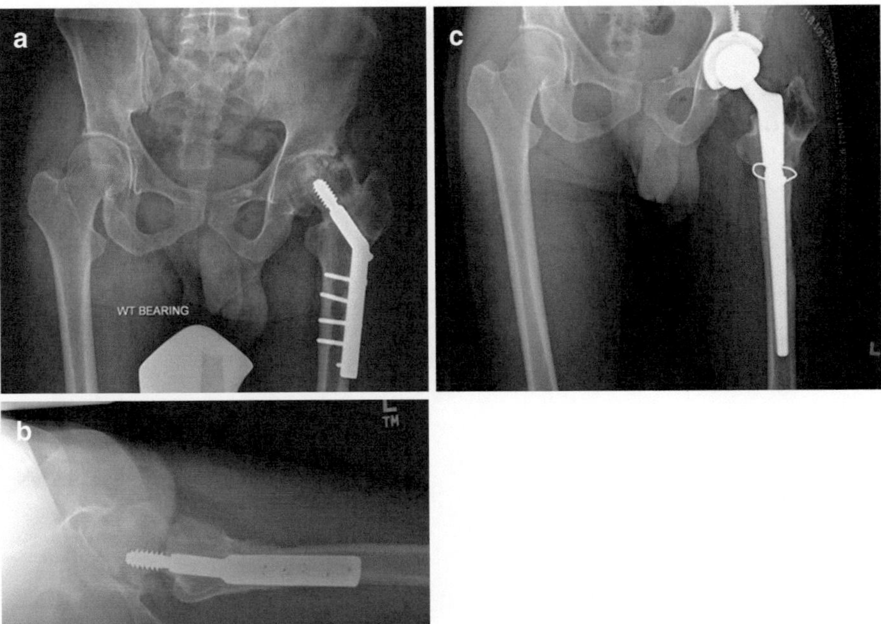

Fig. 3.2 AP (**a**) and lateral (**b**) view of previous intertrochanteric hip fracture treated with a sliding hip screw construct that went on to avascular necrosis. AP pelvis after removal of the sliding hip screw and left total hip arthroplasty treated with a modular diaphyseal engaging stem (**c**)

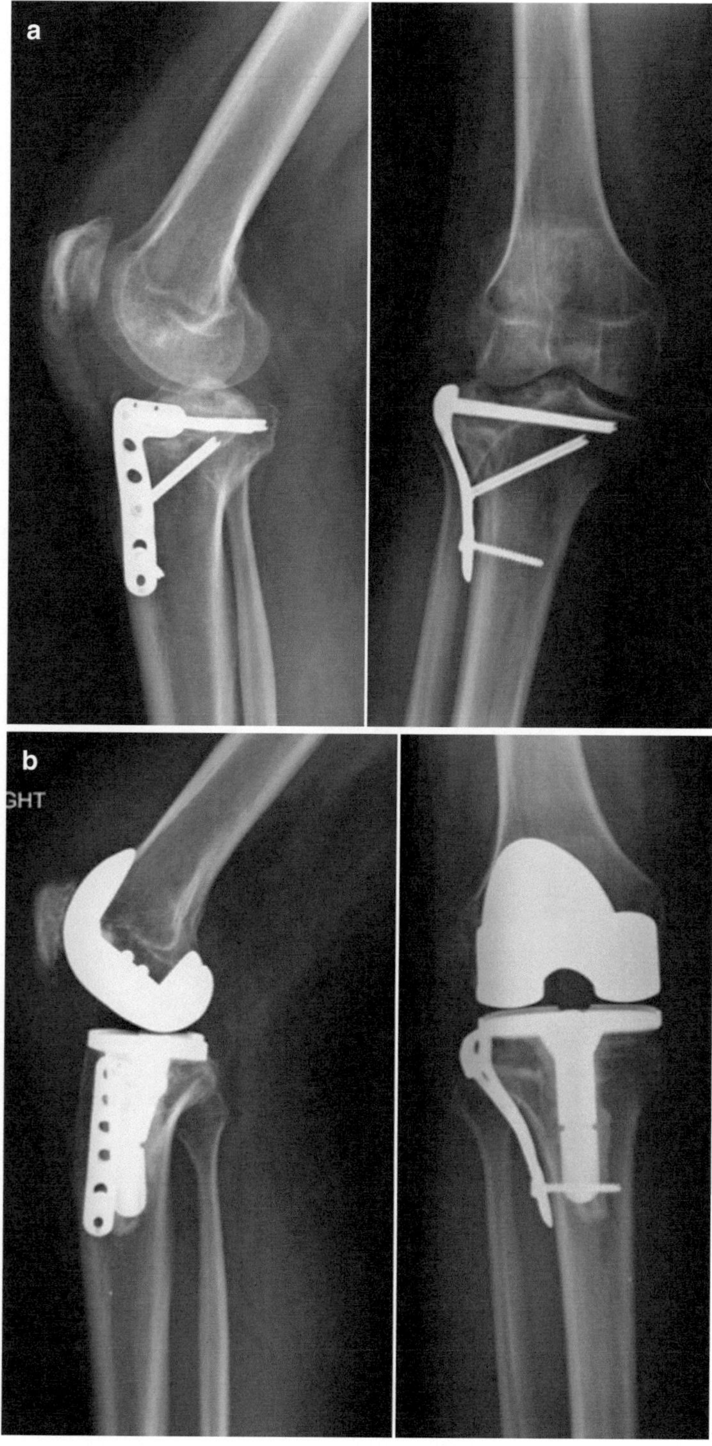

Fig. 3.3 Tibial plateau fracture (**a**) that went on to total knee arthroplasty (**b**). Clinical picture of the complex skin incision associated with reconstruction (**c**)

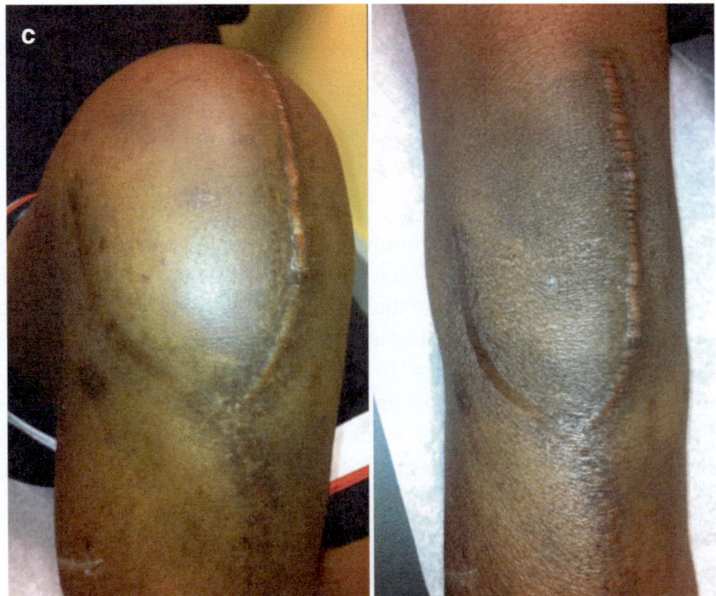

Fig. 3.3 (continued)

Hip Dislocations and Osteonecrosis

Posterior hip dislocations represent about 90% of all traumatic hip dislocations [39], and almost all injuries are a result of motor vehicle collisions. Given the strong association between these two events, young males (16–40 years) are most likely to be affected [40]. Hip dislocations lead to PTOA due to joint incongruity and instability, resulting in chronic inflammation and damage to the articular surface of the hip. In addition, hip dislocations may also result in acetabular fractures and osteonecrosis of the hip head. The overall occurrence rate of PTOA in the hip following posterior hip dislocations ranges from 19% to 55%, with a direct correlation between dislocation severity and the likelihood for future PTOA [41].

Management of PTOA in the Hip

Primary Prevention

Given the nature of the injury mechanism responsible for the majority of hip PTOA, preventing injury to the hip is somewhat more difficult than the knee. Broad measures have been shown to prevent acetabular fractures and hip dislocations which include safe driving practices and stringent adherence to fall precautions in the elderly. If fall precautions are in place, the cause should be investigated by a healthcare provider, medications should be reviewed, strength and balance exercises implemented, and regular vision checkups obtained. Finally, various medical conditions can predispose patients to osteonecrosis and, subsequently, PTOA of the hip. Thus, these high-risk patients may benefit from physician-directed preventative measures.

Secondary Prevention

Once a hip injury has occurred, a number of secondary measures can be implemented in an effort to prevent progression to PTOA. After an acetabular fracture, sufficient anatomic reduction is essential to ensure the joint has the best chance of survival. It should be emphasized that achieving anatomic reduction does not rule out the occurrence of PTOA [42, 43]. When managing hip dislocations, prompt reduction has been correlated with improved outcomes and reduced risk of complications such as the development of avascular necrosis of the femoral head. The orthopedic literature supports hip reduction as soon as possible or within 12 hours following the injury [41].

Tertiary Prevention

Once primary and secondary preventative measures have been exhausted, total hip arthroplasty (THA) may ultimately be indicated. Initially, many of the same nonsurgical management strategies of PTOA of the knee are shared with management of the hip. Once progression of PTOA of the hip can no longer be adequately managed nonoperatively, more invasive interventions including THA may be required (Fig. 3.2). Patients receiving these interventions are usually younger than those receiving THA secondary to primary OA. Although the risk for revision surgery is higher in younger patients, implant durability has improved substantially over the last three decades making THA in younger patients feasible. Despite the improvements, THA in the setting of PTOA has been linked with worse peri- and postoperative outcomes [44]. Thus, the possibility for longer operative times, higher rates of complications, early failures, and revision THA should be discussed with the patient. In rare circumstances, when the arthritic disease in the hip joint is so severe and previous attempts of THA have failed, rarely hip arthrodesis or resection arthroplasty may be indicated. Studies have demonstrated that although patients may be functionally limited, these can be effective procedures for the management of pain. However, arthrodesis has been associated with new onset ipsilateral knee and lower back pain due to the straining forces being placed on the proximal and distal joints. Other concerns associated with arthrodesis include highly variable union rates, likelihood of returning to work, and satisfaction rates, all of which should be discussed at length prior to surgery [45].

Costs Associated with Post-traumatic Osteoarthritis

There has been a robust effort to investigate the economic implications of primary OA and methods of better managing it while minimizing costs. However, the lack of large-scale epidemiologic studies evaluating the prevalence of PTOA has proven to be a major barrier in the development of accurate economic models assessing the financial fingerprint of PTOA on the US healthcare system. Although these two diagnoses share many similarities, PTOA affects a younger more active population, frequently requiring multiple surgical interventions. Thus, it should not be surprising that patients with PTOA have higher direct and indirect medical costs. Moreover, many of these patients are uninsured further complicating management of this debilitating disease. While it is well recognized that OA is one of the leading causes of disability among all diseases, the costs associated with the management of OA are difficult to approximate due to the debilitating nature of the disease and the many modalities of treatment. A recent report by Kotlarz and colleagues [46] utilized data from the Medical Expenditure Panel Survey (MEPS) and estimated that OA costs the US healthcare system $185.5 billion USD annually, of which $149.4 billion USD was expensed to insurers [46]. The report also found that women accounted for nearly two-thirds ($118 billion USD) of the dollars spent on managing OA, further demonstrating the gender discrepancies existing among those diagnosed with OA.

Although the literature surrounding the economic implications of PTOA is limited, a few recent studies have helped provide some perspective on the magnitude of the associated direct costs. Brown and colleagues [2] were the first to utilize a state-based model to estimate the prevalence and disease burden associated with PTOA at a national level. The investigators demonstrated that 6.8% of all patients with OA are due to PTOA of the hip and knee, 0.5% and 6.3%, respectively. Given these reported prevalence rates, the total direct costs associated with PTOA of the hip and knee can be measured at roughly $900 million and $11.7 billion annually (Fig. 3.4). In a separate study by Chin et al. [47], cohorts of patients undergoing primary THA were compared to conversion THA, a common salvage procedure of failed hip fracture fixation secondary to PTOA. The conversion procedures were associated with a significant increase of 26% in total hospital costs over primary OA treatment which, notably, did not account for the commonly occurring postoperative complications and revision procedures following discharge. Despite the paucity of literature comparatively examining postoperative outcomes and resource expenditures associated with PTOA, the available evidence clearly suggests an increased disease burden in patients diagnosed with PTOA compared with primary OA.

The indirect disease burden associated with PTOA is somewhat more concerning, as indirect costs associated with PTOA may be three times greater than direct costs [48]. Given that this population is younger and more active and frequently requires multiple surgical interventions (i.e., ACLR, arthroscopy, fracture fixation,

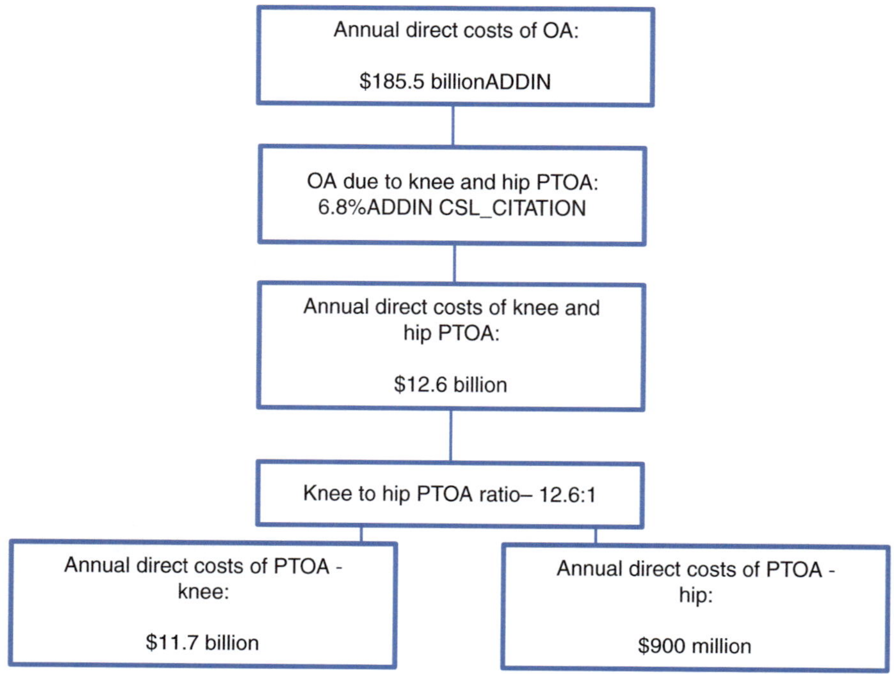

Fig. 3.4 Total direct cost of PTOA of the knee and hip

TJA) dispersed over their lifetime, the burden of PTOA economically and in terms of the individual's quality of life is substantially greater than primary OA. Additionally, many individuals with PTOA are of prime working age with higher rates of absenteeism, and overall work impairment compared with older age groups, [49] and are frequently forced to apply for disability benefits at each treatment juncture. Thus, although difficult to calculate the job-related loss of economic activity due to injuries, indirect costs of PTOA of the hip and knee together may be responsible for more than $35.3 billion annually, far exceeding the direct cost associated with PTOA (Fig. 3.5).

Recommendations

Individuals diagnosed with posttraumatic and primary OA often present with similar symptoms; however, the mechanism of injury varies significantly. Patients with PTOA have had an acute injury subsequently resulting in degenerative changes of the joint, whereas individuals with primary OA have nonspecific wear and inflammation leading to cartilage loss. Given the different mechanisms of injury and goals of treatment, it is crucial that healthcare providers manage PTOA through a

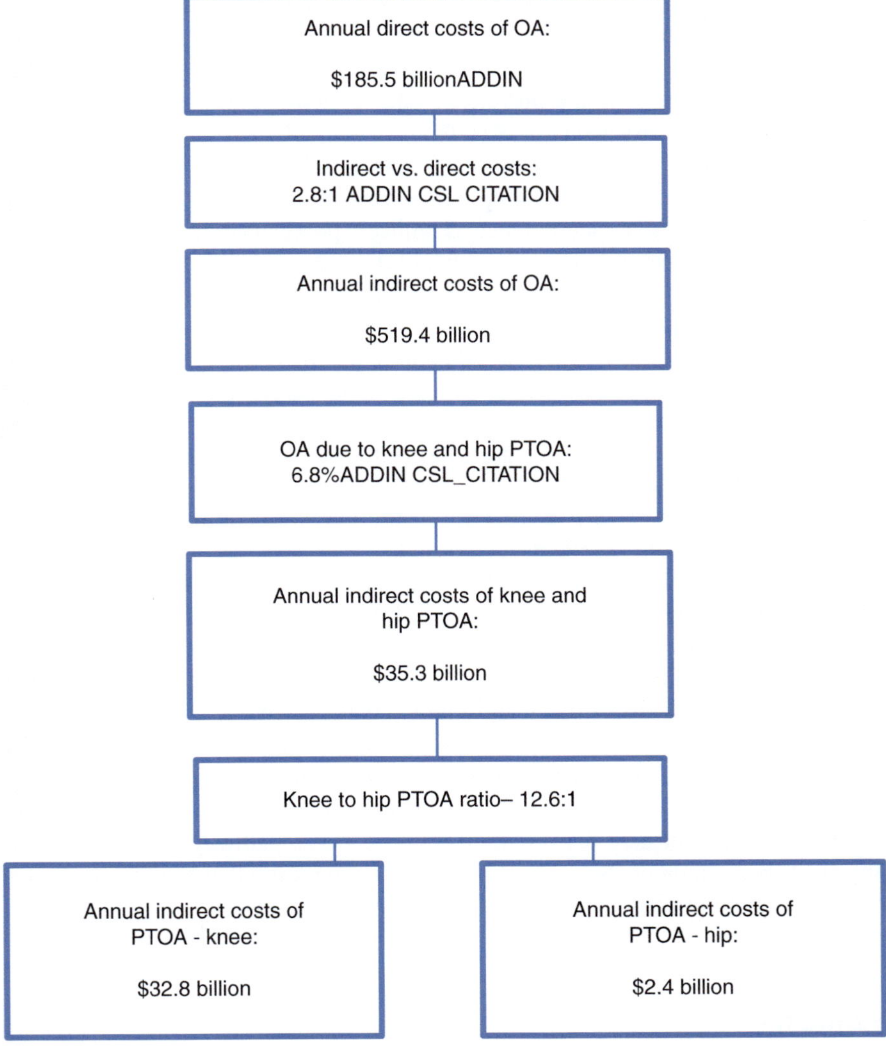

Fig. 3.5 Total indirect cost of PTOA of the knee and hip

designated care pathway (ICP) with the aim of delivering high-quality care while minimizing resource expenditures.

Our review demonstrates the paucity of literature examining postoperative outcomes and resource expenditures associated with the management of PTOA. This is at least in part due to the coding limitations associated with the *International Classification for Disease 9th Edition (ICD-9)*, which fails to differentiate between primary and secondary OA. Fortunately, as of October 2015, the *ICD-10* has been successfully implemented enabling clinicians to diagnose indications for surgery with greater specificity. If the *ICD-10* codes are properly implemented, future investigators may link clinical and billing information to better elucidate resource utilization trends among individuals with OA. However, the utilization of *ICD-10* codes alone is not sufficient as several issues still remain if these diagnostic codes are to be used to estimate the prevalence and economic burdens associated with complex disease processes such as PTOA.

First, the *ICD-10* coding system utilizes nearly 70,000 unique diagnostic codes. It is therefore essential that healthcare providers be familiar with the diagnostic codes within the scope of their practice. Healthcare providers must also avoid "gaming the system" by intentionally using a handful of nonspecific diagnostic codes. To insure that healthcare providers are meaningfully using diagnostic codes, providers should have the opportunity to participate in courses designed to better define the strengths and limitations of the *ICD-10* coding system. Additionally, as mandated by the Affordable Care Act (ACA), healthcare organizations and their providers are responsible for accurately documenting and reporting clinical metrics. Failure to properly do so will likely result in penalties and withheld payments. Thus, we suggest that healthcare organizations periodically audit the diagnostic codes being assigned to episodes of care, improving institution-wide compliance, while also strengthening the quality of the data collected.

Lastly, it is crucial that ICD-10 codes be aligned with CPT and Medicare Severity Diagnosis-Related Groups (MS-DRGs) in order to differentiate arthroplasty procedures by preoperative indication. Disease-specific procedure codes similar to those used in conversion THA and revision arthroplasty may enable investigators to better understand the clinical outcomes and disease burdens unique to PTOA. Without proper coding methodology, it is nearly impossible to distinguish indications for surgery at a macro level, thereby leaving many clinical questions unanswered. Furthermore, proper coding practices would enable investigators to retrospectively evaluate the value of care delivered, ensuring that care pathways are in line with organizational standards. Such an approach will also ensure that healthcare organizations are appropriately compensated for the services rendered.

Summary

Posttraumatic osteoarthritis of the hip and knee is a debilitating disease often affecting younger, more active individuals. Currently an estimated 5.8 million individuals are living with PTOA of the hip and knee at a direct and indirect cost of almost $48.9 billion annually. As Americans continue to live active lifestyles, the number of individuals living with PTOA is projected to steadily grow costing billions more dollars in direct and indirect expenditures. It is therefore critical that healthcare providers lobby for improved diagnostic and procedure codes so that PTOA can be properly monitored and objectively evaluated. Through such an approach, providers will have the resources needed to better address the complexities present in PTOA patients. Once granular coding instruments have been developed and used for these complex patients, the full economic impact of PTOA may be realized.

References

1. Lawrence RC, et al. Estimates of the prevalence of arthritis and other rheumatic conditions in the United States. Part II. Arthritis Rheum. 2008;58(1):26–35.
2. Brown TD, Johnston RC, Saltzman CL, Marsh JL, Buckwalter JA. Posttraumatic osteoarthritis: a first estimate of incidence, prevalence, and burden of disease. J Orthop Trauma. 2006;20(10):739–44.
3. Anderson DD, et al. Post-traumatic osteoarthritis: improved understanding and opportunities for early intervention. J Orthop Res. 2011;29(6):802–9.
4. Buckwalter JA, Brown TD. Joint injury, repair, and remodeling: roles in post-traumatic osteoarthritis. Clin Orthop Relat Res. 2004;423:7–16.
5. Stiebel M, Miller LE, Block JE. Post-traumatic knee osteoarthritis in the young patient: therapeutic dilemmas and emerging technologies. Open Access J Sport Med. 2014;5:73–9.
6. Saltzman CL, et al. Epidemiology of ankle arthritis: report of a consecutive series of 639 patients from a tertiary orthopaedic center. Iowa Orthop J. 2005;25:44–6.
7. Soni A. Top 10 most costly conditions among men and women, 2008: estimates for the U.S. civilian noninstitutionalized adult population, age 18 and older. 2011. 2011.
8. Kester BS, Minhas SV, Vigdorchik JM, Schwarzkopf R. Total knee arthroplasty for posttraumatic osteoarthritis: is it time for a new classification? J Arthroplasty. 2016;31(8):1649–1653.e1.
9. Gelber AC, Hochberg MC, Mead LA, Wang N-YY, Wigley FM, Klag MJ. Joint injury in young adults and risk for subsequent knee and hip osteoarthritis. Ann Intern Med. 2000;133(5):321.
10. Lohmander LS, Englund PM, Dahl LL, Roos EM. The long-term consequence of anterior cruciate ligament and meniscus injuries: osteoarthritis. Am J Sports Med. 2007;35(10):1756–69.
11. Swenson DM, Collins CL, Best TM, Flanigan DC, Fields SK, Comstock RD. Epidemiology of knee injuries among U.S. high school athletes, 2005/2006–2010/2011. Med Sci Sports Exerc. 2013;45(3):462–9.
12. Lebel B, Hulet C, Galaud B, Burdin G, Locker B, Vielpeau C. Arthroscopic reconstruction of the anterior cruciate ligament using bone-patellar tendon-bone autograft: a minimum 10-year follow-up. Am J Sports Med. 2008;36(7):1275–82.
13. Kraus VB, et al. Call for standardized definitions of osteoarthritis and risk stratification for clinical trials and clinical use. Osteoarthr Cartil. 2015;23(8):1233–41.
14. Barenius B, Ponzer S, Shalabi A, Bujak R, Norlén L, Eriksson K. Increased risk of osteoarthritis after anterior cruciate ligament reconstruction: a 14-year follow-up study of a randomized controlled trial. Am J Sports Med. 2014;42(5):1049–57.
15. Roos H, Adalberth T, Dahlberg L, Lohmander LS. Osteoarthritis of the knee after injury to the anterior cruciate ligament or meniscus: the influence of time and age. Osteoarthr Cartil. 1995;3(4):261–7.
16. Badlani JT, Borrero C, Golla S, Harner CD, Irrgang JJ. The effects of meniscus injury on the development of knee osteoarthritis: data from the osteoarthritis initiative. Am J Sports Med. 2013;41(6):1238–44.
17. Rademakers MV, Kerkhoffs GMMJ, Sierevelt IN, Raaymakers ELFB, Marti RK. Operative treatment of 109 Tibial plateau fractures: five- to 27-year follow-up results. J Orthop Trauma. 2007;21(1):5–10.
18. Honkonen SE. Degenerative arthritis after tibial plateau fractures. J Orthop Trauma. 1995;9(4):273–7.
19. Fithian DC, et al. Prospective trial of a treatment algorithm for the management of the anterior cruciate ligament-injured knee. Am J Sports Med. 2005;33(3):335–46.
20. Racine J, Aaron RK. Post-traumatic osteoarthritis after ACL injury. R I Med J (2013). 2014;97(11):25–8.
21. Mandelbaum BR, et al. Effectiveness of a neuromuscular and proprioceptive training program in preventing anterior cruciate ligament injuries in female athletes: 2-year follow-up. Am J Sports Med. 2005;33(7):1003–10.

22. Grindstaff TL, Hammill RR, Tuzson AE, Hertel J. Neuromuscular control training programs and noncontact anterior cruciate ligament injury rates in female athletes: a numbers-needed-to-treat analysis. J Athl Train. 2006;41(4):450–6.
23. Mather RC, et al. Societal and economic impact of anterior cruciate ligament tears. J Bone Joint Surg Am. 2013;95(19):1751–9.
24. Buckwalter JA, Felson DT. Post-traumatic arthritis: definitions and burden of disease. In: Post-traumatic arthritis. Boston: Springer US; 2015. p. 7–15.
25. Riordan EA, Little C, Hunter D. Pathogenesis of post-traumatic OA with a view to intervention. Best Pract Res Clin Rheumatol. 2014;28(1):17–30.
26. Knutsen G, et al. A randomized trial comparing autologous chondrocyte implantation with microfracture. Findings at five years. J Bone Joint Surg Am. 2007;89(10):2105–12.
27. Knutsen G, et al. A randomized multicenter trial comparing autologous chondrocyte implantation with microfracture. J Bone Jt Surg. 2016;98(16):1332–9.
28. Shearer DW, Chow V, Bozic KJ, Liu J, Ries MD. The predictors of outcome in total knee arthroplasty for post-traumatic arthritis. Knee. 2013;20(6):432–6.
29. Georgiadis GM, Skakun FWC. Total knee arthroplasty with retained tibial implants: the role of minimally invasive hardware removal. Am J Orthop. 2016;45(7):E481.
30. Lunebourg A, Parratte S, Gay A, Ollivier M, Garcia-Parra K, Argenson J-N. Lower function, quality of life, and survival rate after total knee arthroplasty for posttraumatic arthritis than for primary arthritis. Acta Orthop. 2015;86(2):189–94.
31. Lustig S, et al. Post-traumatic knee osteoarthritis treated by osteotomy only. Orthop Traumatol Surg Res. 2010;96(8):856–60.
32. Virolainen P, Aro HT. High tibial osteotomy for the treatment of osteoarthritis of the knee: a review of the literature and a meta-analysis of follow-up studies. Arch Orthop Trauma Surg. 2004;124(4):258–61.
33. Chahal J, et al. Outcomes of osteochondral allograft transplantation in the knee. Arthroscopy. 2013;29(3):575–88.
34. Cooper C, et al. Individual risk factors for hip osteoarthritis: obesity, hip injury, and physical activity. Am J Epidemiol. 1998;147(6):516–22.
35. Haidukewych GJ, Rothwell WS, Jacofsky DJ, Torchia ME, Berry DJ. Operative treatment of femoral neck fractures in patients between the ages of fifteen and fifty years. J Bone Jt Surg. 2004;86(8):1711–6.
36. Giannoudis PV, Grotz MRW, Papakostidis C, Dinopoulos H. Operative treatment of displaced fractures of the acetabulum. A meta-analysis. J Bone Joint Surg Br. 2005;87(1):2–9.
37. Mears DC. Surgical treatment of acetabular fractures in elderly patients with osteoporotic bone. J Am Acad Orthop Surg. 1999;7(2):128–41.
38. Butterwick D, et al. Acetabular fractures in the elderly: evaluation and management. J Bone Joint Surg Am. 2015;97(9):758–68.
39. Sowers M, Lachance L, Hochberg M, Jamadar D. Radiographically defined osteoarthritis of the hand and knee in young and middle-aged African American and Caucasian women. Osteoarthr Cartil. 2000;8(2):69–77.
40. Epstein HC. Traumatic dislocations of the hip. Clin Orthop Relat Res. 1973;92:116–42.
41. Kellam P, Ostrum RF. Systematic review and meta-analysis of avascular necrosis and post-traumatic arthritis after traumatic hip dislocation. J Orthop Trauma. 2016;30(1):10–6.
42. Tannast M, Najibi S, Matta JM. Two to twenty-year survivorship of the hip in 810 patients with operatively treated acetabular fractures. J Bone Joint Surg Am. 2012;94(17):1559–67.
43. Meena UK, Tripathy SK, Sen RK, Aggarwal S, Behera P. Predictors of postoperative outcome for acetabular fractures. Orthop Traumatol Surg Res. 2013;99(8):929–35.
44. Srivastav S, Mittal V, Agarwal S. Total hip arthroplasty following failed fixation of proximal hip fractures. Indian J Orthop. 2008;42(3):279–86.
45. Jain S, Giannoudis PV. Arthrodesis of the hip and conversion to total hip arthroplasty: a systematic review. J Arthroplast. 2013;28(9):1596–602.

46. Kotlarz H, Gunnarsson CL, Fang H, Rizzo JA. Insurer and out-of-pocket costs of osteoarthritis in the US: evidence from national survey data. Arthritis Rheum. 2009;60(12):3546–53.
47. Chin G, Wright DJ, Snir N, Schwarzkopf R. Primary vs conversion total hip arthroplasty: a cost analysis. J Arthroplast. 2016;31(2):362–7.
48. Praemer A, Furner S, Rice DP. American Academy of Orthopaedic Surgeons. Musculoskeletal conditions in the United States. American Academy of Orthopaedic Surgeons: Rosemont; 1999.
49. Dibonaventure MD, Gupta S, Mcdonald M, Sadosky A, Pettitt D, Silverman S. Impact of self-rated osteoarthritis in an employed population: cross-sectional analysis of data from the national health and wellness survey. Heal Qual Life Outcomes. 2012;10:30.

Part II
Post-traumatic Arthritis of the Upper Extremity

Chapter 4
Post-traumatic Glenohumeral Arthritis

Uma Srikumaran and Eric Huish

Key Points
- Proximal humerus fractures, glenohumeral instability, and direct cartilaginous trauma are all causes of post-traumatic glenohumeral arthritis.
- Various injury patterns and previous interventions may alter the anatomy of the glenohumeral joint, which must be taken into account when surgical treatment is planned.
- Total shoulder arthroplasty, reverse shoulder arthroplasty, and hemiarthroplasty are all utilized in the treatment of post-traumatic glenohumeral arthritis, each with various benefits and shortcomings.
- Non-arthroplasty options for the treatment of glenohumeral post-traumatic arthritis show transient benefit and may be beneficial in the appropriately selected patient.

Introduction

Post-traumatic arthritis of the shoulder can result from a variety of injuries. Fractures, dislocations, isolated chondral injuries, or rotator cuff pathology may be implicated. As with other arthropathies, there is a broad spectrum of disease ranging from mild discomfort to severe disability with pain, stiffness, and inability to

U. Srikumaran (✉)
The Johns Hopkins University, Division of Shoulder and Elbow Surgery,
Columbia, MD, USA
e-mail: us@jhmi.edu

E. Huish
Stanislaus Orthopaedics & Sports Medicine Clinic, Modesto, CA, USA

© Springer Nature Switzerland AG 2021
S. C. Thakkar, E. A. Hasenboehler (eds.), *Post-Traumatic Arthritis*,
https://doi.org/10.1007/978-3-030-50413-7_4

perform activities of daily living. Appropriate treatment should be based on the initial injury, previous treatment, severity of disease, and patient factors including age, activity level, hand dominance, and goals.

Causes

Fractures

Multiple traumatic etiologies may lead to arthritic changes in the glenohumeral joint. Proximal humerus fractures are among the more commonly implicated injuries with one study showing nearly two-thirds of patients with three- and four-part proximal humerus fractures developed post-traumatic arthritis [50]. This may be due to direct articular damage at the time of injury, malunion with intra-articular step-off, screw cutout, or osteonecrosis (Fig. 4.1). The rate of osteonecrosis reported in the literature varies. A systematic review revealed an overall rate of 2% after nonoperative treatment of all types of proximal humerus fractures [25]. However, nearly half of the included cases in this review were one-part nondisplaced fractures. The three- and four-part subgroups had an osteonecrosis rate of 14%. A separate systematic review looking at proximal humerus fractures treated with open reduction and locked plating showed a 7.9% rate of osteonecrosis [48]. This analysis excluded studies that were limited to two-part fractures but did not give results based on fracture classification. Other studies have shown higher rates of osteonecrosis after open reduction and internal fixation, with up to 35% in one study [19]. Gerber examined the significance of post-traumatic osteonecrosis and showed that all patients with osteonecrosis after proximal humerus fracture had some level of dysfunction compared to a healthy control group. He noted, though, that associated

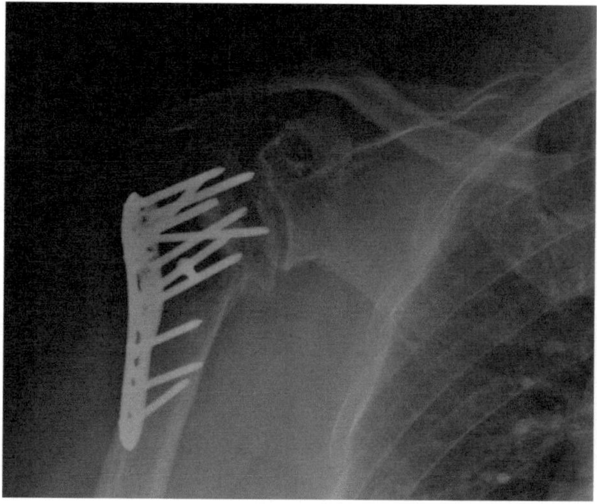

Fig. 4.1 AP radiograph of the shoulder after open reduction and internal fixation of a proximal humerus fracture showing osteonecrosis and collapse of the humeral head with resultant screw protrusion

malunion of the fracture fragments significantly worsened the subjective outcome, pain, forward elevation, and Constant score [20].

Another known complication associated with open reduction and internal fixation is screw cutout, with rates reported as high as 23% overall and up to 43% in patients older than 60 [48, 36]. Articular incongruity has been reported in 67% of malunited proximal humerus fractures [3]. Patients in this study who did not have the incongruity corrected with arthroplasty or shoulder fusion all had unsatisfactory outcomes. Both screw penetration and articular incongruity may alter the contact stresses on remaining intact cartilage leading to post-traumatic arthritis. Further, altered shoulder mechanics or malunion of the tuberosities may also lead to rotator cuff damage and subsequent arthropathy.

While proximal humerus fractures are often implicated in post-traumatic arthritis of the glenohumeral joint, glenoid fractures are less frequently discussed as they are much less common, making up only 10% of scapular fractures, with only 10% of those fractures having significant displacement. Goss recommended 5 mm displacement as a relative indication for treatment with 10 mm as an absolute indication [21]. Fractures with >4 mm step-off were operatively treated, demonstrating good outcomes for DASH scores, SF-36, pain, and return to pre-injury level of activity [1]. Another study with 10-year follow-up after operative treatment had a median Constant score of 94% [42]. Despite good outcomes with intra-articular glenoid fractures and a high tolerance to step-off, recognition of these injuries is still important, as altered glenoid morphology may affect surgical treatment.

Instability

Shoulder dislocations are another potential cause of post-traumatic arthritis (Fig. 4.2a, b). Dislocation arthropathy has been reported to occur at varying rates. One study with 10-year follow-up showed 11% of mild arthropathy with 9% developing moderate to severe arthropathy [23]. Another study showed the presence of arthritis in patients with previous shoulder instability to be 9.2% prior to undergoing surgery [6]. Furthermore, this same study showed development of arthritis in 19.7% of patients after surgery when no arthritis was present preoperatively. It was unclear whether this was a progression from the previous injury or a consequence from surgery. The authors noted that older age at time of first dislocation increased the number of dislocations, and increased follow-up time from surgery were correlated with the development of arthritis. Further, decreased external rotation was also correlated with the development of arthritis. However, it was unknown if this was a cause or a result of the arthritis.

Capsulorrhaphy arthropathy is used to describe arthritis that develops as a result of overtightening the capsule. Matsoukis, who evaluated patients undergoing arthroplasty after previous instability, did not find any significant differences between those with previous surgical treatment of the instability and those without. This finding suggests that dislocation arthropathy and capsulorrhaphy arthropathy may result in similar outcomes after arthroplasty [33].

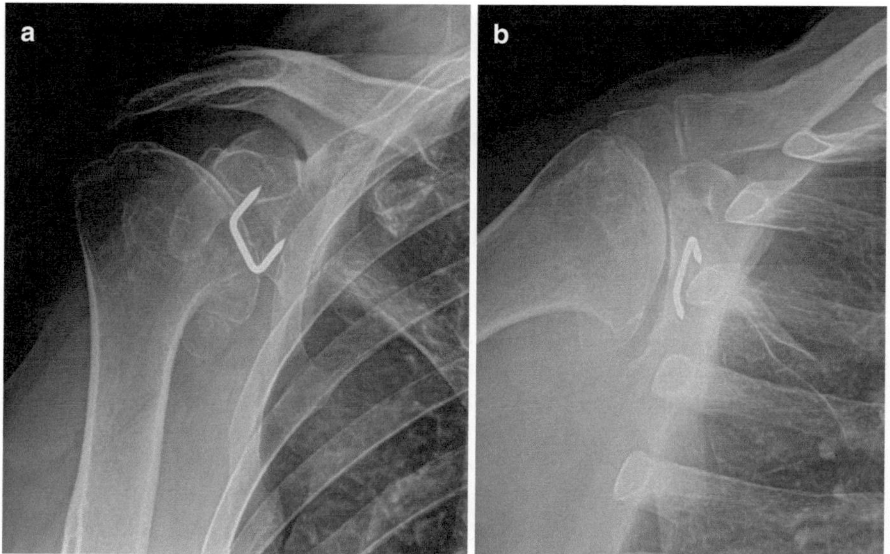

Fig. 4.2 (**a**, **b**) AP and axillary radiographs of a shoulder with post-traumatic arthritis after dislocation and subsequent repair

Other Causes

Other causes of post-traumatic arthritis include isolated chondral or osteochondral injury. Isolated chondral lesions from shearing are rare but have been reported [41], as have osteochondral defects [13]. Arthropathy from rotator cuff tear is more commonly seen in degenerative cases, but may develop after a traumatic tear if ignored. More likely the altered mechanics and anatomy of the joint following trauma may lead to degeneration of the rotator cuff. As with degenerative cases, this pattern is difficult because the lack of rotator cuff function limits treatment options.

Treatment

There are many factors involved in determining the appropriate treatment of post-traumatic glenohumeral arthritis. The surgeon should assess the severity of disease, initial injury, previous treatments, patient age, and functional requirements.

Nonoperative Treatment

The initial treatment of post-traumatic glenohumeral arthritis in all patients should include a trial of nonoperative management. This may include physical therapy, activity modification, medications, or injections. Both corticosteroid and viscosupplementation (hyaluronic acid) injections may be considered, though use of viscosupplementation in the shoulder is off-label. The American Academy of Orthopaedic Surgeons guidelines on the treatment of glenohumeral arthritis are inconclusive on the efficacy of physical therapy, pharmacotherapy, and corticosteroid injections. Further, there was limited evidence found to support viscosupplementation [26]. Only after these modalities have been attempted, surgery should be considered only in a carefully selected patient population, as patients with low demands and multiple medical comorbidities may be best managed with continued observation.

Preoperative Evaluation

Workup prior to possible surgical intervention should be thorough. Standard radiographs should be taken to evaluate joint space, arthritic changes, and other abnormalities including malunion or nonunion of previous fracture and the presence of hardware. Further imaging with CT or MRI may be warranted to evaluate glenoid morphology, rotator cuff integrity, or other soft tissue abnormalities. Careful attention should be paid to a thorough neurological exam as nerve injuries may result from the initial trauma or possibly from previous interventions. In such cases, thorough neurologic exam, an EMG, and NCS may be required.

Any previously operated shoulder should be ruled out for infections and possible source of pain and dysfunction. High rates of positive cultures have been reported in patients undergoing revision shoulder surgery [24]. *Propionibacterium acnes* is often indicated and may be missed unless cultures are held for an extended period of time for this more indolent organism. Preoperative lab work including WBC, ESR, and CRP along with intraoperative frozen sections does not have a high sensitivity for indolent infection [49]. More recently synovial cytokines have been investigated as predictors of periprosthetic joint infections [17] and may lead to improved detection. If infection is discovered, it should be addressed appropriately.

Preoperative planning should include assessment of prior incisions/approaches as well as determination of any hardware that may require removal. The choice of the appropriate surgical procedure is controversial and should be tailored to the individual patient.

Arthroplasty

Total Shoulder Arthroplasty

Arthroplasty is often chosen for treatment of post-traumatic glenohumeral arthritis. In these cases it is important to recognize anatomic changes resulting from previous injury or surgery. Malunited fractures may alter the relationship between the humeral head and shaft making the placement of a humeral stem difficult. Possible solutions include using short stem prostheses (Fig. 4.3a, b) or stemless prostheses. Tuberosity malunion also causes difficulty as arthroplasty components are not designed to address the tuberosities and will not correct malunions that may be a

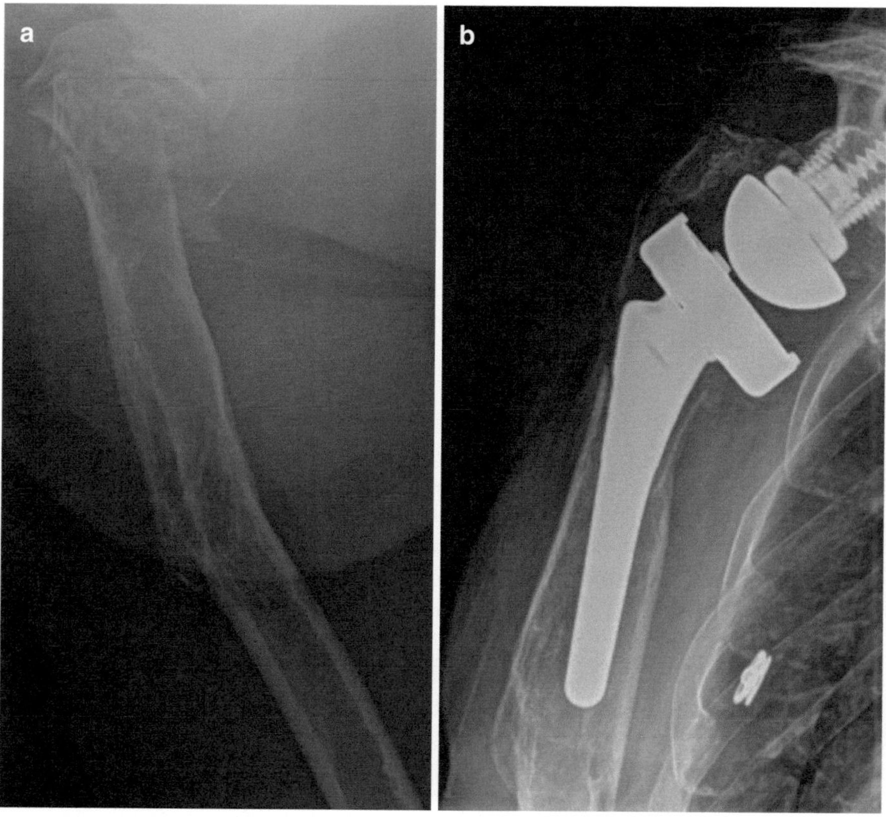

Fig. 4.3 (**a, b**) Preoperative and postoperative radiographs of a humerus with malunion and post-traumatic arthritis treated with reverse shoulder arthroplasty utilizing a short humeral stem

source of impingement and dysfunction. If malunion is severe, osteotomy may be required. The need for tuberosity osteotomy has been shown to result in poorer outcomes [5]. Glenoid degeneration or fracture may also make arthroplasty difficult. Ensuring adequate fixation as well as appropriate version is crucial. Glenoid augments have been developed to treat posterior glenoid wear and recently have been used as an anterior glenoid augment, which may be useful after anterior instability with bony Bankart lesion [28]. Soft tissue changes must also be addressed. Green reported that 65% of patients undergoing arthroplasty after previous instability repair required subscapularis lengthening and anterior capsular release. Eighteen percent required glenoid bone grafting, and one required glenoidplasty [22].

Hemiarthroplasty

Hemiarthroplasty, sometimes used as an acute treatment in trauma, may also be used to treat sequelae of the injury, including arthritis. Since osteonecrosis and malunion are typically limited to the humerus, a hemiarthroplasty may be used to replace the affected surfaces. However, hemiarthroplasty used to treat fracture sequelae showed the lowest survival and highest complication rate when compared to other uses of the implant [18]. Further, studies have shown better pain scores, satisfaction, and survival with a lower reoperation rate after total shoulder arthroplasty than hemiarthroplasty when used specifically for post-traumatic osteonecrosis of the humeral head [44]. Specifically looking at patients younger than 55, total shoulder arthroplasty had outperformed hemiarthroplasty with regard to survivability, pain, motion, and satisfaction [2]. Another study evaluating patients under 50 showed a similar benefit in survival and satisfaction favoring total shoulder arthroplasty [15]. That said, some surgeons try to avoid total shoulder arthroplasty in younger patients despite the known facts of glenoid loosening and increased implant failure over its lifetime [37]. However, the increased survival of total shoulder arthroplasty at 15 years suggests this may be becoming less of a concern [44].

The possibility of poor outcomes with hemiarthroplasty alone coupled with a desire to avoid glenoid instrumentation in young patients has led to a search for variations on the technique that may prove superior. One of these techniques known as the "ream and run" utilizes glenoid reaming without instrumentation at the time of hemiarthroplasty. This, however, is a not widely used and technically difficult procedure with a steep learning curve [32]. Another trialed modification to hemiarthroplasty is biologic resurfacing of the glenoid. Various materials have been used for resurfacing, including meniscus and acellular matrices. Some studies have shown success [31], but high rates of early failure have been reported [39, 47] and the procedure is not routinely performed. Other areas of interest for modifying hemiarthroplasty include use of pyrocarbon implants [8]. Although success has been seen in other joints, studies of its use in the shoulder are lacking.

To this end, the choice between hemiarthroplasty and total shoulder arthroplasty is still debated, especially for young patients.

Humeral Resurfacing

An alternative to hemiarthroplasty is humeral resurfacing. Without addressing the glenoid, the aim is to maintain as much bone as possible so to prevent issues that may arise at the time of revision. Its use has been reported for sequelae of proximal humerus fractures with good results [30, 38]. However, with the advent of stemless humeral prostheses, these are no longer the only bone-conserving option.

Reverse Shoulder Arthroplasty

If the rotator cuff is deficient, in presence of a functional deltoid and adequate bone stock, a reverse shoulder arthroplasty may be considered. Although clinical outcomes for the treatment of fracture sequelae show improvement, results are worse than for acute fractures [10, 14]. To this end, patients who had previous fracture surgery had worse outcomes than those treated initially nonoperatively [10].

Reverse shoulder arthroplasty has also been used with good results as a revision from a failed hemiarthroplasty due to development of glenoid arthritis or rotator cuff failure [29]. However, these results are inferior to those obtained for primary indications.

Reverse shoulder arthroplasty was originally reserved for elderly patients; however, in cases where no other option seems appropriate, reverse shoulder arthroplasty may be an option in a younger patient. Few studies evaluate patients under 60 undergoing reverse shoulder arthroplasty. The current literature shows good early outcomes, but follow-up is limited, and the success rate and patient satisfaction are less than in previous studies looking at an older population [35, 45]. This procedure must be done with caution in a young patient, as long-term outcomes are not yet widely reported with midterm outcomes showing a 15% failure rate, 25% reoperation rate, and 38% complication rate after 5–15 years [16].

Alternative Options

If reverse shoulder arthroplasty is determined to be inappropriate due to patient age, poor glenoid bone stock, nonfunctional rotator cuff, or other reasons, a cuff tear hemiarthroplasty is an alternative. In the most severe cases, where both rotator cuff and deltoid are nonfunctional or where significant brachial plexus injury has occurred, a glenohumeral fusion may be considered. This results in significant impairment compared to normal shoulder function, but remaining scapulothoracic motion may allow for utilization of remaining hand/elbow function in the appropriately selected patient [11].

Non-arthroplasty Surgery

Especially in young patients, non-arthroplasty options may be more attractive to treat post-traumatic glenohumeral arthritis. Arthroscopic debridement has been shown to improve pain and function in 88% of patients with grade IV glenohumeral joint chondral lesions for an average of 28 months [7]. Lesions over 2 cm^2 were associated with failure and recurrence of pain, while microfractures have been shown to improve pain scores, American Shoulder and Elbow Surgeons' scores, and the ability to return to work/activity at 47 months [34]. This study, however, had a 19% failure rate, defined as need for additional surgery. The greatest improvements were seen in isolated humerus lesions. Failure was associated with a larger defect size. Osteochondral autologous transplantation was shown in two cases only by Scheibel to improve Constant scores and have good integration via MRI and by second-look arthroscopy [43]. All patients in this study had evidence of arthritis at latest follow-up, including those with worsening of preexisting arthritis.

Osteochondral allografts have been reported as an alternative solution without the risk of donor site morbidity [27]. Autologous chondrocyte implantation was shown to be effective at 1 year in a case report but has also been reported to cause overgrowth and mechanical damage due to the thin humeral head cartilage [9, 40]. Juvenile cartilage allograft and subchondral calcium phosphate injections have not been described in the literature but may be an area of future research.

Biologic resurfacing of the glenoid is an alternative and not widely used method with a failure rate of up to 28% [12]. That said, as none of these treatments have shown consistent long-term relief of arthritis pain, they may be considered as a temporary solution for patients who are not candidates for arthroplasty due to age, medical condition, or other reasons.

Complications

Postoperative stiffness is a common complication of surgery for post-traumatic arthritis of the glenohumeral joint. Accordingly, attention should be turned to adequate soft tissue release at the time of surgery and an emphasis placed on postoperative physical therapy. Progression of arthritis may also develop after non-arthroplasty surgery or hemiarthroplasty. Component failure is also possible and reported as 5.3% for the glenoid and 1.1% for the humerus in a broad review of shoulder arthroplasty performed for any indication [4]. Long-term studies are lacking for many of our current implants and may change survival data. Other complications in this review include instability in 4.9%, periprosthetic fracture in 1.8%, and nerve injury in 0.8% [4]. Most concerning is infection. The infection rate after revision shoulder arthroplasty has been shown to be 3.15% compared to 0.76% in primary arthroplasties at the same institution [46]. These risks must be considered when selecting the appropriate patient and determining the appropriate treatment.

Summary

The treatment options for post-traumatic arthritis of the glenohumeral joint are as diverse as its causes. Patients are surgical candidates only after failure of nonoperative treatments and thorough preoperative workup. While arthroplasty may be a widely accepted treatment for older or lower-demand patients, there is controversy surrounding the treatment of younger, active patients. In this group, surgical treatment should be individualized after frank discussion of goals and expected outcomes. While significant improvements are seen after surgical intervention, they tend to fall short of expected results for primary procedures with high complication rates. New and emerging implants and techniques may improve treatment in these challenging cases.

Annotated References

1. Anavian J, Gauger EM, Schroder LK, Wijdicks CA, Cole PA. Surgical and functional outcomes after operative management of complex and displaced intra-articular glenoid fractures. J Bone Joint Surg Am. 2012;94(7):645–53. This level IV study examined 33 displaced glenoid fractures with >4mm step off treated surgically. The mean DASH score was 10.8 with 87% of patients pain free and 90% of patients returning to pre-injury level of activity at 27 months follow up.
2. Bartelt R, Sperling JW, Schleck CD, Cofield RH. Shoulder arthroplasty in patients aged fifty-five years or younger with osteoarthritis. J Shoulder Elbow Surg. 2011;20(1):123–30. This level IV study reviewed 46 TSA and 20 Hemiarthroplasties in patients age 55 and under. 10 year survival was 92% for TSA and 72% for hemi with less pain, greater forward elevation, and higher satisfaction in the TSA group.
3. Beredjiklian PK, Iannotti JP, Norris TR, Williams GR. Operative treatment of malunion of a fracture of the proximal aspect of the humerus. J Bone Joint Surg Am. 1998;80(10):1484–97.
4. Bohsali KI, Wirth MA, Rockwood CA Jr. Complications of total shoulder arthroplasty. J Bone Joint Surg Am. 2006;88(10):2279–92.
5. Boileau P, Trojani C, Walch G, Krishnan SG, Romeo A, et al. Shoulder arthroplasty for the treatment of the sequelae of fractures of the proximal humerus. J Shoulder Elb Surg. 2001;10(4):299–308.
6. Buscayret F, Edwards TB, Szabo I, Adeleine P, Coudane H, et al. Glenohumeral arthrosis in anterior instability before and after surgical treatment: incidence and contributing factors. Am J Sports Med. 2004;32(5):1165–72.
7. Cameron BD, Galatz LM, Ramsey ML, Williams GR, Iannotti JP. Non-prosthetic management of grade IV osteochondral lesions of the glenohumeral joint. J Shoulder Elb Surg. 2002;11(1):25–32.
8. Carpenter SR, Urits I, Murthi AM. Porous metals and alternate bearing surfaces in shoulder arthroplasty. Curr Rev Musculoskelet Med. 2016;9(1):59–66. This study discussed the use of trabecular metal, highly cross-linked polyethylene and pyrocarbon as new materials being used in shoulder arthroplasty.
9. Chong PY, Srikumaran U, Kuye IO, Warner JJ. Glenohumeral arthritis in the young patient. J Shoulder Elbow Surg. 2011;20(2 Suppl):S30–40. This review article discusses glenohumeral osteoarthritis in young patients as well as management strategies both operative and non-operative.
10. Cicak N, Klobucar H, Medancic N. Reverse shoulder arthroplasty in acute fractures provides better results than in revision procedures for fracture sequelae. Int Orthop. 2015;39(2):343–8. This study evaluated 37 patients undergoing reverse shoulder arthroplasty for acute fracture or sequelae of fracture. Post-op range of motion was highest in the acute fracture group followed by non-operatively treated fracture sequelae group and finally the previously operated group. Constant score was higher in the group without prior surgery.
11. Cofield RH, Briggs BT. Glenohumeral arthrodesis operative and long-term functional results. J Bone Joint Surg Am. 1979;61(5):668–77.
12. de Beer JF, Bhatia DN, van Rooyen KS, Du Toit DF. Arthroscopic debridement and biological resurfacing of the glenoid in glenohumeral arthritis. Knee Surg Sports Traumatol Arthrosc. 2010;18(12):1767–73.
13. Debeer P, Brys P. Osteochondritis dissecans of the humeral head: clinical and radiological findings. Acta Orthop Belg. 2005;71(4):484–8.
14. Dezfuli B, King JJ, Farmer KW, Struk AM, Wright TW. Outcomes of reverse total shoulder arthroplasty as primary versus revision procedure for proximal humerus fractures. J Shoulder Elbow Surg. 2016;25(7):1133–7. This level III study looked at 49 RSA performed for acute fracture, fracture sequelae, failed hemiarthroplasty, and failed ORIF. At 32 months SPADI, UCLA score, ASES score and Constant score were better in the primary surgery group than the revision surgery group.

15. Eichinger JK, Miller LR, Hartshorn T, Li X, Warner JJ, et al. Evaluation of satisfaction and durability after hemiarthroplasty and total shoulder arthroplasty in a cohort of patients aged 50 years or younger: an analysis of discordance of patient satisfaction and implant survival. J Shoulder Elbow Surg. 2016;25(5):772–80. This level III study examined implant survival and patient satisfaction for hemiarthroplasty and total shoulder arthroplasty in patients 50 and younger. Implant survival was 95% for TSA and 89 for hemi with patient satisfaction 95% VS 71.6% respectively.
16. Ek ET, Neukom L, Catanzaro S, Gerber C. Reverse total shoulder arthroplasty for massive irreparable rotator cuff tears in patients younger than 65 years old: results after five to fifteen years. J Shoulder Elbow Surg. 2013;22(9):1199–208. This level IV study evaluated 40 RSA in patients under 65 with 5–15 year follow up. SSV, forward elevation, pain, and strength all improved but complication rate was 37.5% and failure was 15%.
17. Frangiamore SJ, Saleh A, Grosso MJ, Farias Kovac M, Zhang X, et al. Neer Award 2015: Analysis of cytokine profiles in the diagnosis of periprosthetic joint infections of the shoulder. J Shoulder Elbow Surg. 2016;26(2):186–96. This level III study analyzed the levels of 9 cytokines in synovial fluid in patients with shoulder arthroplasty who were divided into infected and non-infected groups. While many were elevated in the infection cases, a combination of IL-6, TNF-α, and IL-2 showed a sensitivity of 0.80 and specificity of 0.93 for infection.
18. Gadea F, Alami G, Pape G, Boileau P, Favard L. Shoulder hemiarthroplasty: outcomes and long-term survival analysis according to etiology. Orthop Traumatol Surg Res. 2012;98(6):659–65. This level IV study reviewed 272 hemiarthroplasties performed for fracture sequelae, primary OA, cuff tear arthropathy, AVN, RA and other causes with a mean 10 years follow up. Survival in the fracture sequelae group was the lowest of any group at 76.8%.
19. Gerber C, Werner CM, Vienne P. Internal fixation of complex fractures of the proximal humerus. J Bone Joint Surg Br. 2004;86(6):848–55.
20. Gerber C, Hersche O, Berberat C. The clinical relevance of posttraumatic avascular necrosis of the humeral head. J Shoulder Elb Surg. 1998;7(6):586–90.
21. Goss TP. Scapular fractures and dislocations: diagnosis and treatment. J Am Acad Orthop Surg. 1995;3(1):22–33.
22. Green A, Norris TR. Shoulder arthroplasty for advanced glenohumeral arthritis after anterior instability repair. J Shoulder Elb Surg. 2001;10(6):539–45.
23. Hovelius L, Olofsson A, Sandström B, Augustini BG, Krantz L, et al. Nonoperative treatment of primary anterior shoulder dislocation in patients forty years of age and younger a prospective twenty-five-year follow-up. J Bone Joint Surg Am. 2008;90(5):945–52.
24. Itamura JM, Beckett M. Infection rates and frozen sections in revision shoulder and elbow surgery holding cultures 21 days. J Shoulder Elbow Surg. 2013;22:e30–1. This abstract from the ASES 2012 closed meeting examined 109 revision shoulder and elbow cases. 57 patients had at least one positive culture, most commonly P. acnes. The average time to positive culture for P. acnes was 12.5 days.
25. Iyengar JJ, Devcic Z, Sproul RC, Feeley BT. Nonoperative treatment of proximal humerus fractures: a systematic review. J Orthop Trauma. 2011;25(10):612–7. This systematic review looked at 12 studies totaling 650 patients with closed treated proximal humerus fractures at 45.7 months follow up. The overall union rate was 98% and the complication rate was 13% with only 2% AVN.
26. Izquierdo R, Voloshin I, Edwards S, Freehill MQ, Stanwood W, et al. American academy of orthopaedic surgeons clinical practice guideline on: the treatment of glenohumeral joint osteoarthritis. J Bone Joint Surg Am. 2011;93(2):203–5. These AAOS clinical practice guidelines were based on a systematic review of the literature and recommendations are made based on the strength of evidence. These recommendations for treating glenohumeral arthritis were adopted by the AAOS board of directors in December 2009.
27. Johnson DL, Warner JJ. Osteochondritis dissecans of the humeral head: treatment with a matched osteochondral allograft. J Shoulder Elb Surg. 1997;6(2):160–3.

28. Lenart BA, Namdari S, Williams GR. Total shoulder arthroplasty with an augmented component for anterior glenoid bone deficiency. J Shoulder Elbow Surg. 2016;25(3):398–405. This level IV study reported on 5 patients undergoing TSA with an anterior glenoid augment for anterior wear, malunited glenoid fracture, or post-traumatic arthritis. At 33.2 months there were no dislocations or revision surgeries and good patient reported outcomes.

29. Levy J, Frankle M, Mighell M, Pupello D. The use of the reverse shoulder prosthesis for the treatment of failed hemiarthroplasty for proximal humeral fracture. J Bone Joint Surg Am. 2007;89(2):292–300.

30. Levy O, Tsvieli O, Merchant J, Young L, Trimarchi A, et al. Surface replacement arthroplasty for glenohumeral arthropathy in patients aged younger than fifty years: results after a minimum ten-year follow-up. J Shoulder Elbow Surg. 2015;24(7):1049–60. This level IV study reported on 54 humeral resurfacings in patients younger than 50 for various indications including fracture sequelae and dislocation arthropathy. 81.6% survival was seen at 10 years but 18.5% were revised. Constant scores postoperatively were higher in patients undergoing concomitant microfracture of the glenoid.

31. Lo EY, Flanagin BA, Burkhead WZ. Biologic resurfacing arthroplasty with acellular human dermal allograft and platelet-rich plasma (PRP) in young patients with glenohumeral arthritis-average of 60 months of at mid-term follow-up. J Shoulder Elbow Surg. 2016;25(7):e199–207. This level IV study reviewed 55 patients who underwent hemiarthroplasty with human dermal matrix allograft glenoid resurfacing. A significant improvement was seen in the SANE score and 81% of patients were satisfied or highly satisfied with the result. 9.1% were revised to TSA.

32. Matsen FA 3rd. The ream and run: not for every patient, every surgeon or every problem. Int Orthop. 2015;39(2):255–61. This paper discusses the basics of the "ream and run" technique and stresses the importance of patient selection and patient compliance with the postoperative regimen.

33. Matsoukis J, Tabib W, Guiffault P, Mandelbaum A, Walch G, et al. Shoulder arthroplasty in patients with a prior anterior shoulder dislocation results of a multicenter study. J Bone Joint Surg Am. 2003;85-A(8):1417–24.

34. Millett PJ, Huffard BH, Horan MP, Hawkins RJ, Steadman JR. Outcomes of full-thickness articular cartilage injuries of the shoulder treated with microfracture. Arthroscopy. 2009;25(8):856–63.

35. Muh SJ, Streit JJ, Wanner JP, Lenarz CJ, Shishani Y, et al. Early follow-up of reverse total shoulder arthroplasty in patients sixty years of age or younger. J Bone Joint Surg Am. 2013;95(20):1877–83. This level IV study evaluated 67 RSA in patients 60 or younger at 36.5 months post op. Forward elevation, external rotation, ASES score and pain scores all improved from preoperative values with 81% of patients satisfied or very satisfied. Forward elevation greater than 100 degrees was the only predictor of satisfaction.

36. Owsley KC, Gorczyca JT. Fracture displacement and screw cutout after open reduction and locked plate fixation of proximal humeral fractures [corrected]. J Bone Joint Surg Am. 2008;90(2):233–40.

37. Papadonikolakis A, Neradilek MB, Matsen FA 3rd. Failure of the glenoid component in anatomic total shoulder arthroplasty: a systematic review of the English-language literature between 2006 and 2012. J Bone Joint Surg Am. 2013;95(24):2205–12. This level IV systematic review showed rates of radiolucent lines, symptomatic loosening, and revision of the glenoid component in 3853 TSA to be 7.3%, 1.2%, and 0.8% respectively.

38. Pape G, Zeifang F, Bruckner T, Raiss P, Rickert M, et al. Humeral surface replacement for the sequelae of fractures of the proximal humerus. J Bone Joint Surg Br. 2010;92(10):1403–9.

39. Puskas GJ, Meyer DC, Lebschi JA, Gerber C. Unacceptable failure of hemiarthroplasty combined with biological glenoid resurfacing in the treatment of glenohumeral arthritis in the young. J Shoulder Elbow Surg. 2015;24(12):1900–7. This level IV study showed revision to TSA after hemiarthroplasty and biologic glenoid resurfacing with Graftjacket, meniscal allograft, and capsular interposition to be occur at rates of 83.3%, 60%, and 66.7% in a small population of 17 patients with only 16 month follow up.

40. Romeo AA, Cole BJ, Mazzocca AD, Fox JA, Freeman KB, et al. Autologous chondrocyte repair of an articular defect in the humeral head. Arthroscopy. 2002;18(8):925–9.
41. Ruckstuhl H, de Bruin ED, Stussi E, Vanwanseele B. Post-traumatic glenohumeral cartilage lesions: a systematic review. BMC Musculoskelet Disord. 2008;9:107.
42. Schandelmaier P, Blauth M, Schneider C, Krettek C. Fractures of the glenoid treated by operation A 5- to 23-year follow-up of 22 cases. J Bone Joint Surg Br. 2002;84(2):173–7.
43. Scheibel M, Bartl C, Magosch P, Lichtenberg S, Habermeyer P. Osteochondral autologous transplantation for the treatment of full-thickness articular cartilage defects of the shoulder. J Bone Joint Surg Br. 2004;86(7):991–7.
44. Schoch BS, Barlow JD, Schleck C, Cofield RH, Sperling JW. Shoulder arthroplasty for post-traumatic osteonecrosis of the humeral head. J Shoulder Elbow Surg. 2016;25(3):406–12. This level III study examined 37 hemiarthroplasties and 46 TSA for post-traumatic osteonecrosis at 8.9 years post op. The TSA group had less pain and higher satisfaction at last follow up. 15 year survival for hemi was 79.5% vs. 83% for TSA.
45. Sershon RA, Van Thiel GS, Lin EC, McGill KC, Cole BJ, et al. Clinical outcomes of reverse total shoulder arthroplasty in patients aged younger than 60 years. J Shoulder Elbow Surg. 2014;23(3):395–400. This level IV study followed 36 RSA performed in patients younger than 60 for 2.8 years. Improvements were seen in ASES score, SST, SANE, and forward elevation. 25% were considered failures due to ASES score below 50.
46. Sperling JW, Kozak TK, Hanssen AD, Cofield RH. Infection after shoulder arthroplasty. Clin Orthop Relat Res. 2001;382:206–16.
47. Strauss EJ, Verma NN, Salata MJ, McGill KC, Klifto C, et al. The high failure rate of biologic resurfacing of the glenoid in young patients with glenohumeral arthritis. J Shoulder Elbow Surg. 2014;23(3):409–19. This level IV study examined 41 patients who underwent biologic glenoid resurfacing with meniscal allograft or human acellular dermal matrix at 2.8 year follow up. Overall failure rate was 51.2%, 45.2% for meniscus and 70% for dermal matrix. Average time to failure was 3.4 years and 2.2 years for meniscus and dermal matrix respectively.
48. Thanasas C, Kontakis G, Angoules A, Limb D, Giannoudis P. Treatment of proximal humerus fractures with locking plates: a systematic review. J Shoulder Elb Surg. 2009;18(6):837–44.
49. Topolski MS, Chin PY, Sperling JW, Cofield RH. Revision shoulder arthroplasty with positive intraoperative cultures: the value of preoperative studies and intraoperative histology. J Shoulder Elb Surg. 2006;15(4):402–6.
50. Zyto K, Kronberg M, Broström LA. Shoulder function after displaced fractures of the proximal humerus. J Shoulder Elb Surg. 1995;4(5):331–6.

Chapter 5
Post-traumatic Arthritis of the Elbow

Kevin O'Malley, Ryan Churchill, Curtis M. Henn, and Michael W. Kessler

> **Key Points**
> - The risk of post-traumatic arthritis of the elbow is very high after articular injuries.
> - CT arthrography is an excellent modality to assess intra-articular abnormalities.
> - Intra-articular glucocorticoid injections have no efficacy in this population.
> - Several operative options are available in cases of failure of conservative management.

Introduction

Post-traumatic elbow arthritis is relatively common with a reported risk of 44% following articular fractures [1]. Historically, this risk has been well recognized with Dr. Bigelow [2] writing in 1868 "There is no class of injuries so frequently productive of discontent, and perhaps so often the cause of litigation, as traumatic lesions of the elbow joint." Elbow fracture management continues to progress from predominantly nonoperative management to operative treatment in line with principles as shown by Jupiter in 1985 [3]. Treatment of these fractures is complex requiring an understanding of the various nonoperative and operative treatment modalities as well as understanding possible complications such as malunion, nonunion,

K. O'Malley (✉) · R. Churchill · C. M. Henn · M. W. Kessler
Medstar Georgetown University Hospital, Department of Orthopaedics,
Washington, DC, USA
e-mail: Ko257@georgetown.edu; Curtis.M.Henn@gunet.georgetown.edu;
Michael.W.Kessler@gunet.georgetown.edu

© Springer Nature Switzerland AG 2021
S. C. Thakkar, E. A. Hasenboehler (eds.), *Post-Traumatic Arthritis*,
https://doi.org/10.1007/978-3-030-50413-7_5

stiffness, avascular necrosis, heterotopic ossification, and post-traumatic arthritis. In this chapter we will outline the diagnosis and surgical management of post-traumatic elbow arthritis as well as case examples to further describe treatment options and techniques.

Elbow fractures account for 6% of adult fractures with $\frac{1}{3}$ of these fractures involving the distal humerus, $\frac{1}{3}$ to $\frac{1}{2}$ involving the proximal radius, and the remainder involving the proximal ulna. Fractures follow a bimodal age distribution with higher rates seen in young males and elderly females [4].

Post-traumatic osteoarthritis of the elbow is a multifactorial consequence of the initial trauma, the biologic response to the trauma, and the alterations in load distribution that result from articular incongruity and instability [1].

Relatively few studies have analyzed the development of post-traumatic arthritis following elbow injuries. From the available literature, it appears intra-articular distal humerus fractures have the highest rate of post-traumatic arthritis [5–7]. Guitton et al. analyzed radiographs of 139 patients following surgical treatment of an elbow fracture with over 10 years of follow-up. They found mechanisms of injury, age, gender, follow-up duration, occupation, and limb dominance not to be associated with radiographic arthrosis. However, patients with bicolumnar distal humerus, capitellum, and elbow dislocations were more likely to develop post-traumatic radiographic arthrosis [6]. Interestingly, although radiographic arthrosis is present in a high percentage of patients (80% per Doornberg et al.), functional scores do not appear to correlate. Instead, pain, flexion arc, and limb dominance appear to be the most important predictors of functional elbow scores [7, 8]. Notably, none of the 30 patients followed by Doornberg 12 years after intra-articular distal humerus fracture underwent total elbow arthroplasty (TEA) as a consequence of their fracture. Only one patient underwent arthrodesis for symptomatic post-traumatic arthritis [7].

Radial head and neck fractures also show little correlation between radiographic degenerative changes and symptomatic elbow pain [9]. Burkhart showed ulnohumeral arthritis in 12 of 17 patients at an average of 8.8 years following a proximal radius fracture. Again, there was no correlation of radiographic arthrosis to functional scores (Mayo Elbow Performance Score (MEPS) and Disabilities of the Arm, Shoulder and Hand Questionnaire (DASH)) or pain [10].

Long-term data on proximal ulna fractures is limited. Rochet et al. reported on 18 patients with proximal ulna fractures and found 6 to have grade 1 osteoarthritis based on the Broberg and Morrey classification. In comparison to other elbow fractures, olecranon fractures specifically show relatively low rates (20% or less) of post-traumatic arthritis, with articular displacement over 2 mm being the most important risk factor [11, 12].

Classifying post-traumatic elbow arthritis is typically done with the Broberg and Morrey (BM) classification, which is divided into three grades: grade 1 with slight joint space narrowing with minimal osteophyte formation, grade 2 with moderate joint space narrowing and moderate osteophyte formation, and grade 3 showing severe degenerative changes with gross joint destruction [13]. Another classification is the Hasting and Rettig (HR) classification, which like the BM classification is also divided into three grades and has no significant difference in comparison to the

BM classification [14]. Lastly, the Morrey classification can be utilized to describe bone defects of the distal humerus and maybe useful for the preoperative planning [15].

Closely related to post-traumatic elbow arthritis is post-traumatic elbow stiffness. While stiffness specifically is outside the scope of this chapter, it is important to have a basic understanding of post-traumatic stiffness when approaching complex post-traumatic elbow conditions. Our understanding of post-traumatic elbow stiffness continues to grow, and as of today we know that stiff elbows show an increased inflammatory cytokine and myofibroblast infiltration [16]. Stiffness is typically classified into two groups: extrinsic stiffness due to soft tissue and extra-articular processes and intrinsic stiffness secondary to articular pathology [17]. It is important to note the functional arc of the elbow, defined as flexion-extension motion of 30° to 130° and pronosupination of 50° to 50° [18]. Achieving functional range of motion typically occurs in the first 6 months following surgery with minimal range of motion progression after 6 months [19].

History and Physical Exam

Operative planning for post-traumatic elbow arthritis begins with a thorough history and physical. The history should include the initial injury mechanism, initial injuries sustained (fractures and instability), previous operative and nonoperative treatment (especially ulnar nerve management), and any history of infection or soft tissue procedures. Detailed information on symptomatic pain and stiffness should be obtained. For example, pain throughout the range of motion suggests diffuse arthritic changes, while terminal pain suggests impingement by an osteophyte or soft tissue [20]. Pain at rest carries a wider differential diagnosis including infection, cervical spine radiculopathy, soft tissue disease, and reflex sympathetic dystrophy [21]. Patient expectations and lifestyle factors must also be addressed as a manual laborer will have different functional demands and expectations when compared with a sedentary desk worker.

The physical examination should include a thorough inspection of the entire extremity to assess prior surgical incisions for both fracture treatment as well as soft-tissue coverage procedures. Hand thenar musculature should also be assessed (i.e., intrinsic hand wasting). Neurologic evaluation should assess upper extremity sensory and motor function as well as ulnar neuritis specifically. The patient's elbow range of motion should be tested and any painful points should be noted. Collateral ligament stability of the elbow should also be evaluated.

Imaging evaluation should be aimed at obtaining a complete understanding of the degree of arthritis, loose bodies, current hardware, and bone stock. Orthogonal elbow radiographs are the standard initial imaging study. If the patient also complains of wrist pain, full-length forearm and wrist views should be obtained to assess for a potential Essex-Lopresti lesion. Computed tomography (CT) is typically required for further evaluation and is more effective than conventional radiography in assessing osseous causes of elbow stiffness [22]. CT arthrography has been shown to provide improved assessment of intra-articular abnormalities such as osteocartilaginous bodies, hyperplastic synovium, and osteophytes [23]. While three-dimensional (3D) CT has not been evaluated for preoperative planning in this population, we find it extremely helpful for procedures such as arthroscopic or open debridement in patients with large osteophytes and loose bodies. Other diagnostic tests may include electromyographic evaluation in patients with a concerning exam for neuropathy or an entrapment syndrome.

Treatment

Nonsurgical Treatment

Conservative management of post-traumatic elbow arthritis is typically limited to patients with mild arthrosis or low-demand patients. Activity modification, nonsteroidal anti-inflammatory medication, and physical therapy should be considered with an emphasis on maintaining range of motion and reducing painful activities. Intra-articular glucocorticoids may be considered, but have no evidence of efficacy in this population. Viscosupplementation with hyaluronic acid has been shown to result in slight short-term pain relief and activity impairment 3 months following an injection series. However, at 6 months no benefits were shown suggesting it is not useful for long-term treatment [24].

Surgical Treatment

Several operative options are available once nonsurgical measures have been exhausted. Surgical options include arthroscopic or open osteocapsular debridement arthroplasty, interposition arthroplasty, partial joint arthroplasty (e.g., distal humerus hemiarthroplasty or radiocapitellar arthroplasty), total elbow arthroplasty (TEA), and elbow arthrodesis. Sears and colleagues [15] described an algorithmic approach to selecting the appropriate surgical intervention for post-traumatic elbow osteoarthritis. For patients who have pain at the terminal arc of motion, they recommended arthroscopic or open debridement arthroplasty with possible ulnar nerve transposition. For the patient who has pain throughout the entire arc of motion, they describe the use of partial joint arthroplasty for arthritic changes isolated to the radiocapitellar joint or distal humerus and interposition arthroplasty or total elbow arthroplasty for the patient with diffuse osteoarthritic changes. For younger patients who have exhausted most surgical options and do not wish to have 10 pound weight restriction on their extremity from a total elbow arthroplasty, elbow arthrodesis is offered.

Osteocapsular Debridement Arthroplasty

Open and arthroscopic osteocapsular debridement arthroplasties are good options for the patient with mild to moderate arthritis and pain at the terminal aspects of range of motion [25–34]. Open osteocapsular debridement arthroplasty is usually reserved for patients who have a preoperative flexion contractures greater than 90 degrees, preoperative ulnar neuropathy or documented ulnar nerve EMG changes, hardware that needs to be removed, or where arthroscopic debridement is exceptionally difficult [25, 34]. Open procedures include the Outerbridge-Kashiwagi procedure, Morrey ulnohumeral debridement arthroplasty, and the column procedure. In the Outerbridge-Kashiwagi procedure, the patient is positioned in the lateral decubitus with the involved extremity draped free. A posterior midline incision is utilized with a triceps split to visualize the posterior compartment of the elbow. Osteophytes and loose bodies are removed and the capsular undergoes debridement. The olecranon fossa is then fenestrated with a drill to allow limited access to the anterior compartment of the elbow. Loose bodies are removed and any osteophytes about the coronoid are removed. If the patient has a preoperative flexion contracture greater than 90 degrees and less than 90 to 100 degrees of flexion, the posterior band of the medial ulnar collateral ligament (MUCL) should be released, and consideration should be given to transpose the ulnar nerve. If the patient has a preoperative ulnar neuropathy or documented ulnar nerve EMG changes, then the patient should undergo ulnar nerve release and transposition [15, 25]. The column procedure involves utilizing a lateral column approach to the elbow to perform anterior and posterior compartment debridement arthroplasty with care to preserve the lateral ulnar collateral ligament during the procedure. If there is a significant preoperative flexion contracture or ulnar neuropathy, then a separate medial incision is made to address the ulnar nerve and posterior band of the MUCL [25, 35].

Arthroscopic adaptations for osteocapsular debridement have shown good results with the benefit of greater soft tissue preservation and quicker return to activities [26–33, 36]. Relative contraindications to elbow arthroscopy are related to aberrant anatomy of the ulnar and radial nerve from either prior trauma or surgeries. Additionally, in cases where there is severe arthritis arthroscopic debridement may be difficult to complete given the difficulty in gaining access to the joint. In these cases consideration should be given to open identification and protection of the nerve if arthroscopy is undertaken. Savoie and O'Brien[34] described a comprehensive arthroscopic approach to elbow arthritis. To begin, the patient may be positioned prone or lateral decubitus (Fig. 5.1a). A non-sterile or sterile tourniquet may be used. The course of the ulnar nerve is palpated and marked (Fig. 5.1b). The elbow is insufflated utilizing an 18-gauge needle and 20 to 30 milliliters (mL) of sterile saline injected in the area of the soft spot portal or posterior central portal. Next the site of the anteromedial portal is marked 2 centimeters (cm) superior and 2 cm anterior to the medial epicondyle. Only the skin is incised and a 4 millimeter (mm) cannula with a blunt trocar is used to enter the joint. Occasionally this may be difficult and a hemostat may be needed to open the joint capsule. The anterolateral

Fig. 5.1 (**a**, **b**) The photo on the left demonstrates lateral decubitus patient positioning in preparation for elbow arthroscopy. The photo on the right demonstrates landmarks for medial portal placement including the ulnar nerve and the medial epicondyle

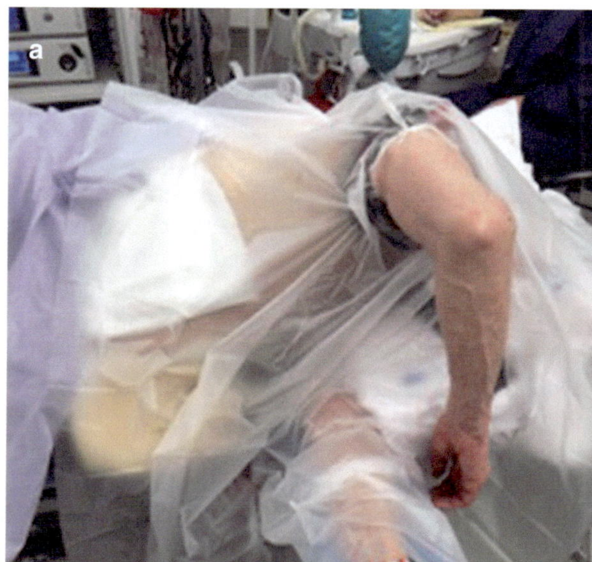

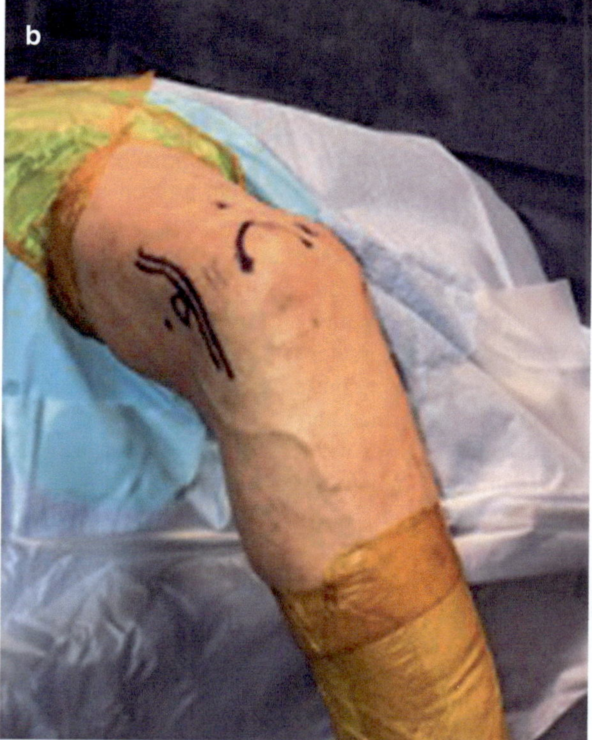

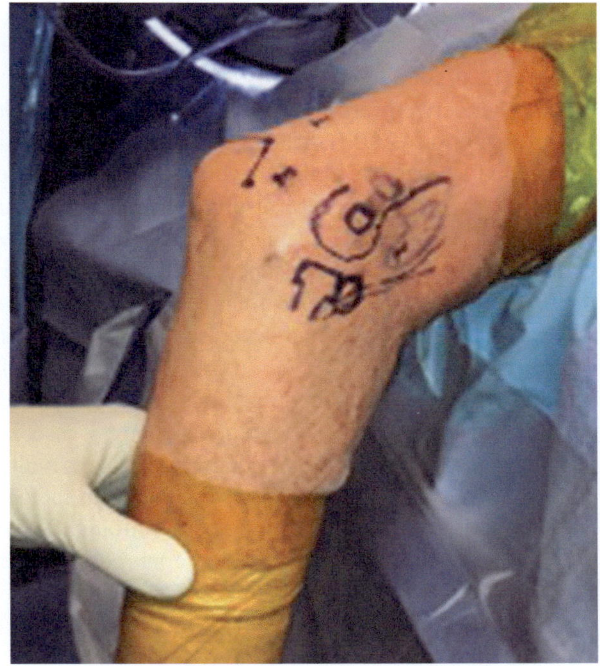

Fig. 5.2 Lateral landmarks for portal placement are drawn out with the overlying incisions for the anterolateral, posterior central, and posterolateral portals shown

portal is then established under direct visualization utilizing a spinal needle. The spot for the portal is typically 2–3 cm anterior the lateral epicondyle and at the superior most aspect of the capitellar cartilage (Fig. 5.2). The procedure proceeds then in a stepwise manner beginning with a diagnostic arthroscopy followed by removal of any loose bodies from the anterior compartment along with osteophytes and synovitis. If the radiocapitellar joint is significantly involved, a radial head resection may be performed through the soft spot portal. Prior to proceeding to the posterior compartment, a fenestration hole is created through the olecranon fossa. Other options include a combined arthroscopic and open procedure with arthroscopic debridement being carried out anteriorly followed by a mini-open posterior elbow debridement. This can be effective when the elbow has more severe arthrosis that may require treatment both laterally and medially in the anterior elbow.

A posterior central portal is created 3 cm proximal to the tip of the olecranon and this serves as the initial viewing portal. A posterolateral portal is made parallel to the posterior central portal just outside the triceps tendon. Once these portals are established, the posterior compartment is debrided, loose bodies removed, and synovectomy performed. The medial and lateral gutters are inspected for loose bodies and plica that may be contributing to the pathology. Finally the tip of olecranon is excised and if necessary the anterior capsule is released. If the patient had preoperative symptoms of ulnar neuropathy, the ulnar nerve may be decompressed in situ. Patients are allowed full range of motion immediately postoperatively without weight-bearing restrictions.

Recent literature has found overall good to excellent results with this procedure in appropriately selected patients with mild to moderate arthritis [25–33, 36]. DeGreef et al. found good results in a cohort of patients with a mean age of 50 years old who underwent arthroscopic osteocapsular debridement with an increase in range of motion (ROM) from 94 to 123 degrees, a significant decrease in pain scores, and an increase in the Mayo Elbow Performance Index (MEPI) by an average of 34 points [37]. These results are reflected in much of the recent literature [25–33, 36]. Galle and colleagues reviewed a consecutive series of 46 patients who underwent arthroscopic osteocapsular debridement. The mean age of the patients in their study was 48 years. They found a significant increase in ROM (final ROM arc 12 degrees to 135 degrees), a decrease in pain, and an increase in the Mayo Elbow Performance Score (MEPS) from 57 preoperatively to 88 postoperatively. Furthermore they had no complications in their cohort of patients [28]. Finally, Lim et al. investigated the preoperative factors associated with outcomes after arthroscopic osteocapsular debridement. Through multivariate analysis they found that preoperative range of motion was the main factor that affected postoperative elbow function and range of motion, and through further analysis preoperative arc of motion greater than 80 degrees was found to be the cutoff for improved postoperative function and arc of motion [30].

Interposition Arthroplasty

Given that the majority of patients with post-traumatic elbow arthritis tend to be younger and of higher demand, interposition arthroplasty serves as a valuable surgical tool in treating this condition in patients who do not wish to have the weight-bearing and activity restrictions associated with TEA. Options for interposition arthroplasty include both autograft (e.g., anconeus, fascia lata) and allograft (e.g., Achilles tendon, fascia lata, dermis) [15, 25]. Contraindications to this procedure include active infection, gross elbow instability or deformity, open physes, no flexor-pronator power, and patients with deficient bone stock about the elbow [25, 38, 39].

As described by Morrey [40], this procedure is performed with the patient positioned in supine or lateral decubitus position. A posterior approach to the elbow is typically utilized. Kocher's interval is then developed between the extensor carpi ulnaris and the anconeus. The lateral ulnar collateral ligament (LUCL) and elbow extensors are released from the lateral epicondyle and tagged. A capsular release is performed and osteophytes are removed. Next the ulnar and humeral articular surfaces are prepared so a congruent articulation is obtained and enough bone is resected so that there is 2–3 mm of laxity to ensure that the joint is not overstuffed. Following this, three to four drill holes are created in the humerus, and the graft is prepared with three to four horizontal mattress sutures that are passed through the drill holes to secure the graft to the distal humerus surface. The joint is then reduced and range of motion assessed for areas of impingement. Finally, the stability of the MUCL is assessed and the LUCL and the extensors are repaired back to the lateral epicondyle. If the LUCL is unable to be repaired, then reconstruction should be performed. Occasionally a hinged external fixator is placed to protect collateral ligament reconstruction when performed. Patients are allowed range of motion on postoperative day 1.

While interposition arthroplasty provides a good option for improved pain and range of motion for the young, active patient, the results tend to be inferior to elbow arthroplasty [25]. Baghdadi et al. reported the results of 39 patients treated with anconeus interposition arthroplasty with an average of 10 years of follow-up. They found 72% of their cohort had good to excellent results with significant improvements in their MEPS. However, they did find a 24% reoperation rate and 7% complication rate in their cohort [39]. Cheng and Morrey described the results of interposition arthroplasty using fascia lata in 13 patients. They found good to excellent results in 62% of the patients with eight complications in six patients and four patients requiring conversion to TEA at an average of 30 months [41]. Furthermore, Larsen and Morrey reported the results of 38 interposition arthroplasties performed with Achilles tendon allograft in a cohort of patients with an average age of 39 years. They found that at an average of 6 years of follow-up, there were significant improvements in range of motion (51° to 97°) and MEPS. Although 29% of patients had a poor result with 18% requiring revision surgery, 88% of all patients reported they would undergo the procedure again. Hence the authors concluded that interposition arthroplasty is a valid salvage procedure for the young patient with severe arthritis, limited motion, and no instability [42].

Radiocapitellar Arthroplasty and Distal Humerus Hemiarthroplasty

There is a relative paucity of literature on radiocapitellar arthroplasty and distal humerus hemiarthroplasty. Currently they are an off-label for treatment of osteoarthritis in the United States, and the situations in which they would be utilized for post-traumatic osteoarthritis are very limited [25]. The studies on distal humerus hemiarthroplasty largely are focused on the use for acute treatment of non-reconstructable elbow fractures. While these studies show relatively good outcomes, they have short-term follow-up and are predominantly in elderly patients [43, 44]. For patients with isolated radiocapitellar arthritis, the use of a radiocapitellar replacement has been described. Heijink and colleagues reported the results of six patients treated with radiocapitellar arthroplasty with an average of 50 months of follow-up. The patients in the study had improvements in range of motion, their DASH scores, MEPS, and pain levels. Overall they had three excellent and three good results with 100% survivorship of implants. An added benefit to radiocapitellar arthroplasty is that it maintains the valgus and external rotation stability of the joint [45]. These results are limited, and further literature and expansion of the recommendations for the use need to occur before this intervention can become standard treatment.

Total Elbow Arthroplasty

Total elbow arthroplasty remains the final operative choice for the majority of patients who have failed other operative interventions. It remains the definitive functional treatment for elderly patients with severe end-stage post-traumatic osteoarthritis. It is not ideal for young active patients with post-traumatic arthritis especially in cases of instability due to increased rates of mechanical wear and the need for early revision [15, 25].

The majority of TEA performed today utilizes a linked semi-constrained prosthesis. In addition to this design, there are unlinked TEA that rely on soft tissue balancing and implant conformity to provide stability. By the nature of being unlinked, these designs result in decreased bone-cement interface stresses and allow load sharing between the implant and the soft tissues. However, an inability to balance the soft tissues is a contraindication to use of this design and as such is not applicable to the majority of patients with post-traumatic osteoarthritis [25].

Procedure

When performing TEA the patient is positioned supine or in lateral decubitus. A sterile tourniquet is routinely used. A variety of deep approaches may be utilized. Originally Bryan and Morrey described elevating the triceps from medial to lateral to expose the joint. This approach can lead to higher rates of postoperative triceps insufficiency, and therefore in recent years, triceps-sparing approaches have seen an increase in utilization. With a triceps-sparing approach, the triceps is left in continuity with windows established medially and laterally for implant placement. After adequate exposure and soft tissue release, the distal humerus and ulna are prepared. This typically includes resection of the tips of the olecranon and coronoid processes. Additionally, the proximal ulna often requires a combination of a bur and bone rasp to allow for entry of trial components. Once trial implants are inserted, bony impingement should be assessed and any sites of impingement resected. Also, in cases where there is concomitant radiocapitellar arthritis, the radial head can be excised with careful resection as the posterior interosseous nerve will be just anterior to the radial head. Once trials are placed and impingement sites addressed, a mini C-arm can be used to confirm appropriate placement. Lastly, in patients with preoperative ulnar nerve symptoms, transposition should be considered. On postoperative day 1, unrestricted range of motion is allowed, but patients are limited to a 1-pound lifting restriction for the first 3 months and nothing heavier than 10 pounds for life.

Studies on TEA in the younger patients suffering from post-traumatic osteoarthritis have been increasing. Schoch et al. recently performed a retrospective review of 11 patients under 50 years old undergoing TEA with a mean follow-up of 3.2 years. They found improvements in pain scores, MEPS, DASH scores, and range of motion. While these are positive results, they reported an 82% complication rate with six mechanical failures (54%) and as such recommended caution when performing TEA in this young patient population [46]. These results correlate to similar complications with mechanical failure and loosening as reported in several earlier studies [47–52].

While there are high complication rates in the young adult population throughout the literature, a successful TEA does improve function and decrease pain. Park et al. reported the results of TEA performed in 23 patients under 40 years old with post-traumatic arthritis with average follow-up of 10.8 years. The authors found significant decreases in pain scores and increased MEPS with improved range of motion with increasing arc of motion from 37.8° to 120.6°. Furthermore, they reported 95% and 89% implants survival rates at 8 and 15 years, respectively [53]. Welsink et al. performed a systematic review of TEA including all indications. Their review included 70 articles with 9379 TEA performed with three different implants. There was an average follow-up time of 81 months of follow-up across all articles. They found for the newer Coonrad-Morrey-style prosthesis that there was an 87.2% survival at 7 years for all indications with a mean range of motion of 30° to 129° with significant improvement in outcomes. They reported an overall 11–38% complication rate with implant loosening being the most common complication (7%) [54]. Furthermore aseptic component loosening is the most common cause for revision TEA (38% of revisions) as demonstrated by Prkic et al. in a systematic review on causes of TEA failure [55].

Elbow Arthrodesis

Elbow arthrodesis remains a treatment option for a very specific patient: the relatively young patient with severe unilateral post-traumatic elbow arthritis who cannot tolerate weight-bearing limitations required for TEA and who is not a candidate for interposition arthroplasty. Historically, elbow arthrodesis has not been tolerated well because the adjacent joints do not compensate well for the motion loss seen with arthrodesis [25].

Arthrodesis may be achieved with compression across the joint utilizing bent plates, Ilizarov frames, compression screws, and cross strut grafts [25, 56, 57]. When performed, the elbow is typically fused at 90° of flexion although arthrodesis at 30° to 45° may be considered for patients who require a specific position for employment or for patients with lower extremity disorders that require the use of the elbow and forearm for transfer. Patient input into the final elbow position can be obtained by placing patients in a hinged elbow brace with varying degrees of flexion. This allows a patient to "try out" the fusion position that will work best for them [40].

Conclusion

Our understanding of post-traumatic elbow arthritis continues to evolve. The development of elbow arthritis is a complex interplay of factors including the initial trauma, the biologic response to the trauma, and the alterations in load distribution over time [1]. Radiographic signs of arthritis are relatively common especially with intra-articular distal humerus fractures. However, patient symptoms and goals need to be appropriately identified and addressed as many patients with radiographic arthritis are relatively asymptomatic and the operative treatment course can result in significant complications and require lifestyle alterations [7]. Conservative management of elbow arthritis includes activity modification, NSAIDs, and physical therapy. Intra-articular injections have little evidence to support long-term efficacy. Surgical treatment includes arthroscopic and open debridement, interposition arthroplasty, partial joint arthroplasty, total elbow arthroplasty, and elbow arthrodesis with each modality having distinct possible benefits and complications.

References

1. Schenker ML, Mauck RL, Ahn J, et al. Pathogenesis and prevention of posttraumatic osteoarthritis after intra-articular fracture. J Am Acad Orthop Surg. 2014;22(1):20–8.
2. Bigelow HJ. Insensibility during surgical operations produced by inhalation. Boston Med Surg J. 1846;35(16):309–17.
3. Kozanek M, Bartonicek J, Chase SM, et al. Treatment of distal humerus fractures in adults: a historical perspective. J Hand Surg Am. 2014;39(12):2481–5.
4. McKee MD. Trauma to the adult elbow and fractures of the distal humerus. Philadelphia: Saunders/Elsevier; 2009.
5. O'Driscoll SW. Elbow arthritis: treatment options. J Am Acad Orthop Surg. 1993;1(2):106–16.
6. Guitton TG, Zurakowski D, van Dijk NC, et al. Incidence and risk factors for the development of radiographic arthrosis after traumatic elbow injuries. J Hand Surg Am. 2010;35(12):1976–80.
7. Doornberg JN, van Duijn PJ, Linzel D, et al. Surgical treatment of intra-articular fractures of the distal part of the humerus. Functional outcome after twelve to thirty years. J Bone Joint Surg Am. 2007;89(7):1524–32.
8. Doornberg JN, Ring D, Fabian LM, et al. Pain dominates measurements of elbow function and health status. J Bone Joint Surg Am. 2005;87(8):1725–31.
9. Herbertsson P, Josefsson PO, Hasserius R, et al. Uncomplicated Mason type-II and III fractures of the radial head and neck in adults. A long-term follow-up study. The Journal of bone and joint surgery American volume 2004;86-a(3):569–74.
10. Burkhart KJ, Mattyasovszky SG, Runkel M, et al. Mid- to long-term results after bipolar radial head arthroplasty. J Shoulder Elb Surg. 2010;19(7):965–72.
11. Eriksson E, Sahlin O, Sandahl U. Late results of conservative and surgical treatment of fracture of the olecranon. Acta Chir Scand. 1957;113(2):153–66.
12. Macko D, Szabo RM. Complications of tension-band wiring of olecranon fractures. J Bone Joint Surg Am. 1985;67(9):1396–401.
13. Broberg MA, Morrey BF. Results of delayed excision of the radial head after fracture. J Bone Joint Surg Am. 1986;68(5):669–74.
14. Amini MH, Sykes JB, Olson ST, et al. Reliability testing of two classification systems for osteoarthritis and post-traumatic arthritis of the elbow. J Shoulder Elb Surg. 2015;24(3):353–7.

15. Sears BW, et al. Posttraumatic elbow osteoarthritis. 5th ed. Philadelphia: Saunders/ Elsevier; 2017.
16. Germscheid NM, Hildebrand KA. Regional variation is present in elbow capsules after injury. Clin Orthop Relat Res. 2006;450:219–24.
17. Morrey BF. The posttraumatic stiff elbow. Clin Orthop Relat Res. 2005;431:26–35.
18. Morrey BF, Askew LJ, Chao EY. A biomechanical study of normal functional elbow motion. J Bone Joint Surg Am. 1981;63(6):872–7.
19. Giannicola G, Polimanti D, Bullitta G, et al. Critical time period for recovery of functional range of motion after surgical treatment of complex elbow instability: prospective study on 76 patients. Injury. 2014;45(3):540–5.
20. Chammas M. Post-traumatic osteoarthritis of the elbow. Orthop Traumatol Surg Res. 2014;100(1 Suppl):S15–24.
21. Cheung EV, Adams R, Morrey BF. Primary osteoarthritis of the elbow: current treatment options. J Am Acad Orthop Surg. 2008;16(2):77–87.
22. Zubler V, Saupe N, Jost B, et al. Elbow stiffness: effectiveness of conventional radiography and CT to explain osseous causes. AJR Am J Roentgenol. 2010;194(6):W515–20.
23. Singson RD, Feldman F, Rosenberg ZS. Elbow joint: assessment with double-contrast CT arthrography. Radiology. 1986;160(1):167–73.
24. van Brakel RW, Eygendaal D. Intra-articular injection of hyaluronic acid is not effective for the treatment of post-traumatic osteoarthritis of the elbow. Arthroscopy. 2006;22(11): 1199–203.
25. Sears BW, Puskas GJ, Morrey ME, et al. Posttraumatic elbow arthritis in the young adult: evaluation and management. J Am Acad Orthop Surg. 2012;20(11):704–14.
26. Kroonen LT, Piper SL, Ghatan AC. Arthroscopic management of elbow osteoarthritis. J Hand Surg Am. 2017;42(8):640–50.
27. Kim SJ, Kim JW, Lee SH, et al. Retrospective comparative analysis of elbow arthroscopy used to treat primary osteoarthritis with and without release of the posterior band of the medial collateral ligament. Arthroscopy. 2017;33(8):1506–11.
28. Galle SE, Beck JD, Burchette RJ, et al. Outcomes of elbow arthroscopic Osteocapsular arthroplasty. J Hand Surg Am. 2016;41(2):184–91.
29. Merolla G, Buononato C, Chillemi C, et al. Arthroscopic joint debridement and capsular release in primary and post-traumatic elbow osteoarthritis: a retrospective blinded cohort study with minimum 24-month follow-up. Musculoskelet Surg. 2015;99(Suppl 1):S83–90.
30. Lim TK, Koh KH, Lee HI, et al. Arthroscopic debridement for primary osteoarthritis of the elbow: analysis of preoperative factors affecting outcome. J Shoulder Elb Surg. 2014;23(9):1381–7.
31. Giannicola G, Bullitta G, Polimanti D, et al. Factors affecting choice of open surgical techniques in elbow stiffness. Musculoskelet Surg. 2014;98(Suppl 1):77–85.
32. Adams JE, Wolff LH 3rd, Merten SM, et al. Osteoarthritis of the elbow: results of arthroscopic osteophyte resection and capsulectomy. J Shoulder Elb Surg. 2008;17(1):126–31.
33. Krishnan SG, Harkins DC, Pennington SD, et al. Arthroscopic ulnohumeral arthroplasty for degenerative arthritis of the elbow in patients under fifty years of age. J Shoulder Elb Surg. 2007;16(4):443–8.
34. Savoie FH 3rd, O'Brien MJ, Field LD. Arthroscopy for arthritis of the elbow. 5th ed. Philadelphia: Saunders/Elsevier; 2017.
35. Mansat P, Morrey BF. The column procedure: a limited lateral approach for extrinsic contracture of the elbow. J Bone Joint Surg Am. 1998;80(11):1603–15.
36. MacLean SB, Oni T, Crawford LA, et al. Medium-term results of arthroscopic debridement and capsulectomy for the treatment of elbow osteoarthritis. J Shoulder Elb Surg. 2013;22(5):653–7.
37. DeGreef I, Samorjai N, De Smet L. The Outerbridge-Kashiwagi procedure in elbow arthroscopy. Acta Orthop Belg. 2010;76(4):468–71.
38. Laubscher M, Vochteloo AJ, Smit AA, et al. A retrospective review of a series of interposition arthroplasties of the elbow. Shoulder Elbow. 2014;6(2):129–33.

39. Baghdadi YM, Morrey BF, Sanchez-Sotelo J. Anconeus interposition arthroplasty: mid- to long-term results. Clin Orthop Relat Res. 2014;472(7):2151–61.
40. Morrey BF. The Elbow and Its Disorders. 5th ed. Philadelphia: Saunders/Elsevier; 2017.
41. Cheng SL, Morrey BF. Treatment of the mobile, painful arthritic elbow by distraction interposition arthroplasty. J Bone Joint Surg. 2000;82(2):233–8.
42. Larson AN, Morrey BF. Interposition arthroplasty with an Achilles tendon allograft as a salvage procedure for the elbow. J Bone Joint Surg Am. 2008;90(12):2714–23.
43. Adolfsson L, Nestorson J. The kudo humeral component as primary hemiarthroplasty in distal humeral fractures. J Shoulder Elb Surg. 2012;21(4):451–5.
44. Steinmann SP. Hemiarthroplasty of the ulnohumeral and radiocapitellar joints. Hand Clin. 2011;27(2):229–32.. vi
45. Heijink A, Vanhees M, van den Ende K, et al. Biomechanical considerations in the pathogenesis of osteoarthritis of the elbow. Knee Surg Sports Traumatol Arthrosc. 2016;24(7):2313–8.
46. Schoch B, Wong J, Abboud J, et al. Results of total elbow arthroplasty in patients less than 50 years old. J Hand Surg Am. 2017;42(10):797–802.
47. Schoch BS, Werthel JD, Sanchez-Sotelo J, et al. Total elbow arthroplasty for primary osteoarthritis. J Shoulder Elb Surg. 2017;26(8):1355–9.
48. Lovy AJ, Keswani A, Dowdell J, et al. Outcomes, complications, utilization trends, and risk factors for primary and revision total elbow replacement. J Shoulder Elb Surg. 2016;25(6):1020–6.
49. Perretta D, van Leeuwen WF, Dyer G, et al. Risk factors for reoperation after total elbow arthroplasty. J Shoulder Elb Surg. 2017;26(5):824–9.
50. Zhou H, Orvets ND, Merlin G, et al. Total elbow arthroplasty in the United States: evaluation of cost, patient demographics, and complication rates. Orthop Rev. 2016;8(1):6113.
51. Giannicola G, Scacchi M, Polimanti D, et al. Discovery elbow system: 2- to 5-year results in distal humerus fractures and posttraumatic conditions: a prospective study on 24 patients. J Hand Surg Am. 2014;39(9):1746–56.
52. Giannicola G, Sacchetti FM, Antonietti G, et al. Radial head, radiocapitellar and total elbow arthroplasties: a review of recent literature. Injury. 2014;45(2):428–36.
53. Park JG, Cho NS, Song JH, et al. Clinical outcomes of semiconstrained total elbow arthroplasty in patients who were forty years of age or younger. J Bone Joint Surg Am. 2015;97(21):1781–91.
54. Welsink CL, Lambers KTA, van Deurzen DFP, et al. Total elbow arthroplasty: a systematic review. JBJS Rev. 2017;5(7):e4.
55. Prkic A, Welsink C, The B, et al. Why does total elbow arthroplasty fail today? A systematic review of recent literature. Arch Orthop Trauma Surg. 2017;137(6):761–9.
56. Kovack TJ, Jacob PB, Mighell MA. Elbow arthrodesis: a novel technique and review of the literature. Orthopedics. 2014;37(5):313–9.
57. Sala F, Catagni M, Pili D, et al. Elbow arthrodesis for post-traumatic sequelae: surgical tactics using the Ilizarov frame. J Shoulder Elb Surg. 2015;24(11):1757–63.

Chapter 6
Post-traumatic Arthritis of the Wrist

Sophia A. Strike and Philip E. Blazar

> **Key Points**
> - Radiocarpal and intercarpal arthritis, when caused by scapholunate ligament injury or scaphoid nonunion, allow for treatment options based on predictable patterns of degenerative change.
> - Radiocarpal, ulnocarpal, and distal radioulnar joint arthritis may be caused by intraarticular fractures of the distal radius or distal radius malunion.
> - Isolated intercarpal arthritis can occur from less common injuries to the carpus and associated ligaments.

Introduction

The wrist joint is a complex structure involving articulation of the eight carpal bones and the forearm. Surrounding ligamentous structures maintain the normal static and dynamic relationships of the osseous components. Alteration of the anatomic relationships through fracture, dislocation, or ligamentous injury can cause abnormal carpal kinematics and, eventually, lead to articular degeneration. Pain, instability, loss of motion, and deformity may negatively impact function. Functional wrist motion has been reported at 5 degrees of flexion, 30 degrees of extension, 10 degrees of radial deviation, and 15 degrees of ulnar deviation [1]. The motion required to

S. A. Strike (✉)
Johns Hopkins University School of Medicine, Baltimore, MD, USA
e-mail: sstrike1@jhmi.edu

P. E. Blazar
Brigham and Women's Hospital, Boston, MA, USA
e-mail: pblazar@partners.org

© Springer Nature Switzerland AG 2021
S. C. Thakkar, E. A. Hasenboehler (eds.), *Post-Traumatic Arthritis*,
https://doi.org/10.1007/978-3-030-50413-7_6

perform daily activities will be unique to each patient based on functional demands and compensatory mechanisms [2]. While traumatic injury remains a common cause of arthritis of the wrist, atraumatic etiologies including inflammatory arthritis, crystalline deposition, hemophilia, and primary osteoarthritis must be considered in the evaluation of these patients [2].

Traumatic etiologies of wrist arthritis include injury to intercarpal, radiocarpal, ulnocarpal, or radioulnar ligaments in isolation or as part of a perilunate injury, nonunion (or malunion) after scaphoid fracture, as well as malunited distal radius fractures [3, 4, 9]. All of these injuries can induce abnormal carpal mechanics and over time cause pain and joint degeneration [3–6].

Posttraumatic arthritis may occur in predictable patterns throughout much of the wrist as will be discussed in the chapter. This allows treatment to be tailored to the stage of degeneration. The natural history of wrist injuries has been described in cases such as scaphoid nonunion and distal radius fracture malunion but is less clear for intercarpal injury such as scapholunate ligament injuries [13–15]. Surgical management of arthritis typically centers on removal or fusion of involved articulations, and the complex structure of the wrist requires a thorough understanding of anatomy and kinematics to select an appropriate treatment for each patient.

Main Text

Wrist Anatomy

The intricate articulation of the osseous structures of the wrist with ligamentous support allows for multiple directions of motion. The combination of intercarpal, radiocarpal, and distal radioulnar joint motions provides multiple degrees of motion: flexion/extension, radial/ulnar deviation, and pronation/supination. The surrounding ligaments of the wrist provide the stability necessary for this wide range of motion [7]. Fractures or ligamentous injury can alter the normal mechanics of motion of these articulations, resulting in abnormal joint loading and subsequent osteoarthritis. This may occur in predictable patterns allowing treatment to be tailored to each patient's stage of arthritic change. Understanding the specific anatomy of the wrist is paramount to understanding these patterns of degeneration.

Carpus and Intercarpal Joints

The carpal bones are customarily described in two carpal rows: proximal and distal. The proximal row consists of, from radial to ulnar, the scaphoid, lunate, triquetrum, and pisiform (Fig. 6.1). This group of carpal bones is also termed the intercalary segment as there are no extrinsic ligamentous connections directly to these structures. The movement of the proximal carpal row is based entirely on their

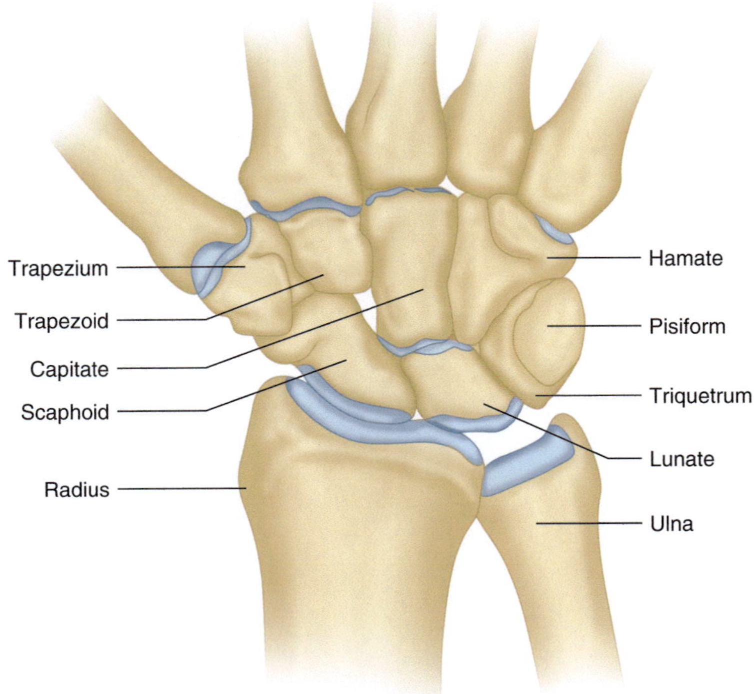

Fig. 6.1 Illustration: Carpus. Proximal row: Scaphoid, lunate, triquetrum, pisiform. Distal row: trapezium, trapezoid, capitate and hamate

articulations with the distal carpal row and the radius and ulna as well as their ligamentous supports [6].

Ligaments of the wrist include palmar and dorsal radiocarpal, ulnocarpal, intercarpal, palmar midcarpal, proximal and distal interosseous, and distal radioulnar ligaments [7]. The proximal interosseous ligaments, the scapholunate and lunotriquetral, provide interconnection between the bones of the proximal carpal row allowing coordinated movement. These interosseous ligaments each contain proximal, volar, and dorsal components with the dorsal aspect of the scapholunate interosseous ligament (SLIL) and the volar component of the lunotriquetral interosseous ligament (LTIL) providing the strongest support for their respective joints [7, 9]. Injury to these ligaments results in atypical patterns of movement between the bones within the carpal row, termed carpal instability dissociative (CID) [3, 6, 8, 9]. The distal carpal row includes, from radial to ulnar, the trapezium, trapezoid, capitate, and hamate (Fig. 6.1). Gelberman reviewed the ring concept of the carpal rows highlighting the interconnected kinematics based on the scaphoid as a stabilizing link between rows and the triquetrum as a pivot point for carpal motion [3]. With radial deviation of the wrist, the distal row moves radially and forces the scaphoid

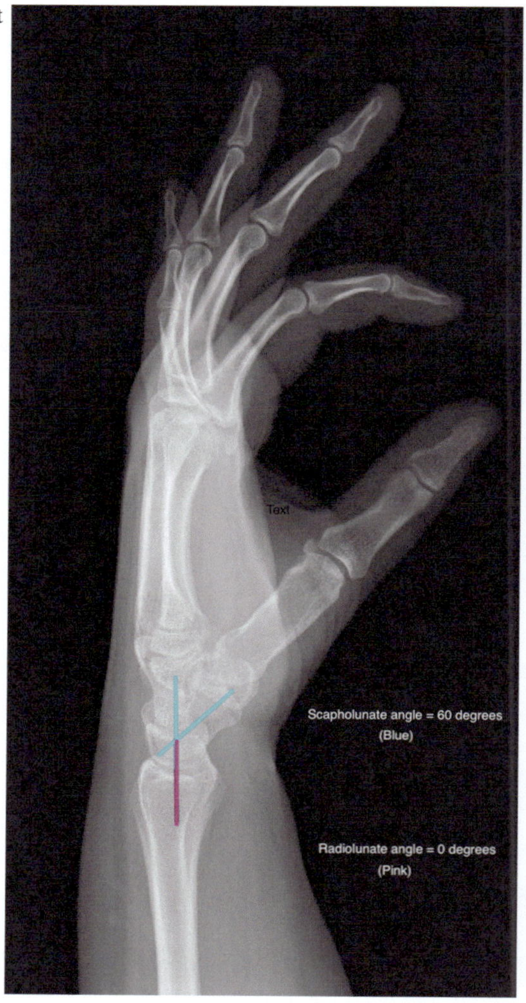

Fig. 6.2 Lateral radiograph of the wrist showing a normal radiolunate angle of zero degrees

and the entire proximal row into flexion to avoid direct impact. The scaphoid rests in a position of slight flexion with a normal radiographic scapholunate angle of less than 70 degrees [6] (Fig. 6.2). The lunate rests in a neutral position, hence the normal radiolunate angle of zero (Fig. 6.2).

Distal Radioulnar Joint

The distal aspects of the radius and ulna form the distal radioulnar joint (DRUJ) that allows the forearm to rotate in pronation and supination in coordination with the proximal radioulnar joint at the elbow. The sigmoid notch of the radius provides a concavity in which the ulna articulates. The surrounding soft tissue structures provide not only stability for the DRUJ but also prevent impingement at the ulnocarpal

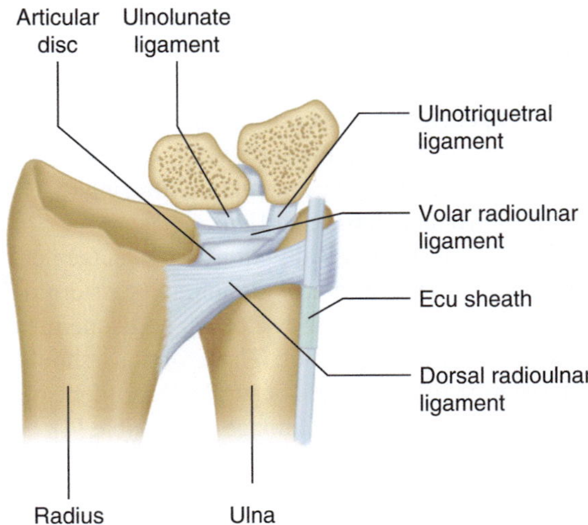

Fig. 6.3 Illustration: Structure of the TFCC

joint. The triangular fibrocartilage complex (TFCC) is composed of fibrocartilage, ligament, and joint capsule and separates the DRUJ from the radiocarpal joint [7]. The TFCC includes the dorsal and palmar radioulnar ligaments, the ECU subsheath, the ulnocarpal ligaments and the triangular articular disc that lies between the dorsal and palmar ligaments [7] (Fig. 6.3).

Wrist Arthritis

Evaluation

Diagnosis of posttraumatic arthritis of the wrist requires a history of trauma; however this is often remote or vague. Tenderness on physical examination is an important clue to the location of injury or arthritis; although, anesthetic and/or cortisone injections may be helpful in localizing pain generators [4]. The scapholunate interval, radial border of the scaphoid, and scaphotrapeziotrapezoidal (STT) joint are important landmarks for palpation although the entirety of the wrist, including all intercarpal joints, should be systematically examined [5, 13]. Dorsal wrist swelling and/or a joint effusion may be present [13]. Pain may be elicited with wrist extension and radial deviation, which loads the radial side of the wrist [9]. Dynamic tests such as the scaphoid shift test should be included in the exam [5, 9]. In this test, scapholunate dissociation may be diagnosed through dorsal subluxation of the scaphoid with palmar-dorsal pressure on the tuberosity during radial deviation causing pain. A clunk will occur as the scaphoid reduces into position with radial deviation and/or removal of pressure [3, 9]. Radiographs are necessary in initial evaluation and should be scrutinized for signs of altered carpal alignment, joint space loss, osteophyte formation, loose bodies, and subchondral sclerosis or cystic change [3, 4, 13]. Standard posteroanterior and lateral views should be obtained in addition to an ulnar-deviated clenched fist, or "scaphoid," view and a 45-degree pronation view [5]. Ulnar variance can only be appropriately assessed with the forearm in neutral rotation, the elbow flexed 90 degrees, and the shoulder at 90 degrees of abduction [5]. The pencil grip view may also demonstrate an increase in ulnar variance as compared to a neutral, non-grip view. Advanced imaging is rarely required for diagnosis; although, magnetic resonance imaging (MRI) may be useful in evaluating the status of articular cartilage [4].

In general, nonsurgical options for management of arthritis of the wrist include immobilization with braces or splints, nonsteroidal antiinflammatory medications (NSAIDs) if tolerated, and selective cortisone injections; although, they often provide only temporary relief. These options should be exhausted prior to surgical intervention [4]. The goals of surgical treatment are to eliminate pain, improve function, and prevent further damage, if possible [4].

Intercarpal and Radiocarpal Arthritis

In contrast to normal kinematics, with carpal ring disruption the bones of the wrist move in a discordant fashion [3]. Injuries causing disruption of the carpal ring may be isolated intercarpal ligament injuries, SLIL injury associated with a distal radius fracture, or multiple intercarpal ligament injuries associated with perilunate instability or dislocation [3, 9]. When associated with an extrinsic cause the resulting deformity is termed carpal instability adaptive (CIA) [3, 6, 9]. When chronic in nature, these injuries may lead to intercarpal and radiocarpal joint degeneration.

Scapholunate Advanced Collapse (SLAC) and Scaphoid Nonunion Advanced Collapse (SNAC)

Chronic SLIL injuries causing carpal instability may lead to subsequent radiocarpal and intercarpal arthritis although the natural history of SL ligament injuries is not well documented [7, 13]. In the pathologic state where the SLIL is compromised, the scaphoid will flex while the lunate will independently fall into extension leading to dorsal angulation of the lunate relative to the radius on a lateral radiographic view, termed dorsal intercalated segment instability (DISI) [3, 5, 6, 9, 13, 15] (Fig. 6.4). As this process progresses the capitate may migrate proximally as well [5]. There are no studies confirming that SL ligament tears, diagnosed with direct visualization through arthroscopy, inevitably lead to arthritis [13]. When degenerative changes do occur, radiographically, they will follow a predictable pattern termed scapholunate advanced collapse, or SLAC, wrist [4, 10, 11]. First described by Watson and Ballet based on their review of 4000 radiographs, of which 210 showed degenerative wrist arthritis, SLAC wrist was the most common pattern affecting 57% of those patients [10]. Initially, changes are noted at the tip of the radial styloid and the distal scaphoid (stage I), followed by involvement of the entire radioscaphoid joint (stage II) (Fig. 6.5). These specific changes result from the

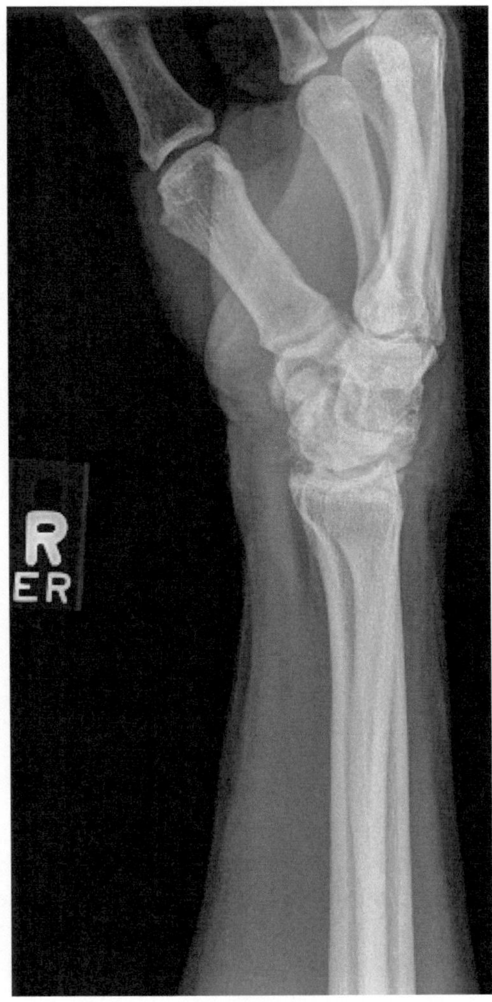

Fig. 6.4 Lateral radiograph demonstrating dorsal intercalated segment instability (DISI) deformity

incongruent geometry of the scaphoid with the radius when the scaphoid falls persistently into flexion [5, 12]. The capitolunate joint is the first midcarpal joint involved (stage III) (Fig. 6.6), and the final stages may include the rest of the carpus although the radiolunate joint is characteristically uninvolved [2, 3, 5, 10–12]. This is thought to be from the highly congruent nature of the lunate in the fossa of the distal radius [10]. It is important to note that patients with a SLAC wrist pattern may be asymptomatic. Further, atraumatic causes such as calcium pyrophosphate deposition must be considered [2, 13]. Radiographs of the contralateral wrist in an asymptomatic patient may also show SLAC changes [13].

Less commonly, nonunion of the scaphoid may lead to a scaphoid nonunion advanced collapse (SNAC) wrist deformity [12, 13] (Fig. 6.7). The SNAC pattern is similar to a SLAC wrist with the anatomic difference being the maintained

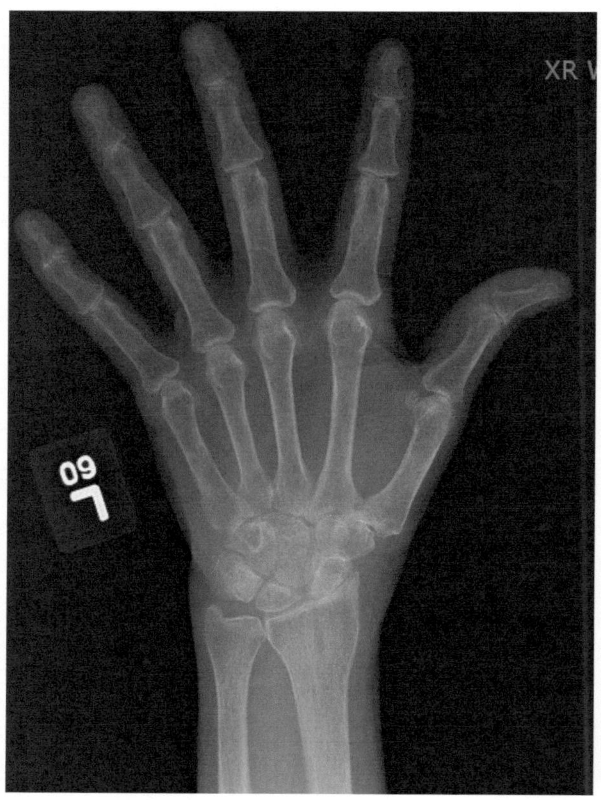

Fig. 6.5 PA radiograph: Stage II SLAC wrist

attachment of the proximal pole of the scaphoid to the lunate via the SLIL and, thus, an arthritis-free articulation between the proximal pole of the scaphoid and the radius [3, 5, 11, 12, 15]. Two reports on the natural history of scaphoid non-unions were published in the 1980s [14, 15]. Mack et al. evaluated 47 scaphoid fractures with a range of five to 53 years of known nonunion and identified three patterns of degeneration. At an average of 8.2 years, patients developed isolated scaphoid sclerosis and cystic changes. By 17.0 years, radioscaphoid arthritis developed, and at an average of 31.6 years generalized arthritis of the wrist developed. Overall they concluded that by 10 years all nonunions were displaced, unstable, or arthritic, and by 20 years, generalized arthritis of the wrist was common. Ruby et al. reviewed their series of 56 scaphoid nonunions and noted a 97% rate of osteo-arthritis at 5 years or greater after injury [15]. These population studies suggest that osteoarthritis is likely to develop in patients with an established scaphoid nonunion, particularly those that are displaced, and thus scaphoid fixation is often recommended for nonunion even in asymptomatic patients, to prevent future degenerative change.

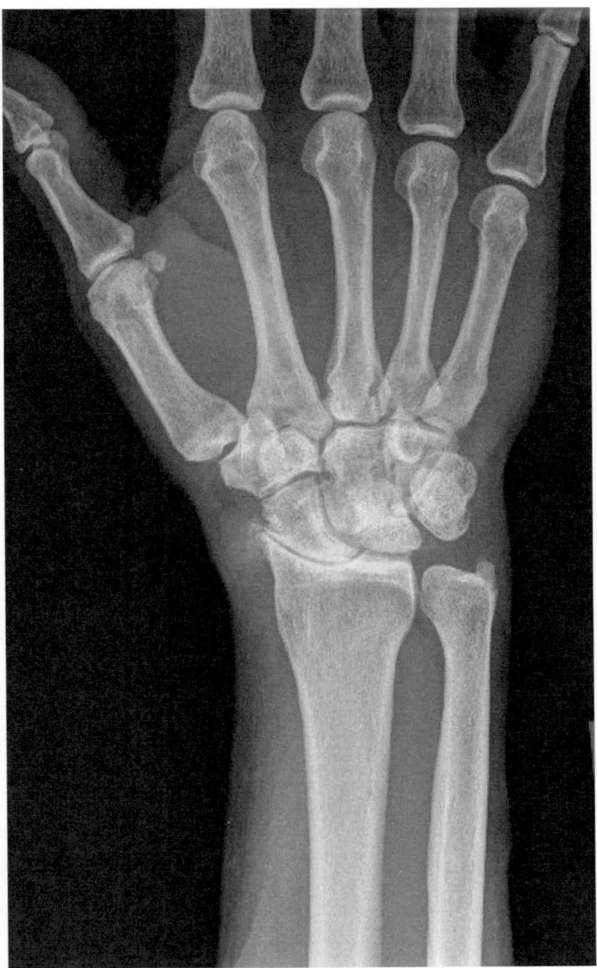

Fig. 6.6 PA radiograph: Stage III SLAC wrist

Management

Nonoperative options are the mainstay of initial treatment although there are no long-term studies evaluating these methods specifically in SLAC/SNAC deformities [4, 13]. As discussed previously, bracing, directed injections, and anti-inflammatory medications may be used in appropriate patients for symptomatic management. Symptoms refractory to conservative management or severe symptoms on presentation warrant consideration of surgical intervention.

Surgical management of SLAC and SNAC wrist is aimed at the stage of involvement. Prior to the development of arthritic changes, direct repair or reconstruction of the scapholunate ligament, with or without radial styloid excision, or treatment of the scaphoid nonunion may be undertaken with the goal of preventing the

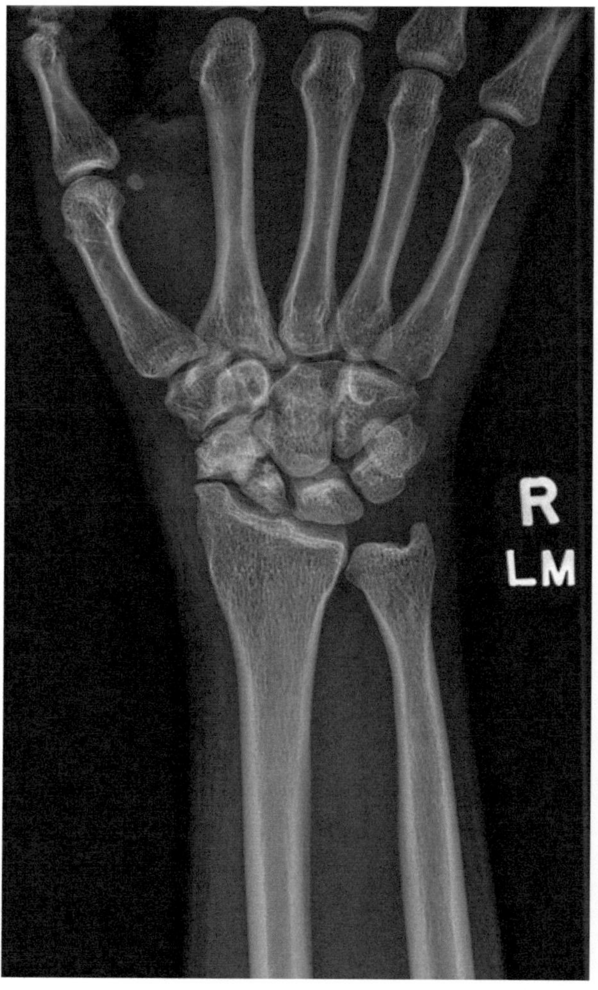

Fig. 6.7 PA radiograph: SNAC wrist

development of end-stage arthritis. Once arthritic changes have occurred, treatment options change significantly [5].

Wrist arthroscopy has a limited role in management but may be useful for evaluation of cartilage surfaces to select an appropriate salvage procedure. For example, arthroscopy allows for direct visualization of the radiocapitate joint to determine if a scaphoidectomy with four-corner fusion (S4CF) is more appropriate than a proximal row carpectomy (PRC), which is contraindicated in the presence of capitolunate arthritis [2, 5]. For stage I SLAC changes, a radial styloidectomy is appropriate to improve pain although this will not inhibit progression of arthritis [5]. Key technical points include protecting the dorsal branches of the radial sensory nerve and resecting less than 3–4 mm to maintain the volar radiocarpal ligaments so as not to induce carpal instability [2, 13]. For more advanced stages of arthritis surgical options include limited wrist fusion, such as a S4CF, scaphocapitate or scaphotrapeziotrapezoidal (STT) arthrodesis, PRC, wrist denervation, total wrist arthroplasty and total wrist arthrodesis [2, 5, 13]. In contrast to total wrist arthrodesis, limited wrist fusions allow for maintenance of wrist motion through preservation of joints unaffected by arthritis [3].

Simple excision of the distal scaphoid may play a role in arthritis management after scaphoid nonunion [3, 5, 13, 16, 17]. Malerich et al. performed a distal scaphoid excision on 19 patients with radioscaphoid arthritis secondary to a scaphoid nonunion, 13 of who sustained pain relief. The procedure is not recommended if capitolunate arthritis is present but has the benefits of minimal ligamentous disruption, and no need for internal fixation or prolonged immobilization [16]. Ruch and Anastasios treated 13 patients with distal scaphoid excision after previous surgery for symptomatic nonunion [17]. At five-year follow-up, only two patients had pain with activity and reported this as mild. Mean wrist flexion and extension increased by 23 and 29 degrees, respectively. In six patients they noted a significant increase in the radiolunate angle, indicating a DISI deformity, but identified no symptomatic correlation [17].

S4CF Versus PRC

A S4CF involves complete removal of the scaphoid with fusion of the remaining capitate, lunate, hamate and the triquetrum [13]. Alternatively, a scaphoidectomy and triquetrectomy can be performed with a three-corner fusion of the capitolunate, capitohamate and hamatolunate joints. Both procedures require undamaged radiolunate articular cartilage, as this joint will remain intact [3, 12]. Correction of a DISI deformity must be performed intra-operatively prior to stabilization or radiocapitate impingement can result dorsally [2, 3, 12]. The radioscaphocapitate and long radiolunate ligament should be preserved to prevent ulnar translation of the carpus [2]. Meticulous surgical technique with preparation of fusion surfaces, removal of debris and proper hardware sizing must be emphasized [13]. Benefits of a S4CF include maintenance of carpal height, preservation of the radiolunate joint and no risk of degeneration at the radiocapitate joint [3]. Risk of nonunion and hardware complications are disadvantages of this procedure [12]. Fusion fixation may be performed with k wires, staples, headless screws or circular plates. K wire fixation is inexpensive but risks pin tract infection, sensory nerve irritation and requires removal [3, 13]. Staples and headless screws provide compression at the expense of possible dorsal impingement with staples, and technical difficulty in placing screws [3, 12]. Multiple studies have shown higher rates of nonunion and complications with circular plate fixation [3, 12, 13]. Saltzmann et al. reviewed seven studies and noted a grouped nonunion rate of seven percent after S4CF [20]. Bain and Watts evaluated clinical outcomes in 35 patients undergoing S4CF at 1, 2, and 10 years and reported pain scores of 0/10 at 1 year, and 22% loss of wrist range of motion. Between 1 and 10 years, there was no significant change in pain, wrist function, patient satisfaction, or arc of wrist motion, suggesting that results are sustainable [18]. Only two patients went on to wrist arthrodesis [18]. Some authors have advocated capitolunate fusion alone, with or without triquetral excision after scaphoidectomy, as outcomes appear similar to a four-corner fusion [2, 13, 19, 43]. In a series of 12 patients undergoing scaphoidectomy and capitolunate arthrodesis with headless compression screws alone, ten patients resumed their prior work activities and the average postoperative grip strength was 81% of the contralateral extremity [19]. The shorter operative time, rapid rate of fusion, preservation of lunotriquetral motion and early rehabilitation are reported benefits of the procedure [19].

Proximal row carpectomy involves resection of the scaphoid, lunate and triquetrum (Fig. 6.8). A new articulation between the capitate and radius is created which requires ensuring that the capitate has intact cartilage proximally prior to committing to this procedure, although there is no data providing guidance on exactly how much cartilage is necessary for a PRC to be successful [2, 3, 12]. Future degeneration of this joint continues to be a risk of PRC particularly in younger patients although it is not clear that these radiographic changes are consistently symptomatic [3, 21]. Pain relief from degeneration of the capitate in the setting of PRC has been obtained with osteochondral resurfacing or interposition procedures however no improvement in range of motion or grip strength is achieved [13]. Preservation of the radioscaphocapitate ligament is necessary to prevent ulnar translation of the capitate off the radius [3]. The benefits of a PRC include a lack of prolonged

Fig. 6.8 PA radiograph after proximal row carpectomy

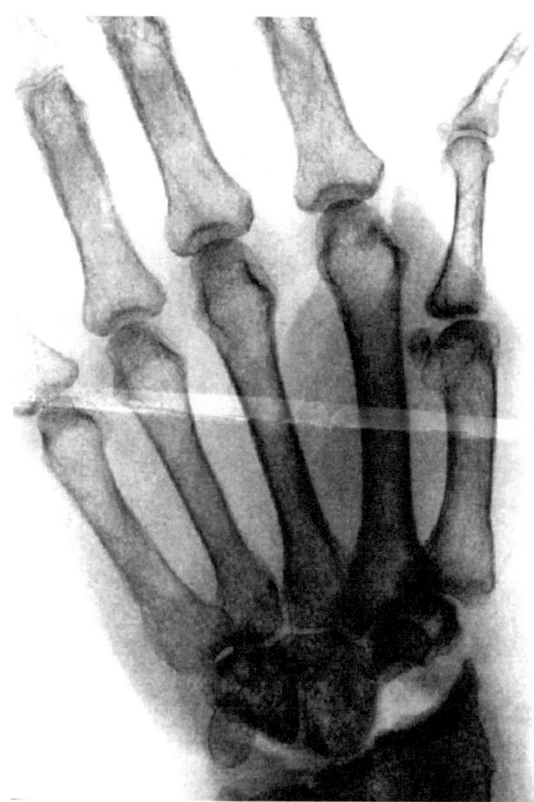

postoperative immobilization, no risk of nonunion or hardware complications, technical ease, greater maintenance of wrist motion and simple conversion to a total wrist arthrodesis or arthroplasty as a salvage option [2, 3, 12, 13, 21].

Multiple studies have examined these two interventions, although randomized controlled trials are limited [5, 44]. In their systematic review, Mulford et al. caution that the current literature lacks unbiased trials and thus interpretation must be made in this context [21]. Both motion-preserving options, S4CF and PRC remain similar in outcomes for SLAC wrist in short-term follow up [13]. Cohen and Kozin performed a cohort study comparing two similar groups, each undergoing either S4CF or PRC at two separate institutions. Pain relief, function, physical score on the SF-36 and patient satisfaction were similar between groups. Greater radial deviation was maintained in the S4CF group [13]. Similar results were noted in a small review of seven studies examining short and medium term outcomes after PRC or 4CF [20]. Grip strength and radial deviation were greater after S4CF while wrist extension and flexion were greater after PRC [20]. In a systematic review of 52 studies examining patients with SLAC or SNAC wrist undergoing either PRC or S4CF, grip strength averaged 70% after PRC and 75% after 4CF. A majority of studies showed a loss of motion after either procedure. Subjective outcomes were "good" 84% of the time after PRC and 85% of the time after 4CF [21]. Grip strength after both is typically reported at 75–80% of the contralateral extremity with a 40–60 degree arc of motion after S4CF and a 60-degree arc of motion after PRC [3]. Kiebhafer recommended PRC for older and less active patients and S4CF in higher demand patients or those less than 35 years old [12]. In general, the procedures are considered equivalent for pain relief, subjective outcomes, grip strength and need for conversion to arthrodesis, in appropriately staged patients [21, 45]. A recent cost-utility analysis identified both S4CF with screw fixation specifically, and PRC as cost effective treatments for management of SLAC/SNAC wrist [46]. The method of fixation in a 4CF alters the cost effectiveness of the intervention, with plate and staple fixation reported as more costly than compression screw fixation [47].

Wrist Denervation

A relatively simple procedure for management of wrist arthritis, denervation remains an option that avoids use of hardware and allows for future salvage options if necessary [13]. Weinstein and Berger reviewed 19 patients undergoing AIN and PIN neurectomies with 2.5 year follow up [22]. Eighty percent of patients reported decreased pain and only two patients went on to arthrodesis with no complications in the group. Overall, 90% of patients would have selected denervation again for their chronic wrist pain [22]. An isolated PIN neurectomy has also been described with 90% of patients satisfied with the procedure [48]. These technically simple procedures can be used as a temporizing measure to delay salvage procedures. Often performed in Europe, complete wrist denervation is an alternative and more extensive option for management of chronic wrist pain. Originally described by Wilhelm, complete wrist denervation involves severance of branches of the PIN,

AIN, palmar cutaneous nerve, sensory branch of the radial nerve, dorsal branch of the ulnar nerve, lateral and medial antebrachial cutaneous nerves and requires five incisions around the wrist [23]. Simon et al. retrospectively reviewed 27 patients undergoing complete wrist denervation by one surgeon. Forty-four percent of patients had complete relief of pain that remained stable in 89%. Grip strength was maintained at 85% of the contralateral arm. Six complications occurred including one case of complex regional pain syndrome and five neuromas with two patients requiring reoperation. Overall 67% of patients were very satisfied [24]. In a longer-term review of 30 complete wrist denervations with average 10 year follow up, 28 patients had improved pain with 22 maintaining this effect through final follow up. Grip strength was reported at 82% of the contralateral extremity [25]. In another review of 71 complete wrist denervations, 22 wrists had complete pain relief and 40 wrists had considerable improvement. Nine patients required reoperation for insufficient pain relief [26]. A more recent study of 39 wrists undergoing total wrist denervation with an average 56 months follow up resulted in pain improvement in 79.5% of cases with four revision procedures and four complications [49]. Complete wrist denervation may provide and maintain sufficient pain relief without sacrificing grip strength or future salvage procedures.

Total Wrist Arthroplasty and Arthrodesis

Severe arthritis of the radiocarpal joint or pancarpal arthritis requires total wrist arthroplasty or arthrodesis [3] (Fig. 6.9). Total wrist arthroplasty removes painful arthritic surfaces and replaces them with a prosthetic option. Early designs included synovitis-inducing silicone implants and unstable prostheses [3]. Newer designs have improved component fixation [3]. Arthroplasty preserves motion when compared to arthrodesis but requires a lifelong lifting restriction, usually of ten pounds or less, and is preferred in low demand patients only [2, 3].

Total wrist arthrodesis is preferred in young laborers and patients who want to continue manual work [3]. Grip strength can be maintained particularly with the wrist fused in slight extension [3]. Arthrodesis is typically performed with commercially available pre-contoured dorsal plates and autogenous bone graft, with cited fusion rates of 93–100% [3, 13]. In a retrospective review of 89 patients undergoing wrist arthrodesis for posttraumatic arthritis, 98% of the 56 patients with plate fixation went on to union, while 82% of those receiving a different form of fixation achieved union [27]. The complication rate after plate fixation was 51%, with 59% of these requiring an additional procedure, while 79% of patients with a different form of fixation had a complication but only 21% of these required an additional procedure [27]. Arthrodesis is thought to be reliable for pain relief and allows patients to perform most activities of daily living through compensation of other joints [2]. Although many studies report patient satisfaction after total wrist arthrodesis, complete pain relief may be less often achieved than perceived based on these series [28]. Jupiter and Adey reported persistent pain in 64% of their series of 22 patients who underwent arthrodesis for posttraumatic arthritis, suggesting that this

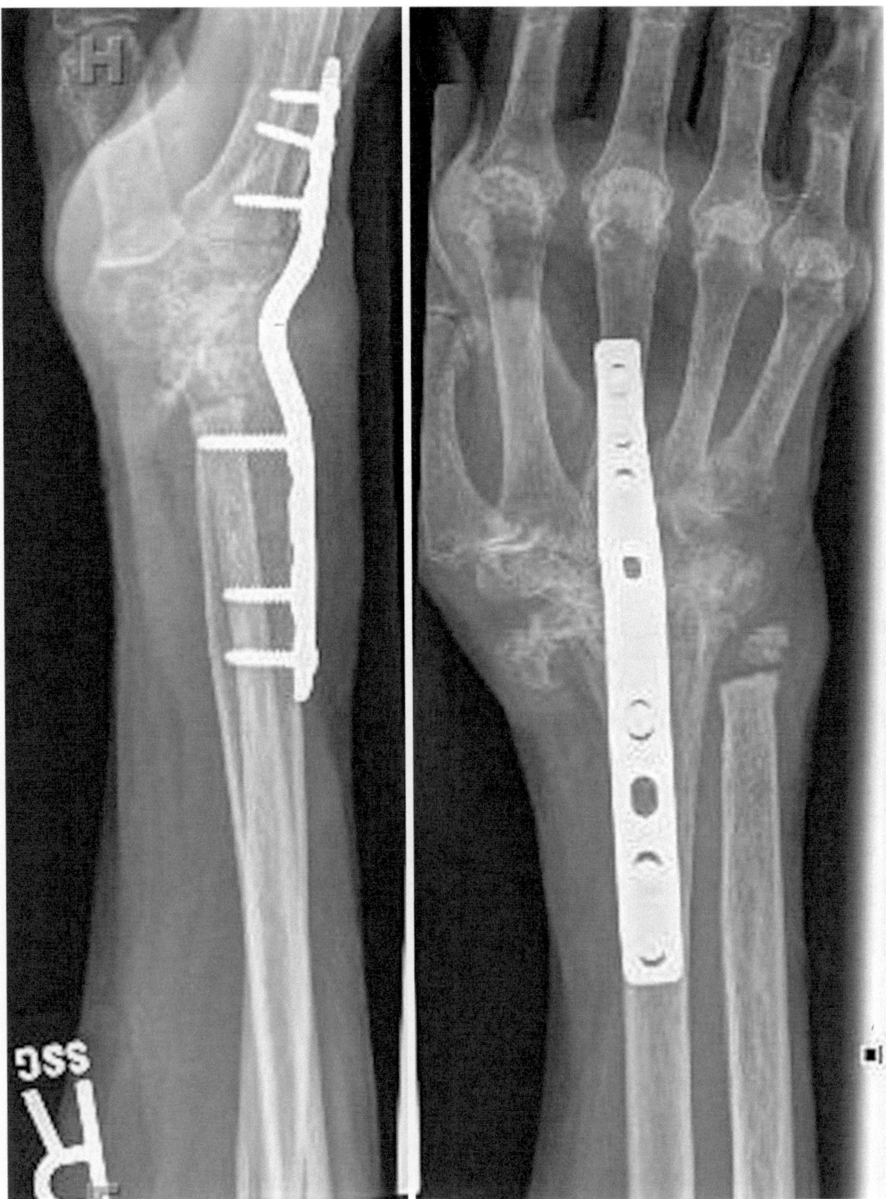

Fig. 6.9 PA and lateral radiographs after total wrist arthrodesis

pain relief procedure may be less predictable than previously thought [28]. De Smet et al. compared PRC to wrist arthrodesis in a nonrandomized retrospective study of 61 patients with posttraumatic osteoarthritis of the radiocarpal joint. While there was no difference in grip strength between groups, functional outcome scores, maintenance of professional activity and complication rates were better in the PRC group [29]. Additional sources of pain must be considered when opting for wrist arthrodesis and should be addressed.

Surgical Technique

A dorsal approach is typically preferred for most salvage procedures. Dissection through the third dorsal compartment with radial transposition of the extensor pollicis longus (EPL) is followed by a longitudinal, step cut or transverse ligament-sparing incision through the dorsal wrist capsule [3]. Lister's tubercle is easily identified in the surgical field and can be removed to obtain distal radius bone graft. For some implants removal of this tubercle allows greater flexibility of plate position and less hardware prominence [3]. Weiss and Rodner recommend a surgical technique that maintains precise capsular incisions to facilitate closure, avoids ligaments of the wrist that are not involved to prevent secondary instability, and uses transverse incisions when possible to preserve motion. Dissection must be performed carefully to protect the sensory branches of radial and ulnar nerves, and excision of the PIN may assist with denervation of the wrist and pain control. Use of autogenous bone graft, preferably from the distal radius or iliac crest, as opposed to resected carpal bone, is recommended [3].

Isolated Radiocarpal Arthritis

Radiocarpal arthritis in the absence of intercarpal arthritis may result after an intra-articular or malunited distal radius fracture [3, 6, 9]. Intra-articular step-off or loss of normal volar tilt, radial height or inclination with malunion may alter points of contact and load leading to degenerative changes.

Management

Radioscapholunate (RSL) arthrodesis may be performed for pain relief at the expense of wrist motion, which is typically 33% of normal. Concomitant excision of the distal scaphoid may increase range of motion to 50–60% of normal [3]. Proponents of scaphoidectomy have postulated that inclusion of the entire scaphoid in an RSL arthrodesis leads to degeneration of the STT joint as the distal row is unable to flex over the proximal row [30]. Garcia-Elias reviewed 15 cases of RSL arthrodesis with distal scaphoidectomy for posttraumatic arthritis from distal radius fractures (13 patients) or perilunate fracture-dislocations (two patients). The midcarpal joints were uninvolved in all patients. Complete pain relief was achieved in ten patients and overall pain relief was noted to be greater than that reported in their previous series of 27 patients who did not have a concomitant distal scaphoidectomy [30]. In comparing their outcomes to the literature on RSL arthrodesis alone, they note greater motion in wrist flexion and radial deviation with distal scaphoidectomy [30].

Isolated Intercarpal Arthritis

Scaphotrapeziotrapezoidal Arthritis

STT arthritis may cause radial-sided wrist pain. The posttraumatic nature of STT arthritis is unclear. While it has been suggested that an isolated SL ligament rupture, without instability or rotatory subluxation of the scaphoid, may cause degeneration of the STT joint, this may be a reflection of the prevalence of STT arthritis as opposed to confirmation that trauma is a common etiology of degeneration at this joint [5].

Management

Management options for STT arthritis include joint debridement, distal scaphoidectomy (open or arthroscopic), trapeziectomy, partial trapezoid resection, STT arthrodesis or arthroplasty [5, 50, 51]. Excisional arthroplasty can be performed for STT arthritis when not associated with dorsal midcarpal instability as distal scaphoid resection could cause collapse into DISI [31]. This technique is technically simple with few complications and does not require prolonged immobilization [31]. Arthrodesis of the STT joint has been extensively although reports often include patients with Kienbock's disease in addition to traumatic etiologies [32]. Radial styloidectomy should be performed at the time of fusion, with postoperative motion expected to be approximately 65% of normal [4]. In a review of multiple studies reporting on a total 238 patients, the average nonunion rate was 13%. The grouped complication rate was 43% and included pin track infection, progressive arthrosis, nerve irritation and osteomyelitis, amongst others [33]. Forty-nine percent of patients reported persistent wrist pain [33]. Alternatively, Pequinot reported a small series of patients undergoing pyrocarbon STT replacements citing a pain relief procedure that preserves carpal stability, has a low complication rate and does not preclude salvage with fusion. Patients had a slight loss of pinch strength and wrist motion with 10 degrees less radial deviation and 15 degrees less wrist extension while grip strength was maintained at 4 year follow up [34].

Lunotriquetral Arthritis

Injury to the LTIL is significantly more rare than SLIL injury and typically occurs from a fall onto an outstretched, supinated and extended wrist [2, 5]. Force transfers from the pisiform into the triquetrum while the lunate remains tethered by the long radiolunate ligament. The contradictory forces lead to rupture of the intervening ligament [2]. These injuries may also occur as part of a perilunate dislocation (stage III). An intact SLIL in the setting of an LTIL rupture will flex the lunate with the scaphoid resulting in a volar intercalated segment instability (VISI) deformity [2, 5, 6, 9]. Ligament rupture with subsequent VISI deformity is not, however, clearly correlated with development of arthritis. In a biomechnical study of ulnar column instability from LTIL tears, cadaveric wrists were loaded in 12 different positions with a pressure sensor film measuring load across the radiocarpal joint in each stage of perilunate injury. No significant differences in pressure were noted in any stage suggesting that a VISI deformity does not necessarily correlate with clinical development of arthritis [35].

Management

After attempting nonoperative interventions, management of lunotriquetral arthritis after an LTIL injury is often with lunotriquetral (LT) fusion. Isolated LT arthrodesis will not improve a static VISI deformity and thus Peterson recommends including the hamate in the fusion or performing a 4CF to correct VISI [5]. Positive ulnar variance must also be corrected with shortening or resection at the time of LT fusion [5]. Kirschenbaum reviewed a series of 14 patients undergoing LT arthrodesis for chronic LT instability. Twelve patients went onto fusion and one pseudarthrosis required a second procedure but healed. Wrist motion ranged from 80% to 88% of the contralateral arm depending on direction of motion tested and grip strength averaged 93% comparatively [36]. LT fusion remains a pain relief operation with reasonable maintenance of motion and grip strength, at least in the short-term [36]. Despite wide use of this procedure, a comparison study of arthrodesis, direct ligament repair and ligament reconstruction reported that the probability of remaining free from a complication at 5 years was less than one percent in the arthrodesis group. This compared to 68.6% and 13.5% for the reconstruction and repair groups, respectively. Results followed the same trend for probability of not requiring further surgery. While DASH scores did not differ, objective measurements and subjective satisfaction scores were significantly higher in the repair and reconstruction groups compared to the arthrodesis group [37]. This study suggests that LT fusion may not be the ideal intervention for degenerative changes due to LTIL injury.

Pisotriquetral Arthritis

This uncommon location of arthritis, when it occurs, is often posttraumatic in nature and may result from acute or chronic injuries [4, 5]. Diagnosis may be suggested by tenderness with loading of the pisotriquetral joint and can be confirmed with a directed injection. A supinated oblique radiographic view allows direct examination of the pisotriquetral joint [5]. Ulnar nerve symptoms or rupture of the small finger flexor profundus are possible with arthritis of this joint, due to the proximity of these structures [5].

Management

As with other forms of arthritis, management with splinting, nonsteroidal antiinflammatory medications or injections, is attempted initially [5]. Simple pisiformectomy with care to preserve the flexor carpi ulnaris insertion is the surgical treatment of choice for cases that do not respond to nonoperative measures [4, 5].

Distal Radioulnar Joint and Ulnocarpal Arthritis

Arthritis of the DRUJ or ulnocarpal joint can have one of many traumatic causes. A fracture of the distal radius with malunion may result in shortening that alters the relative length of the ulna. Normally carrying approximately 20% of the load on the forearm, the ulna is then overloaded inappropriately and ulnocarpal arthritis may result [3, 4]. Furthermore, the relationship of the distal ulnar articulation with the sigmoid notch of the radius may be changed predisposing to DRUJ arthritis [4, 38]. Alternatively, a soft tissue injury such as an injury to the TFCC, which includes the stabilizing ligaments of the DRUJ, can also contribute to the development of post-traumatic arthritis of the DRUJ and/or ulnocarpal joints [4].

Management

Treatment of ulnocarpal arthritis requires offloading the distal ulna. This can be achieved through height restoration with a radial osteotomy, ulnar shortening, wafer procedure or a distal ulnar resection, known as a Darrach procedure.

Arthritis of the DRUJ may be managed with partial or complete distal ulnar resection, hemiresection interposition (HIT) arthroplasty, endoprosthetic replacement or arthrodesis of the DRUJ with pseudarthrosis of the distal ulna, known as the Sauve-Kapandji (SK) procedure [4, 38, 41, 52]. Procedures that maintain the TFCC and ulnar styloid have the benefit of preventing ulnocarpal impingement [4].

Bowers performed a DRUJ HIT arthroplasty in 38 patients with the goal of preserving the ulnocarpal ligament complex. At 2.5 year follow up, 100% of the patients with a traumatic etiology of arthritis had painless range of motion with an average 83 degrees of pronation to 83 degrees of supination and no instability [39]. Nawijn et al. reported higher satisfaction scores in patients undergoing HIT arthroplasty for inflammatory compared to posttraumatic DRUJ arthritis [53]. Santos et al. reported on three patients undergoing DRUJ arthroplasty, two of who had posttraumatic DRUJ arthritis. In the short term, both patients achieved pain relief and had increased motion at the DRUJ [41]. Watson performed a matched ulnar resection in 44 patients, in which a convex resection of the distal ulna is undertaken to match the concave shape of the distal radius with maintenance of the TFCC and ulnocarpal ligaments [40]. Patients were followed for an average 6.5 years and maintained 80.5 degrees of painless pronation and 88.5 degrees of supination [40]. Endoprosthetic replacement with a semiconstrained DRUJ arthroplasty has been utilized in the management of DRUJ arthritis with early reports citing low complication rates and a more recent review reporting further surgery secondary to complications in 29% of patients [54]. Commonly cited soft tissue complications may be more frequent in patients with a history of rheumatoid arthritis or immunosuppression compared to those without [55].

The SK and Darrach procedures are often applicable in similar clinical situations, each with their benefits and complications. The Darrach procedure may be complicated by ulnar translation of the carpus and/or distal ulnar stump instability [4, 40, 41]. The SK procedure may be complicated by a persistently painful pseudarthrosis [40]. Studies on these procedures have been primarily in rheumatoid populations. George et al. published one of the only reports on the use of these procedures in a posttraumatic setting [42]. They retrospectively reviewed the use of the SK or Darrach procedures in patients under age 50 with DRUJ arthrosis after distal radius fracture malunion. Twelve patients after an SK, and 21 patients after a Darrach were included. At final clinical follow up there were no significant differences in subjective pain or functional scores, forearm or wrist rotation, or complication rates between the two groups. One patient required conversion to a Darrach after initial treatment with an SK [42]. The procedures are considered equivalent for treatment of posttraumatic DRUJ arthritis in this group [42]. The SK procedure has been modified to include tenodesis of the ulnar shaft with a distally based portion of the FCU tendon. In a review of 18 patients undergoing this modification, grip strength increased from 36% to 73% of the contralateral upper extremity. Sixteen patients had stable ulnar stumps and overall pain relief was satisfactory [38]. The procedure is recommended in younger patients who place high demands on their wrist or as a salvage procedure in patients with severely limited forearm rotation [38].

Summary

Arthritis of the wrist encompasses degeneration of intercarpal, radiocarpal, ulnocarpal, and distal radioulnar articulations. More common injuries include scapholunate ligament injuries leading to a well-described pattern of arthritis termed a SLAC wrist, and distal radius fractures which can predispose to radiocarpal, ulnocarpal and/or DRUJ arthritis. Evaluation of patients with wrist arthritis requires a thorough history and a physical exam centered on identification of areas of swelling and localizing tenderness on the many articulations of the wrist. Radiographs are often sufficient for diagnosis of arthritis with advanced imaging rarely necessary. Initial treatment with nonoperative interventions such as splinting, injections and NSAIDs are exhausted before surgical intervention. Operative management typically involves debridement, resection, fusion, or replacement of joint surfaces. Most of these interventions in the wrist have proven to be successful pain relief operations at the expense of wrist motion and grip strength although most patients are able to maintain adequate function.

References

1. Palmer AK, Werner FW, Murphy D, Glisson R. Functional wrist motion: a biomechanical study. J Hand Surg Am. 1985;l0A(I):39–46.
2. Wolfe SW, Hotchkiss RN, Pederson WC, Kozin SH. Green's operative hand surgery. Philadelphia: Elsevier/Churchill Livingstone. 6th ed; 2011. p. 429–63.
3. Gelberman RH, Cooney WP, Szabo RM. Carpal instability. J Bone Joint Surg. 2000;82A(4):578–94.
4. Weiss KE, Rodner CM. Osteoarthritis of the wrist. J Hand Surg. 2007;32A(5):725–46.
5. Peterson B, Szabo RM. Carpal osteoarthrosis. Hand Clin. 2006;22(2006):517–28.
6. Linscheid RL, Dobyns JH, Beabout JW, Bryan RS. Traumatic instability of the wrist. Diagnosis, classification, and pathomechanics. J Bone Joint Surg Am. 1972;54(8):1612–32.
7. Berger RA. The anatomy of the ligaments of the wrist and distal radioulnar joints. Clin Orthop Relat Res. 2001;383:32–40.
8. Wolfe SW, Garcia-Elias M, Kitay A. Carpal instability nondissociative. J Am Acad Orthop Surg. 2012;20(9):575–85. Annotation: this review article defines carpal instability nondissociative with a discussion of clinical presentation, pathophysiology and diagnosis. Subtypes of carpal instability nondissociative are described as well as management principles, both nonoperative and surgical.
9. Lee DJ, Elfar JC. Carpal ligament injuries, pathomechanics, and classification. Hand Clin. 2015;31(3):389–98. Annotation: This articles reviews carpal instability, specifically volar and dorsal intercalated segment instability. Normal wrist mechanics as well as pathological deformities are discussed.
10. Watson HK, Ballet FL. The SLAC wrist: scapholunate advanced collapse pattern of degenerative arthritis. J Hand Surg Am. 1984;9(3):358–65.
11. Strauch RJ. Scapholunate advanced collapse and scaphoid nonunion advanced collapse arthritis—update on evaluation and treatment. J Hand Surg Am. 2011;36(4):729–35.
12. Kiefhaber TR. Management of scapholunate advanced collapse pattern of degenerative arthritis of the wrist. J Hand Surg Am. 2009;34(8):1527–30.
13. Cohen MS, Kozin SH. Degenerative arthritis of the wrist: proximal row carpectomy versus scaphoid excision and four-corner arthrodesis. J Hand Surg Am. 2001;26(1):94–104.
14. Mack GR, Bosset MJ, Gelberman R, Yu E. The natural history of scaphoid nonunion. J Bone Joint Surg. 1984;66A(4):504–9.
15. Ruby LK, Stinson J, Belsky MR. The natural history of scaphoid non-union a review of twenty-five cases. J Bone Joint Surg. 1985;67A(3):428–32.
16. Malerich MM, Clifford J, Eaton B, Eaton R, Littler JW. Distal scaphoid resection arthroplasty for the treatment of degenerative arthritis secondary to scaphoid nonunion. J Hand Surg. 1999;24(6):1196–205.
17. Ruch DS, Papadonikolakis A. Resection of the scaphoid distal pole for symptomatic scaphoid nonunion after failed previous surgical treatment. J Hand Surg Am. 2006;31(4):588–93.
18. Bain GI, Watts AC. The outcome of scaphoid excision and four-corner arthrodesis for advanced carpal collapse at a minimum of ten years. J Hand Surg Am. 2010;35(5):719–25.
19. Hegazy G. Capitolunate arthrodesis for treatment of Scaphoid Nonunion Advanced Collapse (SNAC) wrist arthritis. J Hand Microsurg. 2015;7(1):79–86. Annotation: a retrospective review of twelve patients undergoing capitolunate arthrodesis with headless compression screws for

scaphoid nonunion advanced collapse. This study found capitolunate arthrodesis to restore a stable, functional wrist. No level of evidence provided.

20. Saltzman BM, Frank JM, Slikker W, Fernandez JJ, Cohen MS, Wysocki RW. Clinical outcomes of proximal row carpectomy versus four-corner arthrodesis for post-traumatic wrist arthropathy: a systematic review. J Hand Surg Eur Vol. 2015;40(5):450–7. Annotation: A systematic review of seven studies examining clinical outcomes after PRC or S4CF for SLAC/SNAC wrist. Radial deviation and post-operative grip strength were found to be greater after four-corner fusion while PRC had a lower overall complication rate. Level of Evidence III.

21. Mulford JS, Ceulemans LJ, Nam D, Axelrod TS. Proximal row carpectomy vs four corner fusion for Scapholunate (Slac) or Scaphoid Nonunion advanced Collapse (Snac) wrists: a systematic review of outcomes. J Hand Surg Eur Vol. 2009;34(2):256–63.

22. Weinstein LP, Berger RA. Analgesic benefit, functional outcome and patient satisfaction after partial wrist denervation. J Hand Surg Am. 2002;27(5):833–9.

23. Ferreres A, Foucher G, Santiago S. Extensive denervation of the wrist. Tech Hand Up Extrem Surg. 2002;6(1):36–41.

24. Simon E, Zemirline A, Richou J, Hu W, Le Nen D. Complete wrist denervation: a retrospective study of 27 cases with a mean follow-up period of 77 months. Chir Main. 2012;31(2102):306–10. Annotation: a retrospective review of 27 complete wrist denervations performed by one surgeon. Stable pain relief was achieved in 89% of patients with a significant improvement in range of motion of the wrist. Six complications were reported with overall satisfaction in a majority of patients. No level of evidence provided.

25. Hohendorff B, Mühldorfer-Fodor M, Kalb K, Von Schoonhoven J, Prommersberger KJ. Long-term results following denervation of the wrist. [Article in German]. Unfallchirurg. 2012;115(4):343–52. Annotation: A retrospective review of 61 total wrist denervations with an average follow up of ten years. They conclude that total wrist denervation is an option for the chronically painful wrist with long-term satisfaction. No level of evidence provided.

26. Schweizer A, von Känel O, Kammer E, Meuli-Simmen C. Long-term follow-up evaluation of denervation of the wrist. J Hand Surg Am. 2006;31A(4):559–64.

27. Hastings H, Weiss AC, Quenzer D, Wiedeman GP, Hanington KR, Strickland JW. Arthrodesis of the wrist for post-traumatic disorders. J Bone Joint Surg. 1996;78-A(6):897–902.

28. Adey L, Ring D, Jupiter JB. Health status after total wrist arthrodesis for posttraumatic arthritis. J Hand Surg. 2005;30A(5):932–6.

29. De Smet L, Degreef I, Truyen J, Robijns F. Outcome of two salvage procedures for post-traumatic osteoarthritis of the wrist: arthrodesis or proximal row carpectomy. Acta Chir Belg. 2005;105(6):626–30.

30. Garcia-Elias M, Lluch A, Ferreres A, Papini-Zorli I, Rahimtoola ZO. Treatment of radiocarpal degenerative osteoarthritis by radioscapholunate arthrodesis and distal scaphoidectomy. J Hand Surg Am. 2005;30(1):8–15.

31. Garcia-Elias M. Excisional arthroplasty for Scaphotrapeziotrapezoidal osteoarthritis. J Hand Surg Am. 2011;36(3):516–20.

32. Crook T, Warwick D. Avoiding fusion in wrist arthritis. J Bone Joint Surg. 2011:1–5.

33. Siegel JM, Ruby LK. Critical look at intercarpal arthrodesis: review of the literature. J Hand Surg Am. 1996;21(4):717–23.

34. Pequignot JP, D'asnieres De Veigy L, Allieu Y. Arthroplasty for Scaphotrapeziotrapezoidal arthrosis using a pyrolytic carbon implant. Preliminary results. [Article in French]. Chir Main. 2005;24(3–4):148–52.

35. Viegas SF, Patterson RM, Peterson PD, Pogue DJ, Jenkins DK, Sweo TD, et al. Ulnar sided perilunate instability: an anatomic and biomechanical study. J Hand Surg Am. 1990;15(2):268–78.

36. Kirschenbaum D, Coyle MP, Leddy JP, New Brunswick NJ. Chronic lunotriquetral instability: diagnosis and treatment. J Hand Surg Am. 1993;18(6):1107–12.

37. Shin AY, Weinstein LP, Berger RA, Bishop AT. Treatment of isolated injuries of the lunotriquetral ligament. A comparison of arthrodesis, ligament reconstruction and ligament repair. J Bone Joint Surg Br. 2001;83(7):1023–8.

38. Lamey DM, Fernandez DL. Results of the modified Sauve-Kapandji procedure in the treatment of chronic posttraumatic derangement of the distal radioulnar joint. J Bone Joint Surg Am. 1998;80(12):1758–69.
39. Bowers WH. Distal radioulnar joint arthroplasty: the hemiresection-interposition technique. J Hand Surg Am. 1985;10(2):169–78.
40. Watson HK, Ryu J, Burgess RC. Matched distal ulnar resection. J Hand Surg Am. 1986;11(6):812–7.
41. Santos C, Pereira A, Sousa M, Trigeuiros M, Silva C. Indications for distal radioulnar arthroplasty: report on three clinical cases. Rev Bras Ortop. 2015;46(3):321–4. Annotation: A report of three cases in which a metallic prosthesis was used to replace the DRUJ. At one year follow up all three patients had improved pain and range of motion. No level of evidence provided.
42. George MS, Kiefhaber TR, Stern PJ. The Sauve–Kapandji procedure and the Darrach procedure for distal radio–ulnar joint dysfunction after Colles' fracture. J Hand Surg Br. 2004;29(6):608–13.
43. Dargai F, Hoel G, Safieddine M, Payet E, Leonard R, Jaffarbanjee Z, et al. Tenyear radiological and clinical outcomes of capitolunate arthrodesis with scaphoid and triquetrum excision for advanced degenerative arthritis in the wrist: single-center, retrospective case series with 10patients. Hand Surg Rehabil. 2020;39(1):41–7. Epub 2019 Nov 1.
44. Aita MA, Nakano EK, Schaffhausser HL, Fukushima WY, Fujiki EN. Randomized clinical trial between proximal row carpectomy and the four-corner fusion for patients with stage II SNAC. Rev Bras Ortop. 2016;51(5):574–582. eCollection 2016 Sep-Oct.
45. Williams JB, Weiner H, Tyser AR. Long-term outcome and secondary operations after proximal row carpectomy or four-corner arthrodesis. J Wrist Surg. 2018;7(1):51–6. Epub 2017 Jul 27.
46. Daar DA, Shah A, Mirrer JT, Thanik V, Hacquebord J. Proximal row carpectomy versus four-corner arthrodesis for the treatment of SLAC/SNAC wrist: a cost-utility analysis. Plast Reconstr Surg. 2019;143:1432.
47. Kazmers NH, Stephens AR, Presson AP, Xu Y, Feller RJ, Tyser AR. Comparison of direct surgical costs for proximal row carpectomy and four-corner arthrodesis. J Wrist Surg. 2019;8(1):66–71. Epub 2018 Nov 16.
48. Abdelaziz AM, Aldahshan W, El-Sherief FAH, Wahd YESH, Soliman HAG. Posterior interosseous neurectomy alternative for treating chronic wrist pain. J Wrist Surg. 2019;8(3):198–201. Epub 2019 Jan 29.
49. Picart B, Laborie C, Hulet C, Malherbe M. Total wrist denervation: retrospective study of 39 wrists with 56 months' follow-up. Orthop Traumatol Surg Res. 2019;105(8):1607–10. Epub 2019 Sep 5.
50. Catalano LW 3rd, Ryan DJ, Barron OA, Glickel SZ. Surgical management of Scaphotrapeziotrapezoid arthritis. J Am Acad Orthop Surg. 2020;28(6):221–8.
51. Luchetti R, Atzei A, Cozzolino R. Arthroscopic distal scaphoid resection for Scapho-Trapezium-trapezoid arthritis. Hand (N Y). 2019:1558944719864451.
52. Faucher GK, Zimmerman RM, Zimmerman NB. Instability and arthritis of the distal radioulnar joint: a critical analysis review. JBJS Rev. 2016;4(12):01874474-201612000-00001.
53. Nawijn F, Verhiel SHWL, Jupiter JB, Chen NC. Hemiresection interposition arthroplasty of the distal radioulnar joint: a long-term outcome study. Hand (N Y). 2019;13:1558944719873430.
54. Bellevue KD, Thayer MK, Pouliot M, Huang JI, Hanel DP. Complications of semiconstrained distal radioulnar joint arthroplasty. J Hand Surg Am. 2018;43(6):566.e1–9.
55. DeGeorge BR Jr, Berger RA, Shin AY. Constrained implant arthroplasty for distal radioulnar joint arthrosis: evaluation and management of soft tissue complications. J Hand Surg Am. 2019;44(7):614.e1–614.e9. Epub 2018 Oct 18.

Chapter 7
Post-traumatic Arthritis of the Hand

Andrew P. Harris, Thomas J. Kim, and Christopher Got

> **Key Points**
> - The goal standard for interphalangeal joint arthritis is arthrodesis.
> - Thumb MCP joint arthroplasty is a good option for low demand patients.
> - The CMC arthritis treatment algorithm is similar to IP and MCP arthritis.

Introduction

Arthritis of the hand is a common ailment of the general population with a prevalence of approximately 20–30% [1]. Being the second most common location of pain due to osteoarthritis, it is a common condition that hand surgeons must often treat [1, 2]. The scale of the patient's debilitation varies in severity, but the most common complaints involve stiffness, limitations of daily activities, and aesthetic deformity. Unlike large joints such as the knee or hip, where artificial joint replacement has been successful for many years, the small joints of the hand have not enjoyed such long-term success to a similar degree with replacement surgery. This chapter will discuss current treatments and the available literature regarding outcomes of posttraumatic osteoarthritis of the interphalangeal joints of the fingers and thumb as well as of the metacarpophalangeal and carpometacarpal joints.

A. P. Harris
Warren Alpert Medical School of Brown University, Providence, RI, USA
e-mail: andrew_harris@brown.edu

T. J. Kim (✉) · C. Got
Brown University, Warren Alpert Medical School, Providence, RI, USA

© Springer Nature Switzerland AG 2021
S. C. Thakkar, E. A. Hasenboehler (eds.), *Post-Traumatic Arthritis*,
https://doi.org/10.1007/978-3-030-50413-7_7

Distal Interphalangeal Arthritis

Trauma can occur commonly at the distal interphalangeal (DIP) joint as it is located at the most vulnerable distal aspect of the fingers. Fractures at the distal phalanx can occur at the tuft (distal), shaft (middle), or at the articular surface (proximal). Injuries involving the articular surface of the distal phalanx or at the head of the middle phalanx can lead to arthritis at a later time. Bony mallet finger injuries and flexor digitorum profundus avulsion injuries can also involve a significant portion of the DIP joint and can similarly accelerate arthritis.

Treatment for arthritis at the finger joints is similar in algorithm to that of the large joints. Conservative treatment is the first choice consisting of antiinflammatory medications and occupational therapy. In contrast to larger joints, immobilization may be implemented in finger and thumb osteoarthritis. This is often achieved in the thumb with 1st CMC braces. Steroid injections are also an option but due to the small volume of the joint, correctly injecting an intraarticular dose is challenging. A steroid injection can often provide temporary relief for some patients. When these conservative measures have failed, surgical treatment options can be considered, including arthrodesis or arthroplasty. The gold standard for symptomatic end-stage arthritis at this joint is an arthrodesis [3]. There are many different techniques but the principle remains the same: removal of any remaining articular surface and sclerotic bone on both sides of the joint, and creation of a stable fusion bed using hardware such as a simple Kirschner wires (K-wire) or a compression screw (Fig. 7.1).

The compression screw is usually a cannulated screw which is usually placed in retrograde fashion. After exposing the joint and preparing the joint surfaces, a K-wire is advanced antegrade from the distal phalanx. As the wire tents the skin, a stab incision is made over the wire, and the wire is advanced until it protrudes just beneath the surface of the proximal aspect of the distal phalanx. The fusion surfaces are then reduced, and the wire is advanced retrograde across the fusion surface under direct visualization into the center of the middle phalanx. Then, while the fusion surfaces are held in compression, the screw is advanced over the wire. There are two main designs of compression screw that use the concept of variable thread pitch to achieve compression when the screw is advanced. The Herbert-type compression screw has a smooth center shaft with different thread pitches at the leading and trailing ends. The other screw design is fully threaded where the pitch varies along its entire length. Both types serve the same purpose in creating a compression force across the fusion bed (Fig. 7.2). Rates of union, reported to be from 80% to 100%, are high regardless of technique (Fig. 7.3) [3, 4].

Complications from DIP arthrodesis can include nonunion, failure of hardware, fracture of the distal phalanx, and infection. Stern et al. reported a nonunion rate of 11% for DIP joint arthrodesis [5]. In the event of a symptomatic nonunion, techniques have been described to remove the screw, curette out the nonunion site, and place a cortico-cancellous graft either from the distal radius or from the iliac crest [6]. There are no large series reporting outcomes for revision arthrodesis; however, the few cases reported have achieved successful revision arthrodesis with these

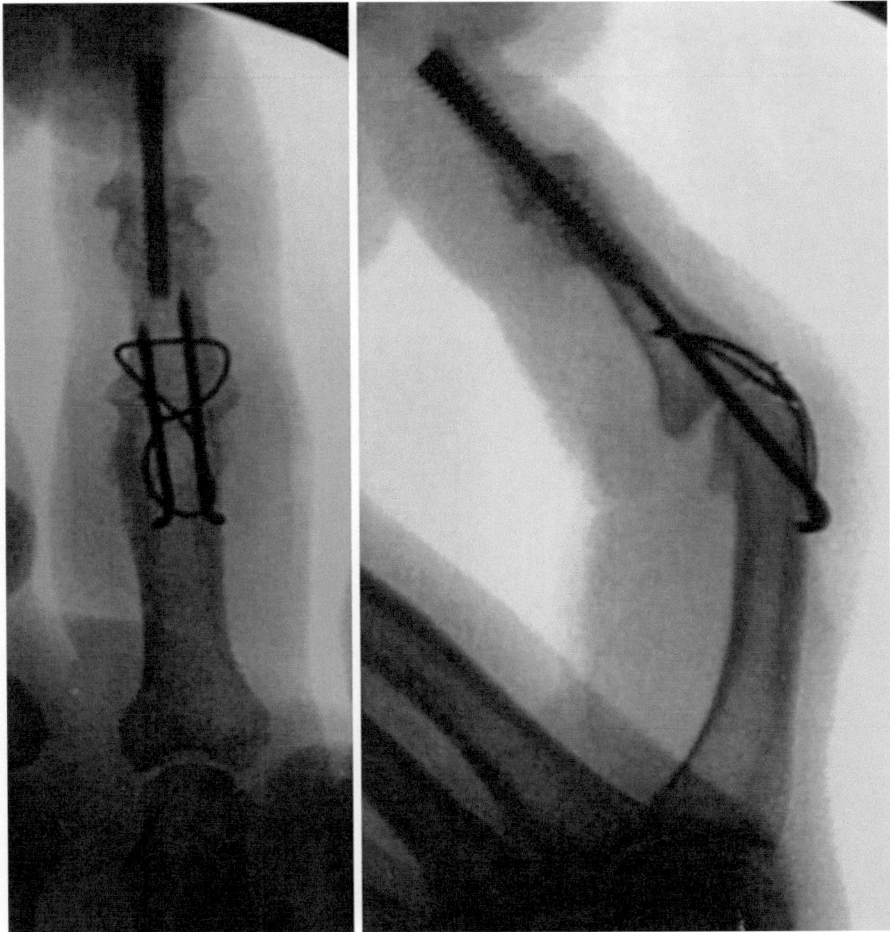

Fig. 7.1 Distal interphalangeal joint fusion with a compression screw and a proximal interphalangeal joint fusion with cerclage wire and Kirschner wires (AP and lateral views)

techniques [6]. Fractures of the distal phalanx can also occur as the average antero-posterior diameter of the distal phalanx is 3.5 mm while the trailing thread diameter of a Herbert standard screw is 3.9 mm, Acutrak Mini screw is 3.6 mm, and Stryker TwinFix screw is 4.1 mm [7, 8]. This can lead to disruption of the dorsal cortex of the distal phalanx and pressure on the germinal matrix, which can cause nail deformities [9]. Thus, it is important to select a proper size screw that will fit both the middle phalanx and the distal phalanx. Herbert compression screws usually range from 2.5 mm to 3.0 mm with no smaller diameters available. Smaller screw sizes have been developed, with Acutrak Micro (Regina, Canada) providing diameters ranging from 2.0 mm to 2.4 mm.

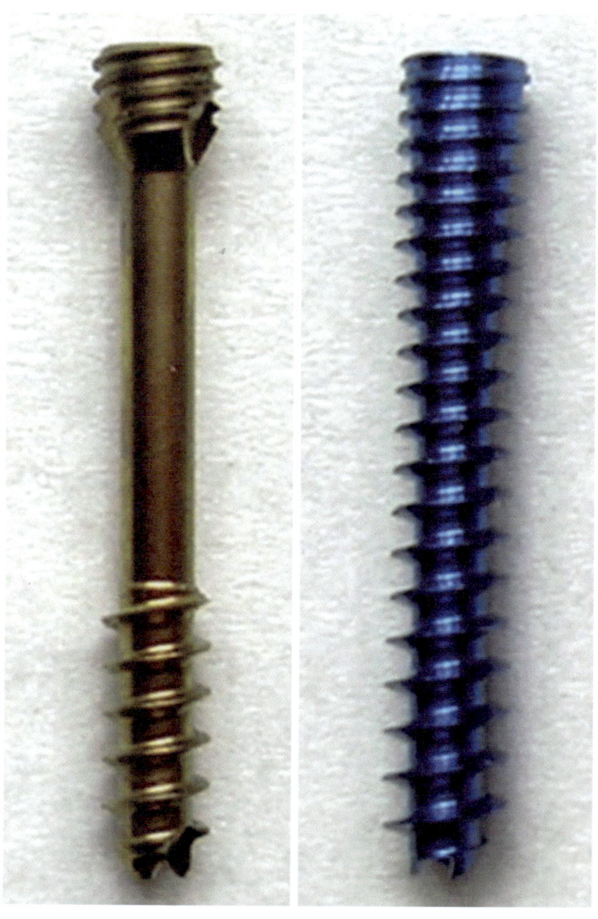

Fig. 7.2 Herbert compression screw versus fully threaded variable pitch screw

DIP arthroplasty is indicated in a select patient population. In musicians or other patients with a similar demand for fine dexterity at the fingertips, preserving motion at the DIP joint is preferred. In contrast, arthrodesis eliminates all motion at site of fusion and is more suitable for patients requiring increased demand such as heavy laborers. Fusion, in general, is the most reliable option for pain relief and avoids complications related to implant loosening and breakage [10]. Silicone arthroplasty has been reported to be performed for a small number of patients with varying but similar complication rates compared to arthrodesis at 1–10% [11, 3].

Proximal Interphalangeal Joint Arthritis

Proximal interphalangeal (PIP) joint injuries are notorious for the subsequent stiffness and arthritis that can occur. It is still a problem that has not yet been solved and because of this, there are many different treatment options. The anatomy of the PIP

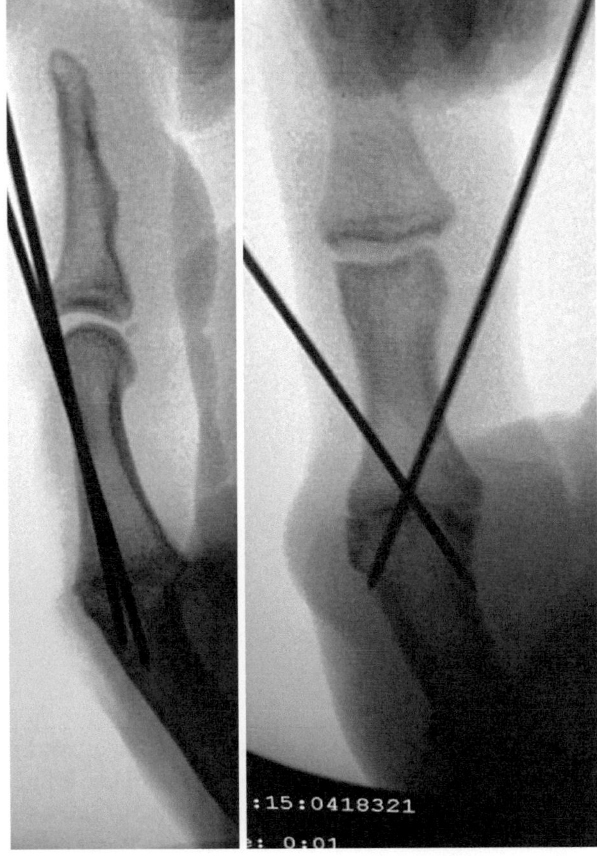

Fig. 7.3 AP and lateral view of a thumb interphalangeal joint fusion with Kirschner wires

joint can be considered as a box with the volar plate forming the floor of the box, the collateral ligaments forming the sides, and the extensor mechanism forming the roof. At least two sides of the box must be disrupted for the box to become unstable. The joint is in a vulnerable position away from the palm but has enough of a lever arm so that when forces are applied from the fingertip, it can create significant injury.

Treatment options start with hand therapy, splinting, and antiinflammatories. Because posttraumatic arthritis and stiffness in the PIP joint involves much more than just the bony articular surface, therapy is essential. The soft tissue structures that contract respond well to serial digital casting, ultrasound, heat, and stretching [12–14]. Patient compliance is of utmost importance as it is a long and tedious process. Surgical options include arthroplasty and arthrodesis. The gold standard for symptomatic end-stage posttraumatic arthritis is arthrodesis. This is especially true for the index finger where pinch strength is desired and for manual laborers with increased demands on their hands. Other options for PIP joint arthrodesis are similar to the DIP joint with a tension band, compression screw, and plating commonly utilized (Fig. 7.4).

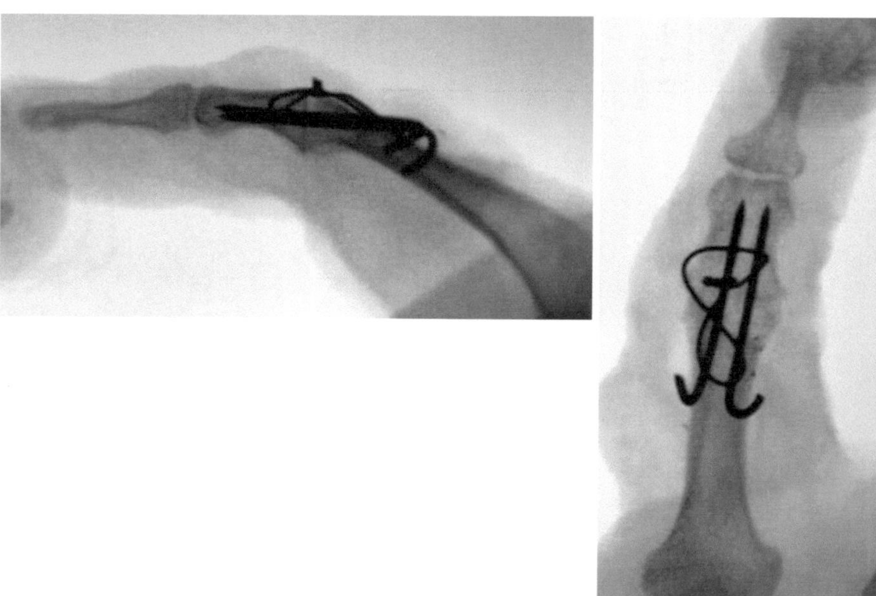

Fig. 7.4 Proximal interphalangeal joint arthrodesis with Kirschner wires and tension band (AP and lateral view)

Arthroplasty techniques include volar plate arthroplasty, silicone arthroplasty, and surface replacement arthroplasty. Volar plate arthroplasty was initially a procedure for acute fracture-dislocations of the PIP joint for which the native articular surfaces were unable to be reconstructed [15]. It has since then become a procedure that can be used for posttraumatic arthritis of the PIP joint with decent success [16, 17]. The procedure involves resection of the non-reconstructable/arthritic portions of the remaining articular surfaces and contouring those to fit one another. The volar plate is then detached distally off of the middle phalanx and transposed into the joint. Lin and colleagues performed a modified version of this procedure in seven patients with posttraumatic PIP joint arthritis. They found a decrease in pain scores and an increase in the average arc of motion by 64 degrees at a 2 year follow-up [16]. Dionysian et al. followed 17 patients for an average of 11.5 years with range of motion ranging from 30 to 110 degrees [15]. Only four patients demonstrated mild joint narrowing [15]. Silicone arthroplasty has been used to relieve pain and maintain joint motion since the 1960s [18]. They serve as spacers that allow the soft tissues to form a capsule and a pain-free stable joint. Studies have found good to excellent pain relief with no significant change in range of motion [19, 20]. Complications include implant fracture, lateral instability, silicone synovitis, and bony erosion with a reported 10–14% revision rate [21]. Because of these potential issues, there have been a number of different surface replacement arthroplasties developed.

The two most widely used joint replacements are currently the titanium-polyethylene and pyrocarbon implants. The titanium-polyethylene implants typically consist of proximal and distal titanium shafts, an alloyed proximal joint surface, and an ultra-high-molecular-weight polyethylene distal joint surface. The pyrocarbon implants consist of a radiopaque graphite core with a radiolucent pyrolitic carbon coating. This implant material has a modulus of elasticity that is similar to cortical bone. Both the titanium and pyrocarbon implants are unlinked, condylar constrained, noncemented devices. The joint stability is maintained by the joint surface geometry and the preserved collateral ligaments. A prospective randomized trial studied the differences between silicone arthroplasty, titanium arthroplasty, and pyrocarbon arthroplasty. Pain reduction and grip strength were similar in all groups. Range of motion was superior only temporarily in the titanium and pyrocarbon groups compared to the silicone group. The complications were more frequent and severe in the surface replacement groups. The titanium devices group had 27% removed and eventually replaced by silicone implants. The pyrocarbon group had 39% removed and replaced. Based on this and more recent studies that have demonstrated poor outcomes with surface replacement arthroplasty, posttraumatic arthritis is still an unsolved problem [21]. New techniques to gain stronger bone implant fixation to avoid this all too common complication of loosening with joint surface replacement are currently being investigated.

Arthrodesis is the gold standard for posttraumatic arthritis of the PIP joint. There are multiple techniques to fuse the PIP joint, including screw fixation, K-wires, tension band, and plate fixation. All three techniques are commonly used and are often dictated by surgeon preference; however, a study performed by Leibovic and Strickland demonstrated screw fixation provided the lowest nonunion rate [22]. The PIP is fused in the position of optimal function. The index and middle fingers are usually more functional in 15–30 degrees of flexion as they are used in fine pinch. The ulnar digits are more functional in 30–45 degrees of flexion as they are used in grip. Obtaining these optimal fusion angles are key to retaining maximal hand function.

Metacarpophalangeal Joint Arthritis

The hand contains five metacarpophalangeal (MCP) joints consisting of articulations with the metacarpal and first phalanx of each digit. The MCP joints are prone to trauma, especially in the setting of striking an inanimate object with a closed fist. The 2nd through 5th are the most distally based articulation when viewing a clenched hand, making them vulnerable to intraarticular damage. Crush injuries and blunt force trauma, like the other articulations of the hand, are other common mechanisms of injury.

Initial treatment of MCP posttraumatic arthritis is similar to other joints of the hand. Conservative treatment involves a multimodal approach and is generally initiated with nonsteroidal antiinflammatory medications (NSAIDS), commonly consisting of ibuprofen, celebrex, naproxen, or meloxicam. Topical treatments such as voltaren gel can be implemented. Occupational therapy or hand therapy can provide significant benefit in terms of strength and range of motion, depending on the severity of arthritis. Splinting may also be employed at the risk of increasing stiffness but providing comfort by immobilizing the affected joint. The thumb MCP joint is more amenable to maintaining function while splinted as compared to the digits 2 through 5. As with other larger articulations, the MCP joint may also undergo a trial of corticosteroid injection. Timing of injection is important because if near-future operative intervention is possible, the authors of this chapter recommend the last injection to be a minimum 3 months prior to prevent risk of infection with a maximum trial of three injections spaced at least 3 months apart [23, 24].

When conservative treatments have been exhausted, failing to provide relief and restoration of function to the affected hand, surgical options may be considered. MCP joint arthroplasty is one of the most frequently applied surgical interventions for low demand patients. Early arthroplasty designs were of the constrained hinged variety but commonly failed due to loosening or fracture [25]. Today's MCP arthroplasty components consist of either silicone or pyrocarbon. Chung et al. reported significantly improved patient reported outcomes at 1 year for patients receiving the Swanson MCP joint arthroplasty for rheumatoid arthritis [26]. In 1999, Cook et al. studied 53 predominately rheumatoid patients receiving 151 MCP pyrocarbon arthroplasties, reporting a 12% revision rate and 81.4% survival rate at 10 years [27]. Houdek et al. showed excellent results for patients with open traumatic non-reconstructable articular MCP injuries treated initially with pyrocarbon arthroplasty.

For higher demand patients or patients who have failed MCP arthroplasty, fusion of the MCP joint can be considered an initial surgical treatment or salvage procedure. Arthrodesis is effective at eliminating pain, but fusion at the correct flexion angle is necessary to provide maximum function given the limited mobility. Bicknell et al. retrospectively reviewed 27 patients that underwent thumb MCP joint fusion patients, reporting high patient satisfaction, a low complication rate, and small losses in dexterity, strength, and motion [28]. No consensus has been reached for the exact optimal position of fusion. Steiger et al. determined the optimum fusion angle of the thumb MCP to be 15 degrees of flexion and 10 degrees of pronation in contrast to a study by Saldana et al. recommending fusion for men 25 degrees and for women at 20 degrees. The angles of fusion were based on each patient's needs at the time of surgery [29, 30]. The angles of fusion of the 2nd through 5th MCP joints are generally 10, 20, 30, and 40 degrees respectively, which is the average resting positions these joints [30]. As shown by Ledgard et al., reporting improved function of patients treated with simultaneous fusion of the 2nd through 5th MCP joints for posttraumatic arthritis, the hand is able to retain excellent function if joints are fused in the appropriate position [31].

Carpometacarpal Arthritis

Carpometacarpal (CMC) joints are susceptible to trauma much like the MCP, PIP, and DIP articulations. The hand contains five CMC articulations, with the thumb CMC articulation being the most complex and important in consideration of hand function. Much like the MCP joints, the CMC joints of digits are more prone to injury and dislocation during a clenched fist strike with direct transfer of force to these articulations. The thumb CMC has two well-known intraarticular fracture pattern eponyms known as the "Rolando" and "Bennett" with the most common mechanism of axially directed force to the thumb [32]. The Rolando fracture pattern is characterized by intraarticular comminution of the 1st proximal metacarpal [33]. The Bennett fracture is characterized by a volar split of the proximal 1st metacarpal, where the volar oblique ligament inserts on the fracture fragment [34]. Aside from posttraumatic arthritis, idiopathic osteoarthritis of the thumb CMC is one of the most commonly treated conditions for practicing hand surgeons.

Even after periarticular fracture fixation of the CMC joints, posttraumatic arthritis may occur. The treatment algorithm employed is very similar to the MCP, PIP, and DIP joints. Treatment begins with conservative management, consisting of nonsteroidal antiinflammatory drugs (NSAIDS), splinting, and hand therapy or occupational therapy. Splints specifically constructed for the thumb CMC have been shown to provide significant improvement in hand function and pain relief and are often employed early in treatment. Splinting of the CMC joints 2 through 5, however, is difficult to accomplish while maintaining hand function. Corticosteroid injection is often instituted in the setting of thumb CMC arthritis but is considered a temporary solution as the duration of symptom relief has been shown to be dependent on severity of arthritis [35]. Meenagh et al., in a randomized controlled trial, showed no clinical benefit of corticosteroid injection versus placebo for patients with moderate to severe arthritis [36]. Injection of CMC joints 2 through 5 may also be attempted; although, posttraumatic arthritis to these joints is much less common than to the thumb [37].

After conservative modalities of treatment have been exhausted and pain and function have not improved to the satisfaction of the patient, surgical intervention may be warranted. Surgical options for the thumb include trapeziectomy (excisional arthroplasty) with or without suspensionplasty or ligament reconstruction, CMC fusion, and joint replacement [38, 39]. Excisional arthroplasty is considered the gold standard treatment for relatively active patients [38]. Patients who are young, healthy, or high demand and laborers may benefit from CMC fusion [39]. Low demand patients may be considered for joint replacement. Silicone thumb CMC joint replacements initially showed excellent results but were later found to be fraught with complications including synovitis, silicone wear, subluxation, cold creep, and bony erosion [38]. Early studies of pyrocarbon interpositional thumb CMC implants have shown promising results for selected low-demand patients [40]. CMC articulations 2 through 5 have relatively small amounts of motion compared to the thumb and generally respond well to fusion. However, Yong et al. have shown promising early results using the Dupert's arthroplasty technique for the 5th CMC joint, which involves resection of the base of the 5th metacarpal and fusion of the proximal shaft to the 4th metacarpal [41].

Conclusion

Posttraumatic arthritis of the hand is a common condition treated by hand surgeons. Even with proper fixation of fractures, posttraumatic arthritis may be inevitable due to the nature of the original injury. Treatment options are relative to each patient's activity demands, but, in general, conservative measures consisting of NSAIDs, immobilization, and steroid injections are trialed early on. When conservative measures have failed to alleviate discomfort and pain, surgical intervention with joint replacement, excisional arthroplasty, or arthrodesis may be warranted depending on the joints involved.

References

1. Lawrence RC, Helmick CG, Arnett FC, et al. Estimates of the prevalence of arthritis and selected musculoskeletal disorders in the United States. Arthritis Rheum. 1998;41(5):778–99. https://doi.org/10.1002/1529-0131(199805)41:5<778::AID-ART4>3.0.CO;2-V.
2. Oliveria SA, Felson DT, Reed JI, Cirillo PA, Walker AM. Incidence of symptomatic hand, hip, and knee osteoarthritis among patients in a health maintenance organization. Arthritis Rheum. 1995;38(8):1134–41.
3. Leibovic SJ. Instructional Course Lecture. Arthrodesis of the interphalangeal joints with headless compression screws. J Hand Surg. 2007;32(7):1113–9. https://doi.org/10.1016/j.jhsa.2007.06.010.
4. Brutus J-P, Palmer AK, Mosher JF, Harley BJ, Loftus JB. Use of a headless compressive screw for distal interphalangeal joint arthrodesis in digits: clinical outcome and review of complications. J Hand Surg. 2006;31(1):85–9. https://doi.org/10.1016/j.jhsa.2005.09.009.
5. Stern PJ, Fulton DB. Distal interphalangeal joint arthrodesis: an analysis of complications. J Hand Surg. 1992;17(6):1139–45.
6. Owusu A, Isaacs J. Revision of failed distal interphalangeal arthrodesis complicated by retained headless screw. J Hand Surg. 2013;38(7):1408–13. https://doi.org/10.1016/j.jhsa.2013.04.018.
7. Wyrsch B, Dawson J, Aufranc S, Weikert D, Milek M. Distal interphalangeal joint arthrodesis comparing tension-band wire and Herbert screw: a biomechanical and dimensional analysis. J Hand Surg. 1996;21(3):438–43. https://doi.org/10.1016/S0363-5023(96)80360-1.
8. Darowish M, Brenneman R, Bigger J. Dimensional analysis of the distal phalanx with consideration of distal interphalangeal joint arthrodesis using a headless compression screw. Hand (N Y). 2015;10(1):100–4. https://doi.org/10.1007/s11552-014-9679-x.
9. Dickson DR, Mehta SS, Nuttall D, Ng CY. A systematic review of distal interphalangeal joint arthrodesis. J Hand Microsurg. 2014;6(2):74–84. https://doi.org/10.1007/s12593-014-0163-1.
10. Drake ML, Segalman KA. Complications of small joint arthroplasty. Hand Clin. 2010;26(2):205–12. https://doi.org/10.1016/j.hcl.2010.01.003.

11. Sierakowski A, Zweifel C, Sirotakova M, Sauerland S, Elliot D. Joint replacement in 131 painful osteoarthritic and post-traumatic distal interphalangeal joints. J Hand Surg Eur Vol. 2012;37(4):304–9. https://doi.org/10.1177/1753193411422679.

12. Hunter E, Laverty J, Pollock R, Birch R. Nonoperative treatment of fixed flexion deformity of the proximal interphalangeal joint. J Hand Surg Edinb Scotl. 1999;24(3):281–3. https://doi.org/10.1054/jhsb.1999.0111.

13. Houshian S, Jing SS, Chikkamuniyappa C, Kazemian GH, Emami-Moghaddam-Tehrani M. Management of posttraumatic proximal interphalangeal joint contracture. J Hand Surg. 2013;38(8):1651–8. https://doi.org/10.1016/j.jhsa.2013.03.014.

14. Nunley RM, Boyer MI, Goldfarb CA. Pyrolytic carbon arthroplasty for posttraumatic arthritis of the proximal interphalangeal joint. J Hand Surg. 2006;31(9):1468–74. https://doi.org/10.1016/j.jhsa.2006.07.017.

15. Dionysian E, Eaton RG. The long-term outcome of volar plate arthroplasty of the proximal interphalangeal joint. J Hand Surg. 2000;25(3):429–37.

16. Lin S-Y, Chuo C-Y, Lin G-T, Ho M-L, Tien Y-C, Fu Y-C. Volar plate interposition arthroplasty for posttraumatic arthritis of the finger joints. J Hand Surg. 2008;33(1):35–9. https://doi.org/10.1016/j.jhsa.2007.10.020.

17. Burton RI, Campolattaro RM, Ronchetti PJ. Volar plate arthroplasty for osteoarthritis of the proximal interphalangeal joint: a preliminary report. J Hand Surg. 2002;27(6):1065–72. https://doi.org/10.1053/jhsu.2002.35871.

18. Swanson AB, de Groot Swanson G. Flexible implant resection arthroplasty of the proximal interphalangeal joint. Hand Clin. 1994;10(2):261–6.

19. Bales JG, Wall LB, Stern PJ. Long-term results of Swanson silicone arthroplasty for proximal interphalangeal joint osteoarthritis. J Hand Surg. 2014;39(3):455–61. https://doi.org/10.1016/j.jhsa.2013.11.008.

20. Swanson AB, Maupin BK, Gajjar NV, Swanson GD. Flexible implant arthroplasty in the proximal interphalangeal joint of the hand. J Hand Surg. 1985;10(6 Pt 1):796–805.

21. Daecke W, Kaszap B, Martini AK, Hagena FW, Rieck B, Jung M. A prospective, randomized comparison of 3 types of proximal interphalangeal joint arthroplasty. J Hand Surg. 2012;37(9):1770–1779.e1-e3. https://doi.org/10.1016/j.jhsa.2012.06.006.

22. Leibovic SJ, Strickland JW. Arthrodesis of the proximal interphalangeal joint of the finger: comparison of the use of the Herbert screw with other fixation methods. J Hand Surg. 1994;19(2):181–8. https://doi.org/10.1016/0363-5023(94)90002-7.

23. Woon CY-L, Phoon E-S, Lee JY-L, Ng S-W, Teoh L-C. Hazards of steroid injection: suppurative extensor tendon rupture. Indian J Plast Surg. 2010;43(1):97–100. https://doi.org/10.4103/0970-0358.63971.

24. Lu H, Yang H, Shen H, Ye G, Lin X-J. The clinical effect of tendon repair for tendon spontaneous rupture after corticosteroid injection in hands. Medicine (Baltimore). 2016;95(41) https://doi.org/10.1097/MD.0000000000005145.

25. Adkinson JM, Chung KC. Advances in small joint arthroplasty of the hand. Plast Reconstr Surg. 2014;134(6):1260–8. https://doi.org/10.1097/PRS.0000000000000733.

26. Chung KC, Kotsis SV, Kim HM. A prospective outcomes study of Swanson metacarpophalangeal joint arthroplasty for the rheumatoid hand. J Hand Surg. 2004;29(4):646–53. https://doi.org/10.1016/j.jhsa.2004.03.004.

27. Cook SD, Beckenbaugh RD, Redondo J, Popich LS, Klawitter JJ, Linscheid RL. Long-term follow-up of pyrolytic carbon metacarpophalangeal implants. J Bone Joint Surg Am. 1999;81(5):635–48.

28. Bicknell RT, MacDermid J, Roth JH. Assessment of thumb metacarpophalangeal joint arthrodesis using a single longitudinal K-wire. J Hand Surg. 2007;32(5):677–84. https://doi.org/10.1016/j.jhsa.2007.02.010.

29. Steiger R, Segmüller G. Arthrodesis of the metacarpophalangeal joint of the thumb. Indications, technic, arthrodesis angle and functional effect. Handchir Mikrochir Plast Chir Organ Deutschsprachigen Arbeitsgemeinschaft Handchir Organ Deutschsprachigen

Arbeitsgemeinschaft Mikrochir Peripher Nerven Gefasse Organ V. 1989;21(1): 18–22.

30. Saldana MJ, Clark EN, Aulicino PL. The optimal position for arthrodesis of the metacarpophalangeal joint of the thumb: a clinical study. J Hand Surg Edinb Scotl. 1987;12(2):256–9.

31. Ledgard JP, Tonkin MA. Simultaneous four finger metacarpophalangeal joint fusions - indications and results. Hand Surg Int J Devoted Hand Up Limb Surg Relat Res J Asia-Pac Fed Soc Surg Hand. 2014;19(1):69–76. https://doi.org/10.1142/S0218810414500129.

32. Haughton D, Jordan D, Malahias M, Hindocha S, Khan W. Principles of hand fracture management. Open Orthop J. 2012;6:43–53. https://doi.org/10.2174/1874325001206010043.

33. Mumtaz MU, Ahmad F, Kawoosa AA, Hussain I, Wani I. Treatment of rolando fractures by open reduction and internal fixation using mini T-plate and screws. J Hand Microsurg. 2016;8(2):80–5. https://doi.org/10.1055/s-0036-1583300.

34. Ladd AL, Lee J, Hagert E. Macroscopic and microscopic analysis of the thumb carpometacarpal ligaments. J Bone Joint Surg Am. 2012;94(16):1468–77. https://doi.org/10.2106/JBJS.K.00329.

35. Khan M, Waseem M, Raza A, Derham D. Quantitative assessment of improvement with single corticosteroid injection in thumb CMC joint osteoarthritis? Open Orthop J. 2009;3:48–51. https://doi.org/10.2174/1874325000903010048.

36. Meenagh G, Patton J, Kynes C, Wright G. A randomised controlled trial of intra-articular corticosteroid injection of the carpometacarpal joint of the thumb in osteoarthritis. Ann Rheum Dis. 2004;63(10):1260–3. https://doi.org/10.1136/ard.2003.015438.

37. Hunt TR. Degenerative and post-traumatic arthritis affecting the carpometacarpal joints of the fingers. Hand Clin. 2006;22(2):221–8. https://doi.org/10.1016/j.hcl.2006.02.004.

38. Matullo KS, Ilyas A, Thoder JJ. CMC arthroplasty of the thumb: a review. Hand (N Y). 2007;2(4):232–9. https://doi.org/10.1007/s11552-007-9068-9.

39. Zhang X, Wang T, Wan S. Minimally invasive thumb carpometacarpal joint arthrodesis with headless screws and arthroscopic assistance. J Hand Surg. 2015;40(1):152–8. https://doi.org/10.1016/j.jhsa.2014.10.020.

40. Odella S, Querenghi AM, Sartore R, DE Felice A, Dacatra U. Trapeziometacarpal osteoarthritis: pyrocarbon interposition implants. Joints. 2014;2(4):154–8.

41. Yang Y, Scheker LR, Kumar KK. Arthroplasty for fifth carpometacarpal joint arthritis. J Wrist Surg. 2015;4(2):110–4. https://doi.org/10.1055/s-0035-1549291.

Part III
Post-traumatic Arthritis of the Lower Extremity

Chapter 8
Post-traumatic Arthritis of the Acetabulum

Savyasachi C. Thakkar, Erik A. Hasenboehler,
and Chandrashekhar J. Thakkar

> **Key Points**
> - Articular step-off greater than 2mm significantly increases the risk of post-traumatic arthritis.
> - The high failure rate of cemented acetabular components has made uncemented implants the mainstay for reconstruction in cases of posttraumatic arthritis.
> - The results of THA after acetabular fracture are humbling at 10 years when compared to THA for cases unrelated to posttraumatic arthritis.
> - The overall revision rates after THA following acetabular fractures are substantially higher than those following a conventional primary THA and, hence, a multispecialty treatment approach of these challenging injuries is essential.

S. C. Thakkar (✉)
Hip & Knee Reconstruction Surgery, Johns Hopkins Department of Orthopaedic Surgery,
Columbia, MD, USA
e-mail: savya@jhmi.edu

E. A. Hasenboehler
Department of Orthopaedic Surgery, Adult Trauma Service,
The Johns Hopkins Medical Institution, Baltimore, MD, USA
e-mail: ehasenb1@jhmi.edu

C. J. Thakkar
Joints Masters Institute, Mumbai, Maharashtra, India

Breach Candy Hospital, Mumbai, Maharashtra, India

Lilavati Hospital, Mumbai, Maharashtra, India

Hinduja Hospital, Mumbai, Maharashtra, India

© Springer Nature Switzerland AG 2021
S. C. Thakkar, E. A. Hasenboehler (eds.), *Post-Traumatic Arthritis*,
https://doi.org/10.1007/978-3-030-50413-7_8

Introduction

Acetabular fractures are challenging injuries that require careful planning and specific fixation for each fracture pattern. These injuries typically demonstrate a bimodal distribution – young patients with high-energy trauma and old patients with osteoporotic bone from low-energy falls [15]. Despite accurate open reduction and internal fixation of challenging acetabular fractures, there is an undeniable risk of developing posttraumatic arthritis that can compromise patient outcomes [19]. Certain select fracture types with significant comminution in poor bone quality require activity modification and weight-bearing restrictions as open reduction and anatomic fixation would not be successful. However, the majority of the fractures require anatomic restoration of the articular surface, especially in young patients. Elderly patients with poor bone quality may be treated conservatively allowing imperfect articular surface congruency, followed by total hip arthroplasty (THA) [20].

The incidence of posttraumatic arthritis is 13% in cases where the articular congruity has been adequately restored (less than 2 mm). There is a marked increase in posttraumatic arthritis to 44% when the step-off between acetabular articular fragments is greater than 2 mm [6]. However, the reported incidence of posttraumatic arthritis can be as high as 67% per some reports [17, 23]. Most cases of posttraumatic arthritis after acetabular fractures require THA as the mainstay of treatment. Usually, such patients can fall into one of the following three categories [12]:

- Category I – Patients with hip degeneration due to the initial injury or because of complications associated with prior treatments. Such patients may present with osteonecrosis of the femoral head, fracture mal-union, or nonunion and remnant fracture fragments.
- Category II – Comminuted fractures in elderly patients with osteoporosis that are not amenable to primary open reduction internal fixation and must rely on healing by secondary congruence. In these cases, patients can either receive a THA for an acute fracture or delayed arthroplasty for secondary congruence.
- Category III – The nature of the fracture precludes a good result with initial anatomic fixation. Impacted and multifragmentary fractures through the weight-bearing dome of the acetabulum are usually not amenable to good function even after excellent open reduction and internal fixation leading to posttraumatic arthritis.

THA remains the main treatment for posttraumatic arthritis after acetabular fractures. However, it remains inferior when compared to THA for nonfracture-related arthritis [7, 19, 21]. Increased failure in posttraumatic situations can be attributed to cemented acetabular components, initial method of fracture fixation, preexisting hardware, increased propensity for infection, younger age of the patient, abnormal anatomy, sclerotic bone bed, and decreased acetabular bone stock [15]. Conversely, cementless acetabular reconstruction has improved survivorship and has become the preferred implant choice for posttraumatic arthritis of the acetabulum [1].

In this chapter, we will outline our treatment algorithm for posttraumatic arthritis of the acetabulum including surgical planning, implant selection, and surgical technique, and we will also present some representative cases highlighting key principles. In addition, we will review current outcomes associated with THA for posttraumatic arthritis of the acetabulum.

Surgical Planning

Planning for surgery involves a thorough understanding of the patho-anatomy associated with the original fracture and possible fixation constructs used initially. A complete history and physical examination is imperative, and in acute cases, it is imperative to check the patient's soft tissue to exclude degloving injuries such as the Morel-Lavallée lesion [3]. Prior incisions must be examined to understand which approach to the hip has been previously used. Previous wounds must be examined for infections such as erythema, fluctuance, drainage, and sinus tracts. Chronic wounds with exposed bone or hardware will likely require muscle flap coverage and plastic surgeon consultation. Skin bridges between old and new incisions should be maximized in order to preserve skin blood supply.

A detailed neurovascular examination must be documented including the motor, sensory, and peripheral vascular status. Acetabular fractures may be associated with neurovascular compromise due to the mechanism of injury or subsequent surgical procedures. Nerve conduction studies, electromyography (EMG), and vascular studies may be considered preoperatively if the status is compromised. Our preference is to use the posterolateral approach to the hip which is extensile and allows adequate exposure to the acetabulum and the femur.

From the surgical perspective, we can classify the patients in to three types [20]:

- Type I – Patients requiring a conventional primary THA. In these cases, there is adequate bony support for the cup, and the hip center of rotation is preserved in its native anatomic location with no need for structural reconstruction. Such patients typically display posttraumatic arthritis in well-reduced fractures and osteonecrosis of the femoral head.
- Type II - Patients require fracture stabilization along with THA. In the majority of cases a primary THA implant would suffice, but, occasionally, there is inadequate bony support for an acetabular cup due to the unstable fracture pattern of present nonunion. Such patients will require cup support with additional internal fixation.
- Type III – Patients that require significant reconstruction; these are challenging situations due to significant alterations in the joint anatomy. With such cases, it is essential to restore the hip center of rotation with revision THA principles including bone graft or augments, cage or cup-cage constructs, and, possibly, even custom tri-flange components. Examples include cases with an absent wall, defective column, or cases with acetabular protrusio.

Radiographic evaluation begins with radiographs consisting of anteroposterior views of the pelvis and both hips along with Judet views, and inlet-outlet views of the pelvis [8]. In addition, we typically perform computed tomography (CT) scans with three-dimensional (3D) reconstruction [9, 14]. These images help with evaluating the adequacy of bony support for cup fixation at the appropriate location. We prefer classifying acetabular defects using the Paprosky classification system [16]. The images also help with evaluating the preexistent internal fixation that may or may not need to be removed to perform a THA. It is also essential to evaluate the need for supplementary fixation of walls and columns and the need for structural enhancement by bone grafts, prosthetic augments, cup-cage constructs, or custom tri-flange implants [2, 5]. This approach will help with the reconstruction of the hip center of rotation while determining adequate bony coverage of the uncemented cup over at least 80% of its outer diameter [12].

Implant Selection

The high failure rate of cemented acetabular components has made uncemented implants the mainstay for reconstruction in cases of posttraumatic arthritis [1, 5, 13]. Uncemented multihole porous metal cups allow the surgeon to plan screw trajectories in the available host bone, while the porous metal surface can achieve initial scratch fit for primary stability. Based on the type of bone defect created due to the initial injury and subsequent surgeries, it is also advisable, especially for complex reconstructions, to have various porous metal augments and cages available. Custom tri-flange components typically require 3D CT reconstructions and subsequent manufacturing from the implant company. In such cases implants should be ordered several weeks in advance.

Surgical Technique

Hypotensive anesthesia is essential to reduce blood loss in such challenging surgeries. We prefer the extensile posterolateral approach to the hip for these surgeries for excellent visualization of the acetabulum and the femur. It is important to securely fix the patient in the lateral decubitus position using either a peg board or a hip positioning device. This is because the surgeon must rely on external landmarks for appropriate cup placement, as internal structures such as the posterior wall, transverse acetabular ligament, and weight-bearing roof may not be in the native anatomic position. Intraoperative fluoroscopy must be available as well to confirm cup placement and restoration of hip center of rotation.

In cases with prior internal fixation hardware, the position of the implants may be used to locate the correct placement of the cup. We usually do not remove the previously placed implants unless they obstruct cup placement. Adequate, careful soft tissue dissection is required to visualize the acetabulum in its entirety. Release of the insertion of the gluteus maximus tendon from the linea aspera should be performed to allow the femur to be shifted anteriorly. Also, removal of the anterior capsule and scar tissue allows for a pocket to be created for the femur to be translated anteriorly. A supra-acetabular Steinmann pin or a 90-degree bent Gelpi retractor, a right angle Hohmann retractor on the posterior column, a ball-spike pusher to shift the femoral shaft anteriorly, and a blunt Hohmann retractor at the inferior border of acetabulum usually suffice for a clear 360-degree view of the socket.

Placing the cup in adequate anteversion and abduction is critical to the patient's function and implant longevity. With porous metal implants, it is essential to coat the exposed surface of the implant to avoid excessive fibrosis. While closing the incision, it is essential to not leave any dead space, and the use of drains with meticulous soft tissue closure must be ascertained. Postoperative care resembles the protocol for THA such as posterior-hip precautions and physical therapy. However, the weight-bearing status may vary depending on the stability of the reconstruction construct and it may have to be modified on an individual basis. In the next section, we will present several cases that reinforce the aforementioned principles.

Case Examples

We present case examples based on the three types of patients [20] described in the surgical planning section of the chapter:

- Type I – Patients requiring a conventional total hip arthroplasty. Figures 8.1, 8.2, and 8.3 are case examples of patients that had prior acetabular fractures which had united with sufficient bone stock for primary total hip arthroplasty without additional acetabular reconstruction.
- Type II – Patients requiring fracture stabilization along with THA. Figures 8.4, 8.5, and 8.6 are case examples of patients requiring acute fracture fixation and concurrent THA to ensure adequate support for the implants.
- Type III – Patients requiring significant acetabular reconstruction to restore the center of rotation. Figures 8.7, 8.8, and 8.9 are case examples of patients that rely upon revision hip replacement principles to ensure optimal outcome.

Outcomes

We review several studies that report on the mid-term and long-term outcomes for THA in cases of posttraumatic arthritis after acetabular fractures. A recent study from the Mayo Clinic reported their mid-term results on 30 primary THAs that were performed with a porous metal acetabular component after open reduction internal fixation (ORIF) of acetabular fractures from 1999 through 2010 [22]. From these

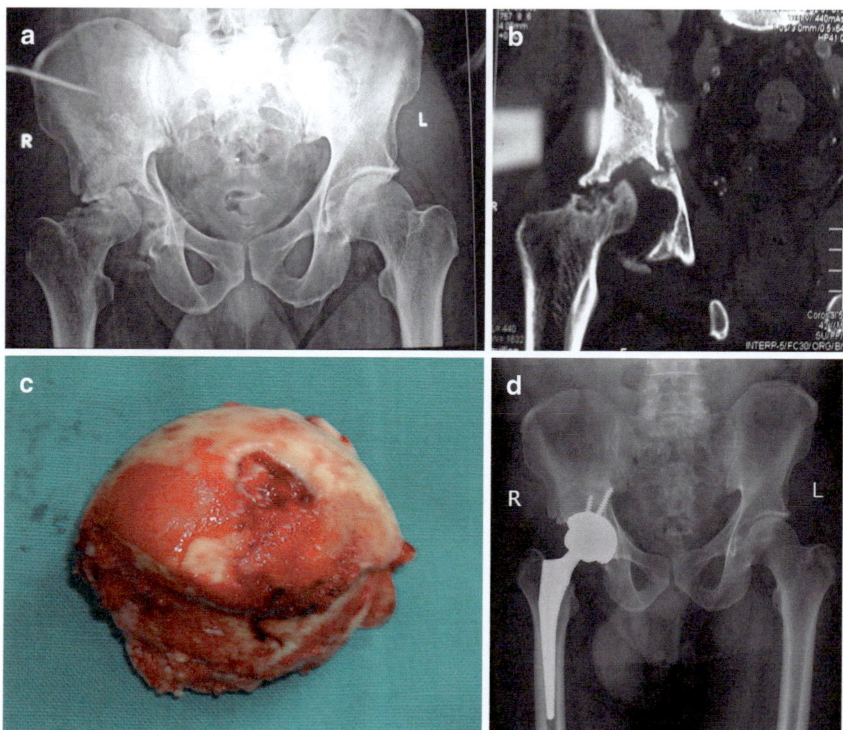

Fig. 8.1 (**a**) Pre-operative AP Pelvis radiograph of a 42 year-old male with an old acetabular fracture leading to post-traumatic arthritis secondary to femoral head osteonecrosis. (**b**) Pre-operative CT scan showing the incarcerated head fragment. (**c**) Intra-operative photograph of the incarcerated femoral head. (**d**) Post-operative AP pelvis radiograph displaying press-fit acetabular and femoral components

Fig. 8.2 (**a**) Pre-operative AP pelvis radiograph of a patient with a chronic mal-united acetabular fracture and pelvic ring injury. (**b**) 3D CT reconstructions of a patient with a chronic mal-united acetabular fracture and pelvic ring injury. (**c**) Post-operative AP pelvis radiograph displaying press-fit acetabular and femoral components

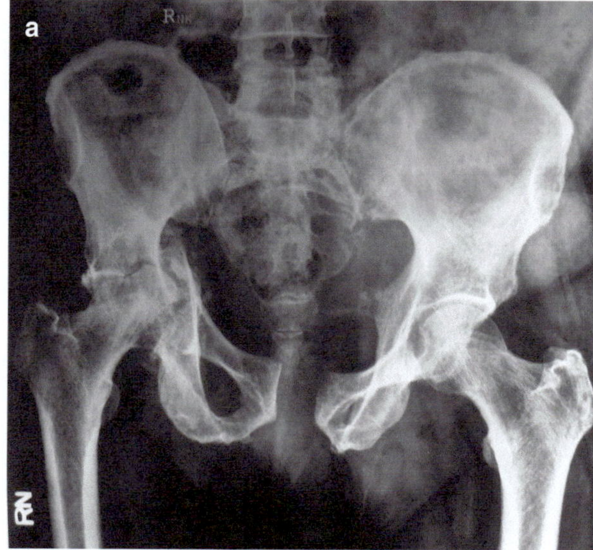

Fig. 8.2 (continued)

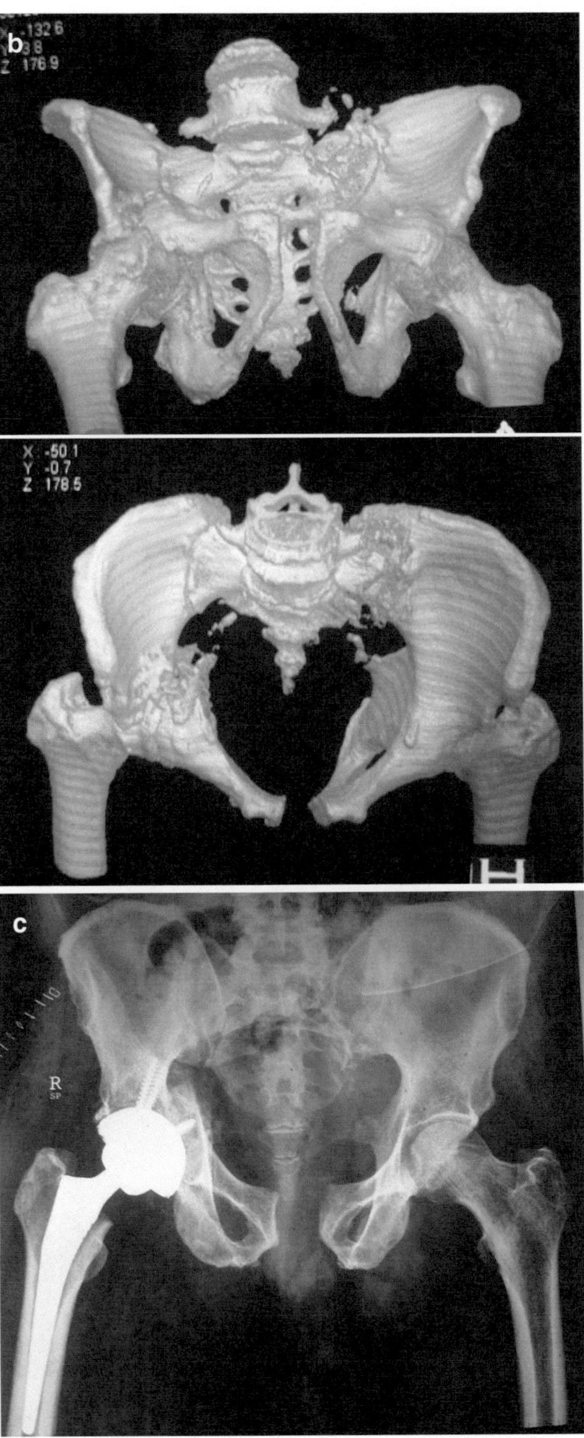

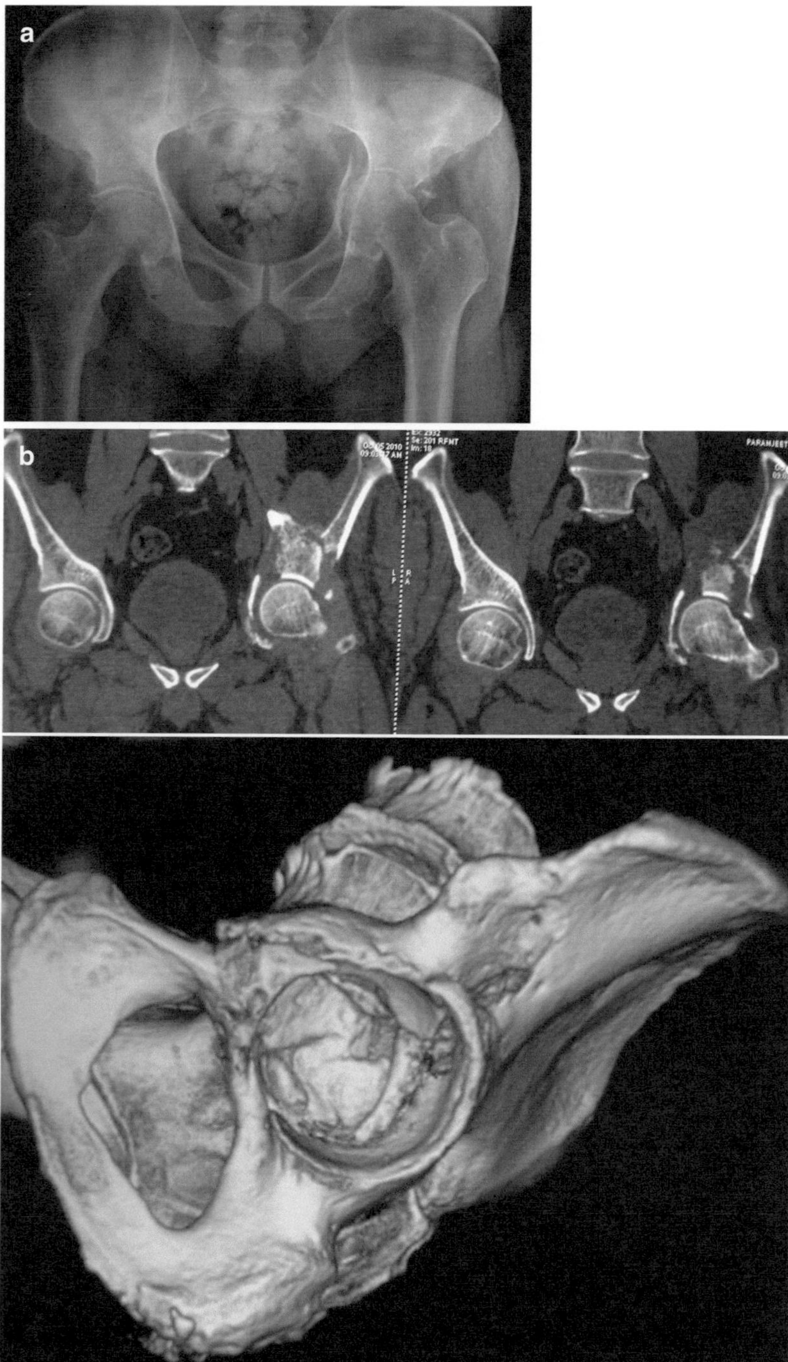

Fig. 8.3 (**a**) Pre-operative AP pelvis radiograph of a patient with a chronic acetabular fracture and medial protrusion of the femoral head. (**b**) 3D CT reconstructions of a patient with a chronic acetabular fracture and medial protrusion of the femoral head. (**c**) Post-operative AP pelvis radiograph displaying press-fit acetabular and femoral components with medial bone graft

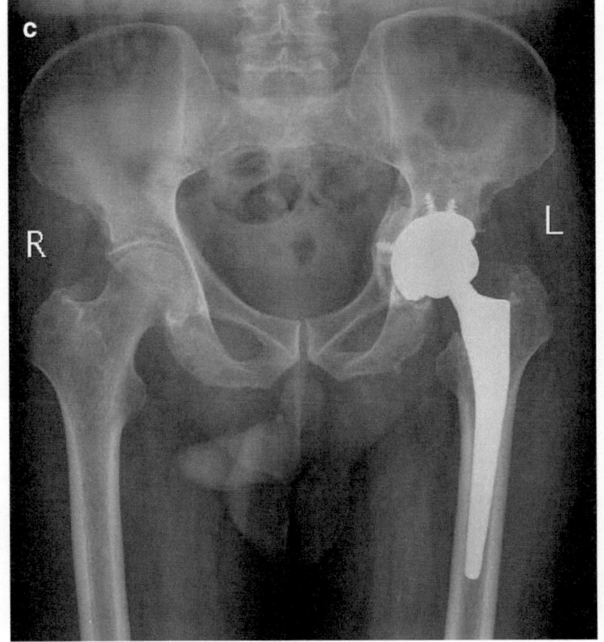

Fig. 8.3 (continued)

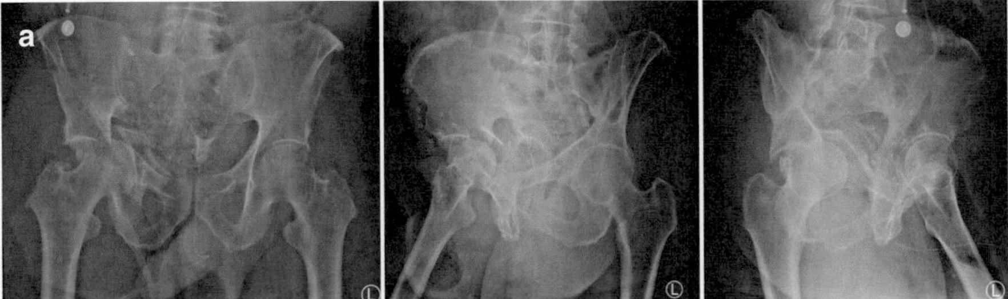

Fig. 8.4 (**a**) Pre-operative radiographs of a 67 year old patient with a both columns acetabular fracture and antecedent hip pain associated with osteoarthritis. (**b**) 3D CT reconstruction of a 67 year old patient with a both columns acetabular fracture and antecedent hip pain associated with osteoarthritis. (**c**) Post-operative AP pelvis radiograph displaying press-fit acetabular and femoral components with medial bone graft and posterior column and wall fixation

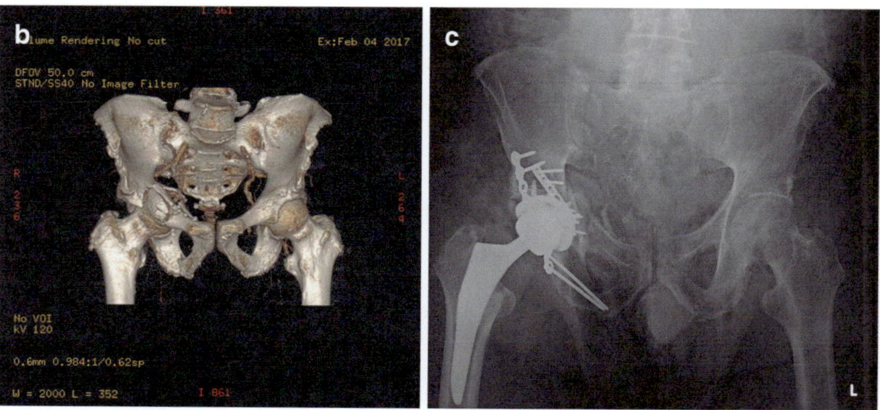

Fig. 8.4 (continued)

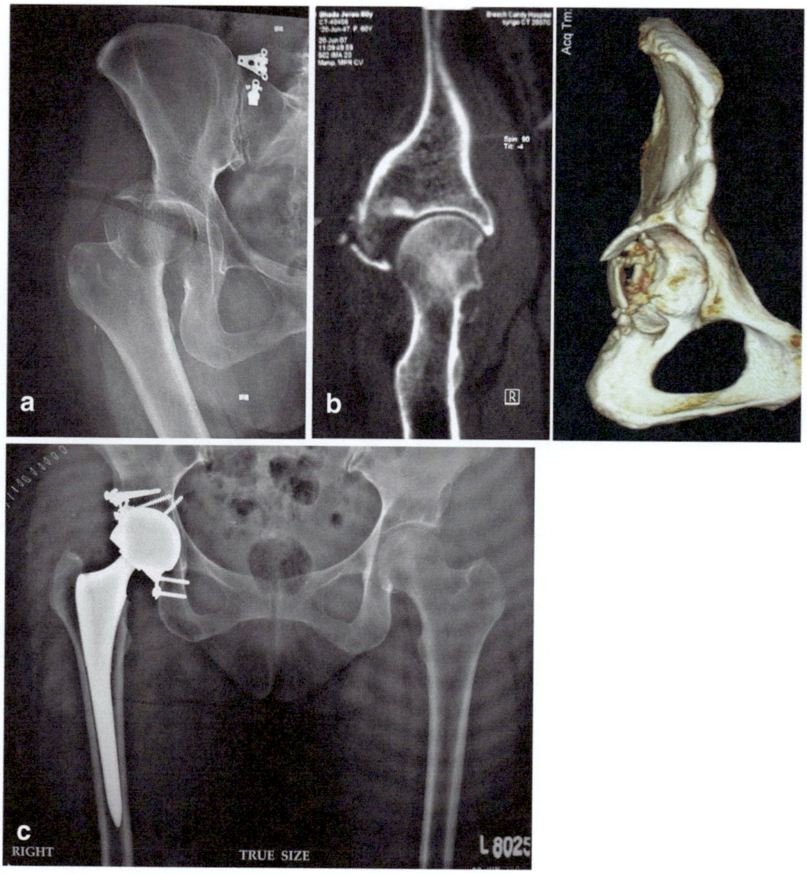

Fig. 8.5 (**a**) Pre-operative AP right hip radiograph of a 60 year-old gynecologist who sustained a fracture-dislocation of her left hip after a fall. (**b**) 3D CT reconstructions of a 60 year-old patient with the fracture dislocation. (**c**) Post-operative AP pelvis radiograph displaying press-fit acetabular and femoral components with posterior wall fixation

Fig. 8.6 (**a**) Pre-operative AP right hip radiograph of a 65 year-old male treated non-operatively for a right acetabular fracture. (**b**) CT reconstruction showing posterior wall erosion and femoral head subluxation. (**c**) Intra-operative pictures showing the acetabular defect and reconstruction with a segment of the femoral head fixed with inter-fragmentary screws and supported by a buttress plate, restoring the socket. A cemented hip replacement was performed. (**d**) Post-operative AP pelvis radiographs showing a cemented total hip replacement with posterior wall and column fixation

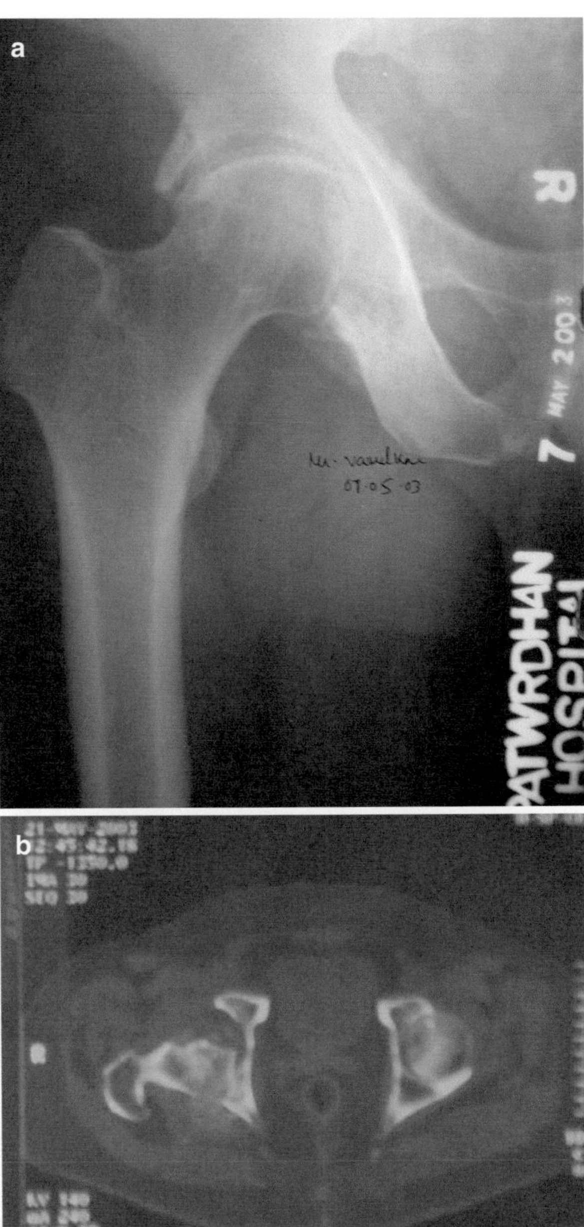

S. C. Thakkar et al.

Fig. 8.6 (continued)

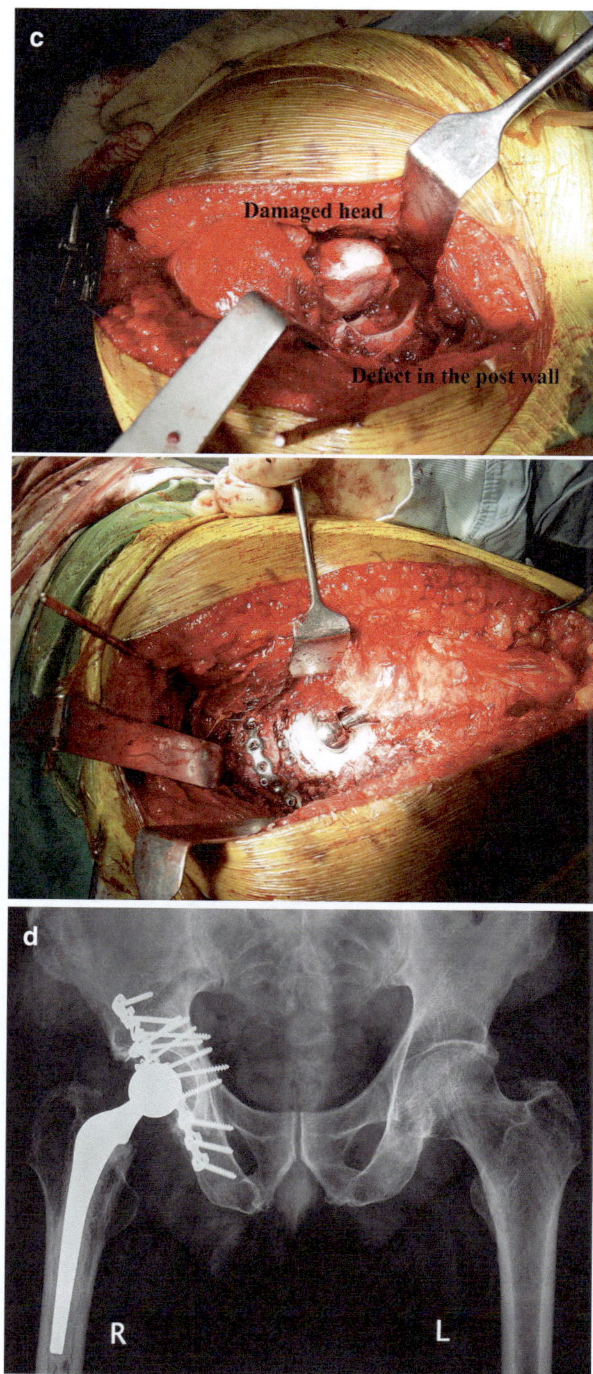

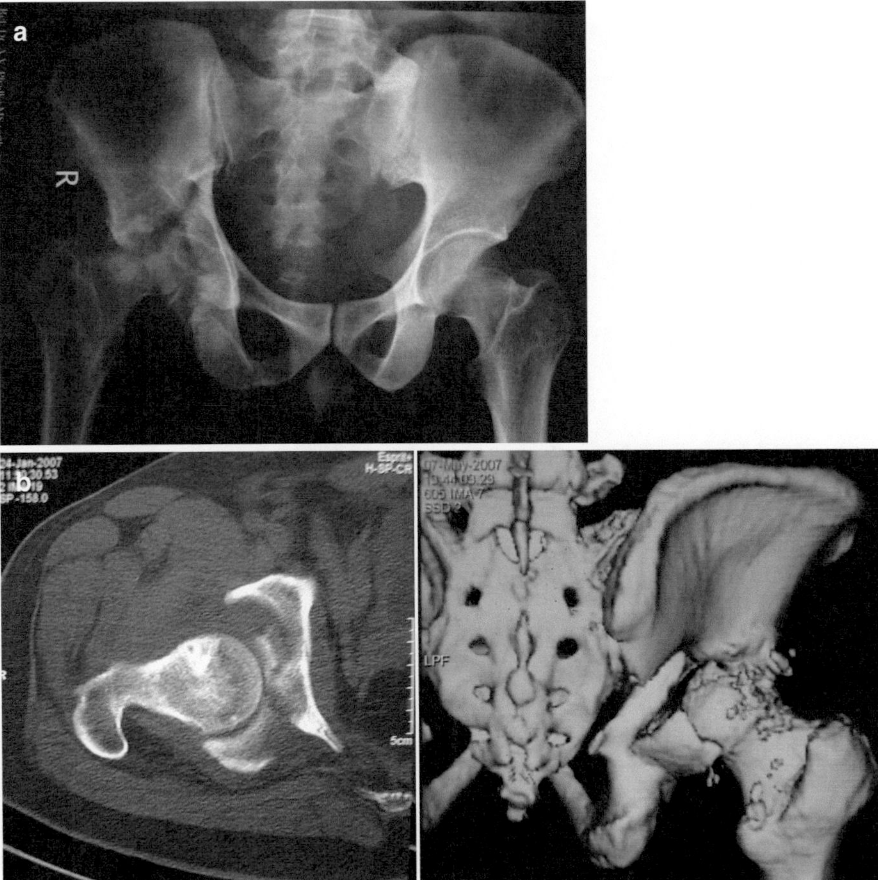

Fig. 8.7 (**a**) Pre-operative AP pelvis radiograph of a 32 year-old patient with a both-columns acetabular fracture. (**b**) 3D CT reconstructions of the fracture pattern. (**c**) Post-operative AP pelvis radiograph showing a cage-cup construct with fixation of the posterior column. A trochanteric osteotomy had to be performed to access the acetabulum during the procedure

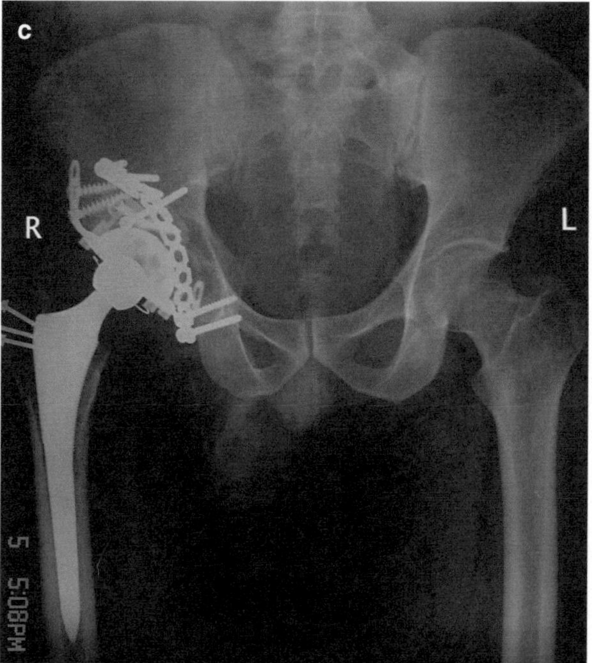

Fig. 8.7 (continued)

cases, 28 (93%) THAs had a minimum follow-up of 2 years. The authors reported that the fracture pattern was of the elementary type in 8 of 30 hips (27%, posterior wall fracture in 6 hips, transverse fracture in 2 hips) and associated type in 13 of 30 hips (43%, T-type fracture in 5 hips, transverse-posterior wall fracture in 4 hips, posterior column/posterior wall in 3 hips, and associated both column in 1 hip). The fracture pattern was unknown in 9 of 30 hips. Nine of 30 hips (30%) had radiographic evidence of osteonecrosis of the femoral head, and 6 of those had confirmed traumatic dislocations at the time of their initial injury. A majority of patients underwent the anterolateral approach, and only 9 of 30 hips were performed using the posterolateral approach. No acetabular components were revised for aseptic loosening. Five-year survival with revision for any reason as the endpoint was 88% (95% confidence interval, 0.70–0.96). Failures were related to infection. Three hips (11%) underwent resection for infection, with all being treated with two-stage arthroplasty. Harris hip scores improved from a median of 39 preoperatively (range, 3–87) to 82 at the most recent follow-up (range, 21–100; $p < 0.01$). Fifteen of 28 hips (54%) had a good or excellent result, 3 (11%) had a fair result, and 10 (35%) had a poor result. Two patients (7%) experienced at least one dislocation postoperatively. Both were treated with a closed reduction and hip abduction brace treatment.

Fig. 8.8 (**a**) Pre-operative AP pelvis radiograph of a patient with failed acetabular fracture fixation. (**b**) Intra-operative images showing fixation of a cage and the femoral head autograft. (**c**) Post-operative images displaying the cage-cup construct and restoration of the hip center of rotation

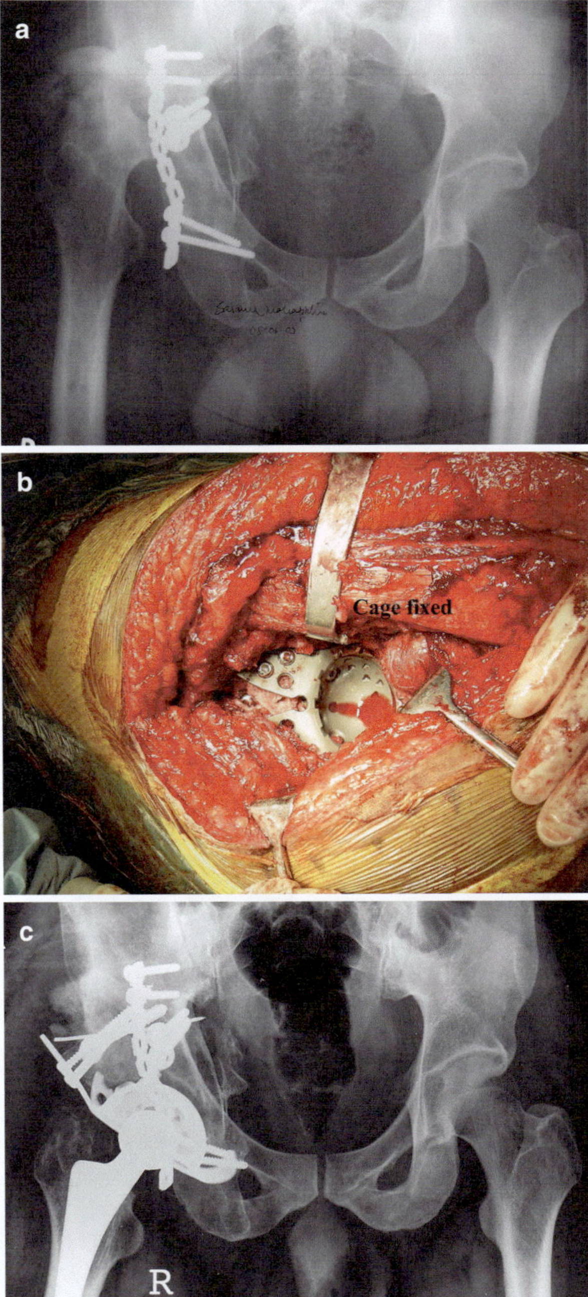

Fig. 8.9 (**a**) Pre-operative AP pelvis radiograph of a comminuted both columns fracture. (**b**) 3D CT reconstruction of the fracture pattern. (**c**) Post-operative radiographs showing posterior column fixation and cage cup construct

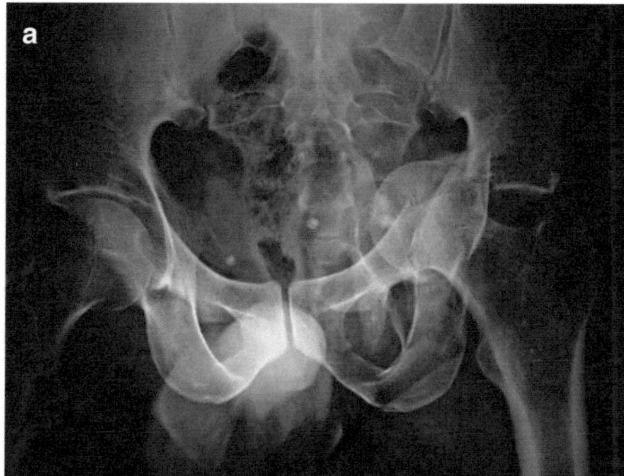

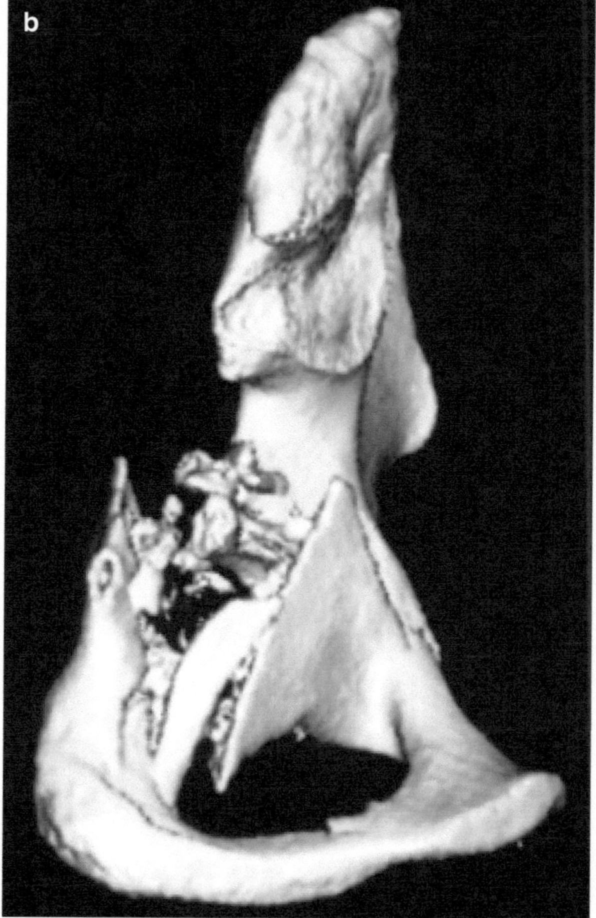

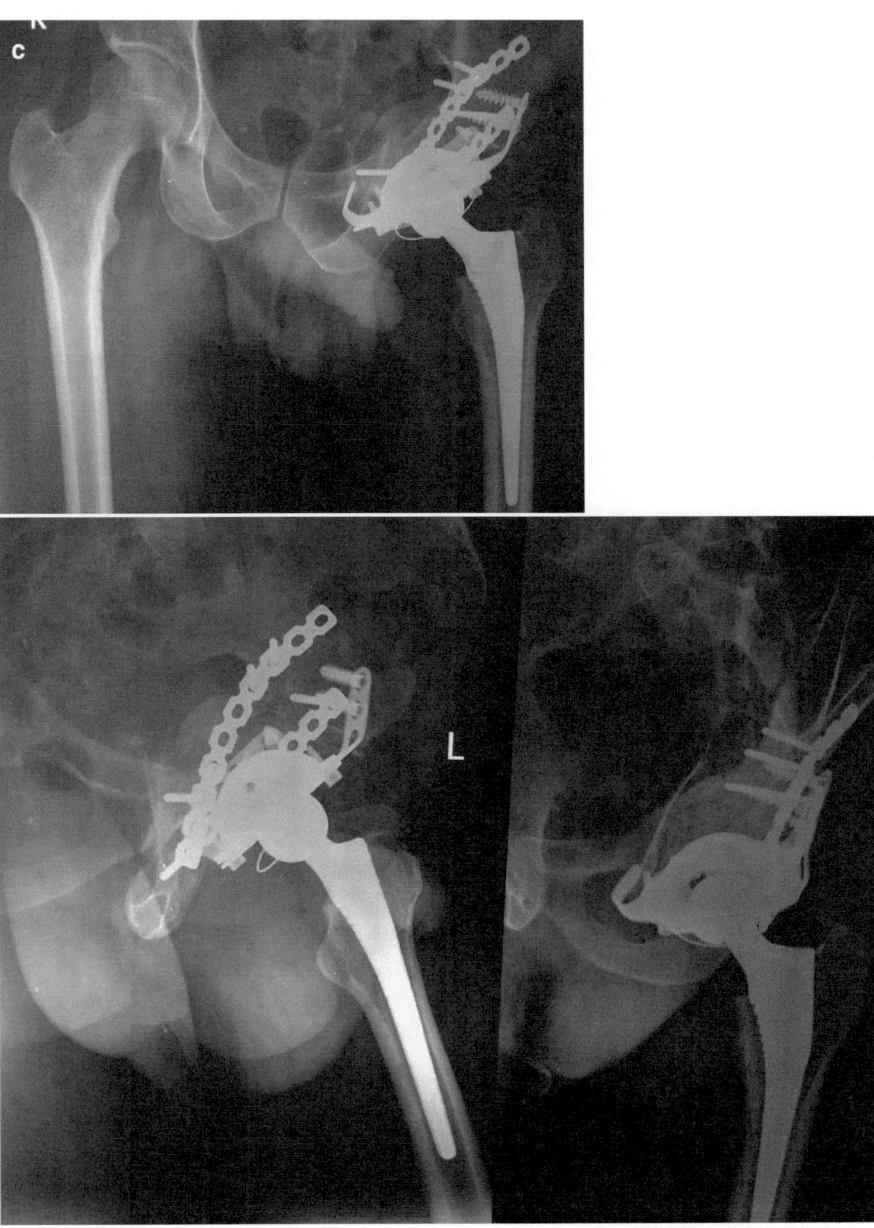

Fig. 8.9 (continued)

Another promising study from the Hospital for Special Surgery describes their results with 32 THAs performed for posttraumatic arthritis after acetabular fractures; 24 patients were treated with a prior ORIF, and 8 were managed conservatively [18]. Average time from fracture to THA was 36 months (range, 6–227 months). The average follow-up was 4.7 years (range, 2.0–9.7 years). With regard to fracture classification, 16 patients (50%) had simple fracture patterns, and 16 patients (50%) had associated patterns. One patient had a concomitant pelvic fracture. The most common fracture patterns were isolated posterior wall fractures in 13 (41%) cases, both-column fractures in 4 (13%) cases, and posterior column–posterior wall in 5 (16%) cases. Cementless acetabular components were used in all 32 cases. The authors reported 79% 5-year end point survival for revision, loosening, dislocation, or infection. Survival for aseptic acetabular loosening was 97%. Six (19%) revision surgeries were necessary due to infection (two cases), aseptic acetabular loosening (one case), aseptic femoral component loosening (two cases), and a liner exchange for dislocation (one case). Revision surgery correlated with nonanatomic restoration of the hip center and a history of infection ($P < 0.05$). Two other patients also had at least one dislocation, but they both responded to conservative treatment with closed reduction and bracing, which resulted in a dislocation rate of 9%. Harris hip scores increased from 28 (0–56) to 82 points (20–100).

Studies from China have reviewed outcomes at 5 years and 6.3 years after THA for acetabular fractures. Zhang et al. retrospectively analyzed 53 patients (55 hips) who underwent THA because of failed treatment for acetabular fractures. The mean duration of follow-up was 64 months (range, 32–123 months) in 49 patients [23]. Thirty-three hips (60%) had simple fracture patterns, and 22 (40%) had complex patterns. The most common patterns were posterior wall fractures in 28 (51%) hips, transverse-posterior wall fractures in 13 (23%) hips, and fractures of the posterior column and posterior wall in 6 (11%) hips. Patients treated without ORIF underwent a posterolateral approach to the hip. However, in patients with prior fixation, a posterolateral approach was used in 28 hips, while a direct lateral approach and a posterolateral plus anterolateral approach were used for removal of hardware in 2 hips, respectively. The authors used cement-less cups in 48 of 55 hips, and cemented cups in 7 hips with 5 of them in combination with acetabular reinforcement rings (ARRs). The authors report that with revision or definite radiographic loosening as the end-point, the 5-year survival in their study was 100%. Three cement-less acetabular components had a partial radiolucency (zones 2 and 3 [4]); in 2, the radiolucency was less than 1 mm wide, and in 1, it was more than 2 mm wide. All of them were associated with a good or excellent Harris hip score and were considered stable. A complete radiolucency, from zones 1 to 3, more than 2 mm wide, was seen in 1 cemented cup. None of the acetabular cups or ARRs showed any evidence of migration. All bone grafts completely incorporated without any complications. Complications included 1 dislocation and 3 sciatic nerve injuries. No instances of deep wound infection were present. The dislocation was successfully treated with closed reduction with no recurrence. The mean duration of follow-up was 64 months (range, 32–123 months) in 49 patients (51 hips); 4 patients were lost to follow up. The average Harris hip score increased from 49.5 (range, 22–78) before surgery to

90.1 (range, 56–100) at the latest follow-up examination ($P < 0.001$). Results were excellent for 36 hips, good for 11, fair for 2, and poor for another 2. In the ORIF group, the average Harris hip score increased from 9.5 (range, 30–78) to 90.1 (range, 56–100) ($P < 0.001$), and in the non-ORIF group, it increased from 54.3 (range, 22–76) to 92.4 (range, 56–100) ($P < 0.001$). Moreover, the average postoperative Harris score was significantly higher in the ORIF group than in the non-ORIF group ($P < 0.05$). Similar significant improvements in average Harris hip scores were also seen both in patients with cement-less acetabular reconstructions and in those with cemented cups ($P < 0.001$). Another study from China evaluated outcomes of cement-less acetabular components at 6.3 years (range, 3.1–8.4 years) after surgery in 31 hips with posttraumatic arthritis after acetabular fractures [10]. Of the 31patients, 19 (65%) had undergone ORIF (open-reduction group), and 12 (35%) had received conservative treatment for the acetabular fractures (conservative-treatment group). 14 patients (45%) had elementary fracture patterns while 17 patients (55%) had associated fracture types. The posterolateral approach to the hip was used in all patients. At the follow-up of 6.1 years, the authors reported no infection and no revision surgery. The rate of anatomical restoration of center of hip rotation was 100% (19/19) in the open-reduction group, and 67% (8/12) in the conservative-treatment group ($P = 0.02$), compared with 93% (13/14) in the simple group and 82% (14/17) in the complex group ($P = 0.61$). Anatomical restoration was positively related to fracture treatment ($r = 0.48$; $P = 0.006$), but it had no relation to fracture pattern ($r = 0.16$; $P = 0.40$). By the final follow-up evaluation, six acetabular components had partial radiolucent lines at the bone implant interface, all 1 mm or less; and they occurred in zone 1 in five hips and in zone 3 in one hip. Osteolysis was not observed in any patient. Of the patients with structural bone graft, only one had minor graft resorption. Four patients (13%) had complications after THA. One patient whose complex fracture was treated conservatively fell 4 years after surgery, causing posterior hip dislocation. Another patient whose complex fracture was treated with ORIF had posterior hip dislocation 14 days after surgery because of failure to adhere to posterior hip precautions. Both patients were successfully treated with closed reduction; neither patient had a recurrent dislocation until the latest follow-up evaluation. The sciatic nerve was injured during THA in one patient in the open-reduction group who had a complex fracture. The patient had dorsal pedal numbness and drop foot after surgery. The average Harris hip score increased from 49 ± 15 before surgery to 89 ± 5 after surgery, and 29 patients (94%) had either excellent or good results. The average Harris hip score for the open-reduction and conservative-treatment groups increased to 87 ± 6 and 91 ± 3 ($P = 0.07$), respectively, after surgery; for the complex and simple groups, it increased to 88 ± 6 and 90 ± 4 ($P = 0.25$), respectively. There was no significant difference between the open-reduction and conservative-treatment groups or between the complex and simple groups regarding the number of hips with excellent and good results.

The results of THA after acetabular fracture are humbling at 10 years when compared to THA for cases unrelated to posttraumatic arthritis. Morrison et al. performed a retrospective case-control study for patients at their institute between 1987 and 2011 [15]. During this period, the authors performed 95 THAs after acetabular fracture; of those, 74 (78%) met inclusion criteria and had documented follow-up beyond 2 years in their institutional registry. They also selected 74 matched patients based on an algorithm that matched patients based on preoperative diagnosis, date of operation, age, gender, and type of prosthesis. All surgeries were performed through the posterolateral approach. The primary outcomes were revision and incidence of complications. Secondary outcomes were radiographic signs of heterotopic ossification or implant loosening. The majority of acetabular fractures were treated by ORIF (58 of 74 [78%]), whereas 16 of 74 (22%) were treated nonoperatively. The most frequent type of fracture involved the posterior wall, accounting for 31% of all injuries. Fractures involving both columns were seen in 16%, whereas other fracture types were less common and were observed in less than 10% of patients. 49% of patients had elementary fracture types while 51% of patients had associated patterns. The 10-year survivorship after THA was lower in patients with a previous acetabular fracture than in the matched cohort (70%, 95% confidence interval [CI] 64–78% versus 90%, 95% CI 86–95%; $p < 0.001$). Younger patients (<60 years) had worse THA survivorship after acetabular fractures than did older patients (60%, 95% CI 51–69% versus 83%, 95% CI 72–94%; $p < 0.038$), and both had inferior survivorship to the matched cohort (92%, CI 87–97% and 96%CI 92–99%; $p < 0.001$). The 10-year survival for THA after a simple acetabular fracture was 83% (95% CI 77–89%) as compared with 60% (95% CI, 52–68%; $p = 0.032$) for associated fractures. Patients with previous acetabular fracture had a higher likelihood of developing infection (7% [five of 74] versus 0% [zero of 74]; odds ratio [OR], 11.79; $p = 0.028$), dislocation (11% [eight of 74] versus 3% [two of 74]; OR, 4.36; $p = 0.048$), or heterotopic ossification (43% [32 of 74] versus 16% [12 of 74]; OR, 3.93; $p < 0.001$). In patients with previous acetabular fracture, 13 patients (20%) were revised for loose acetabular component, 6 patients for wear and joint instability (8%), 2 for infection, and 1 each for femur fracture, loose femoral component, and recurrent dislocation. Revisions for the matched cohort included 11 patients for cup loosening and one patient for recurrent dislocations.

Of the 51 patients in the acetabular fracture group, who did not have a revision, 6 had no radiographs available, 46 had well-fixed components, and none had cup loosening. Of the 62 control patients without revision, 3 had no radiographs available, 59 had well-fixed components, and none had cup loosening.

To summarize the outcomes of THA in posttraumatic arthritis after acetabular fractures, Makridis et al. performed a systematic review in 2014 [11]. In total 654 patients were reviewed (659 hips) with a median follow-up of 5.4 years (range 12 months – 20 years). Median follow-up was 3.9 years (range 12 months–12 years) in the acute THA group and 6.3 years (range 12 months – 20 years) in the delayed THA group. A large majority of fractures were posterior wall fractures (140 patients; 21.4%) followed by transverse/posterior wall fractures (63 patients; 9.6%), posterior column-posterior wall fractures (51 patients; 7.8%), and both column fractures (49 patients; 7.5%). Treatment of acetabular fractures was only described in 625 fractures of which 473 fractures (75.7%) were treated with ORIF and 152 fractures (24.3%) nonoperatively. The majority of the studies reviewed by the authors reported no failure of initial treatment of acetabular fractures. 237 patients (36%)

were treated with acute total hip arthroplasty. Delayed total hip arthroplasty was performed in the remainder of the reviewed patients following either operative or nonoperative management of the initial acetabular fracture. In the early-THA cases, the median interval between time of injury and total hip arthroplasty was 10 days (1–29). In the delayed cases, the average time from injury to THA was 6.6 years (2 months–45 years).

With regard to acetabular components, an uncemented acetabular component was used in 484 patients (80.1%) and a cemented one in 120 patients (19.9%). For femoral components, the data was available in 569 hips with 340 patients (59.8%) receiving an uncemented and 229 patients (40.2%) a cemented femoral component. An antiprotrusion acetabular cage was rarely used, and acetabular bone graft was used in all cases. Anterolateral and posterolateral surgical approaches were used in a majority of the cases. In the early THA group, Kaplan–Meier survivorship analysis with any loosening, osteolysis, or revision as the end-point revealed that the 10-year cup survival was 81%. In the late THA group, this percentage was 76%. The log-rank test showed that this difference was not significant ($P = 0.287$). In the late THA group where the proportion of uncemented and cemented implants were available, Kaplan–Meier survivorship analysis with any loosening, osteolysis, or revision as the end-point revealed that the 10-year survival was 86.7% for the uncemented cups and 81% for the cemented. The log-rank test showed that this difference was not significant ($P = 0.163$). In the early THA group, 13 cups (7.5%) out of 173 implants were revised. Four cups were revised for aseptic loosening, one for traumatic loosening, six for dislocation, and two for infection. It was unclear how many of these cups were cemented and how many were uncemented. In the late THA group, 35 cups (9.6%) out of 365 implants were revised. Sixteen cups (45.7%) were uncemented (13 were revised for aseptic loosening, 1 for traumatic loosening, and 2 for infection). Nineteen cups (54.3%) were cemented (17 were revised for aseptic loosening, 1 for dislocation, and 1 for infection). The three most common complications were heterotopic ossification, infection, and dislocation which occurred in a total of 292 out of 654 patients (44.6%). The Harris hip score was used to describe the functional outcome with a median value of 88 points. Regardless of the type of treatment, and according to the Harris hip score, younger patients achieved better clinical outcomes than older patients (92.94 ± 4.48 versus 81.68 ± 4.58, respectively) ($P < 0.001$). Almost all of the studies did not compare Harris hip scores for acute versus delayed THA. Thirty-three patients died, and the overall mortality rate was 5%. No patient died in the acute perioperative phase. The minimum time of postoperative mortality was 4 months after surgery and maximum within 10 years after surgery.

In conclusion, THA for posttraumatic arthritis associated with acetabular fractures shows promising results and satisfactory functional and radiological outcomes. However, there are no prospective studies to compare directly the outcomes following acute or delayed total hip arthroplasty secondary to acetabular fractures. The largely retrospective data available in the literature indicate that the clinical outcomes, revision rates, and implant survivorship do not differ when either an early or a late THA is performed. The overall revision rates after THA following acetabular fractures are substantially higher than those following a conventional primary THA, and, hence, a multispecialty treatment approach of these challenging injuries is essential.

References

1. Bellabarba C, et al. Cementless acetabular reconstruction after acetabular fracture. J Bone Joint Surg Am. 2001;83:868–76.
2. Bone and Joint Trauma Study Group [GETRAUM]. Indications and technical challenges of total hip arthroplasty in the elderly after acetabular fracture. Orthop Traumatol Surg Res. 2014;100:193–7.
3. Chokshi FH, Jose J, Clifford PD. Morel-Lavallee lesion. Am J Orthop. 2010;39:252–3.
4. DeLee JG, Charnley J. Radiological demarcation of cemented sockets in total hip replacement. Clin Orthop. 1976;121:20–32.
5. Enocson A, Blomfeldt R. Acetabular fractures in the elderly treated with a primary Burch-Schneider reinforcement ring, autologous bone graft and a total hip arthroplasty. A prospective study with a 4-year follow-up. J Orthop Trauma. 2014;28:330–7.
6. Giannoudis PV, Grotz MR, Papakostidis C, Dinopoulos H. Operative treatment of displaced fractures of the acetabulum. A meta-analysis. J Bone Joint Surg Br. 2005;87:2–9.
7. Huo MH, et al. Total hip replacements done without cement after acetabular fractures: a 4- to 8-year follow-up study. J Arthroplasty. 1999;14:827–31.
8. Judet R, Judet J, Letournel E. Fractures of the acetabulum: classification and surgical approaches for open reduction. Preliminary report. J Bone Joint Surg Am. 1964;46:1615–46.
9. Kendoff D, et al. Value of 3D fluoroscopic imaging of acetabular fractures comparison to 2D fluoroscopy and CT imaging. Arch Orthop Trauma Surg. 2008;128:599–605.
10. Lai O, et al. Midterm results of uncemented acetabular reconstruction for posttraumatic arthritis secondary to acetabular fracture. J Arthroplast. 2011;26(7):1008–13.
11. Makridis KG, et al. Total hip arthroplasty after acetabular fracture: incidence of complications, reoperation rates and functional outcomes: evidence today. J Arthroplast. 2014;29:1983–90.
12. Mears DC, Velyvis JH, Chang CP. Displaced acetabular fractures managed operatively: indicators of outcome. Clin Orthop Relat Res. 2003;407:173–86.
13. Mears CD, Velyvis JH. Primary total hip arthroplasty after acetabular fracture. Instr Course Lect. 2001;50:335–54.
14. Moed, et al. Computed tomographic assessment of fractures of the posterior wall of the acetabulum after operative treatment. J Bone Joint Surg Am. 2003;85-A:512–22.
15. Morrison Z, et al. Total hip arthroplasty after acetabular fracture is associated with lower survivorship and more complications. Clin Orthop Relat Res. 2016;474:392–8.
16. Paprosky WG, Perona PG, Lawrence JM. Acetabular defect classification and surgical reconstruction in revision arthroplasty: a 6-year follow-up evaluation. J Arthroplast. 1994;9:33–44.
17. Ragnarsson B, Mjöberg B. Arthrosis after surgically treated acetabular fractures. A retrospective study of 60 cases. Acta Orthop Scand. 1992;63:511.
18. Ranawat A, et al. Total hip arthroplasty for posttraumatic arthritis after acetabular fracture. J Arthroplast. 2009;24(5):759–67.
19. Romness DW, Lewallen DG. Total hip arthroplasty after fracture of the acetabulum. Long-term results. J Bone Joint Surg Br. 1990;72:761–4.
20. Thakkar Chandrashekhar J, Rajshekhar KT, Thakkar SC. Total hip arthroplasty after acetabular fractures. Arthropaedia. 2014;1:105–14.
21. Weber M, Berry DJ, Harmsen WS. Total hip arthroplasty after operative treatment of an acetabular fracture. J Bone Joint Surg Am. 1998;80:1295–305.

22. Yuan BJ, Lewallen DG, Hanssen AD. Porous metal acetabular components have a low rate of mechanical failure in THA after operatively treated acetabular fracture. Clin Orthop Relat Res. 2015;473:536–42.
23. Zhang L, et al. Total hip arthroplasty for failed treatment of acetabular fractures. J Arthroplast. 2011;26(8):1189–93.

Chapter 9
Post-traumatic Arthritis of the Proximal Femur

Raj M. Amin, Erik A. Hasenboehler, and Babar Shafiq

> **Key Points**
> - Optimal treatment for posttraumatic arthritis of the proximal femur is patient specific.
> - Hip arthroscopy is on the forefront of treatment modalities.
> - Arthroplasty for proximal femur fractures is increasingly indicated during the index fracture.
> - Varus malunion is a common mode of failure following treatment of femoral neck fractures.

Introduction

Epidemiology

Symptomatic posttraumatic osteoarthritis (PTOA) occurs in approximately 12% proximal femur fracture patients [1–3]. In addition to causing substantial patient burden, PTOA is an expensive problem that accounts for $3.1 billion in annual treatment spending in the United States [3]. With an increasingly elderly population and advances in medical care which have improved overall longevity, the incidence of

R. M. Amin · B. Shafiq (✉)
Department of Orthopaedic Surgery, The Johns Hopkins Medical Institutions,
Baltimore, MD, USA
e-mail: ramin6@jhmi.edu; bshafiq2@jhmi.edu

E. A. Hasenboehler
Department of Orthopaedic Surgery, Adult Trauma Service,
The Johns Hopkins Medical Institution, Baltimore, MD, USA
e-mail: ehasenb1@jhmi.edu

© Springer Nature Switzerland AG 2021
S. C. Thakkar, E. A. Hasenboehler (eds.), *Post-Traumatic Arthritis*,
https://doi.org/10.1007/978-3-030-50413-7_9

PTOA figures will increase [4]. As such, an understanding of the disease and treatment options currently available is a key component of the treating musculoskeletal practitioners skill set.

Pathophysiology of Failure

Though traumatic osteoarthritis is thought of as a long-term consequence after proximal femur fracture, it begins immediately after injury. The amount of chondral damage occurring during this time period is difficult to quantify and is due to a number of factors including acute inflammation, pressure necrosis, and direct injury.

Given the significant amount of soft tissue disruption and local hemorrhage, the postfracture milieu contains a high proportion of chondrotoxic mediators. In the newly fractured proximal femur, this provides an opportunity for cytokines, matrix metalloproteinases, interleukins, neutrophils, and reactive oxygen species to cause articular disruption [5]. Additionally, in fracture patterns where the joint capsule is not violated, a pressure necrosis phenomenon from fracture hematoma may accelerate chondrocyte apoptosis. This has been likened to a "compartment syndrome of the hip." As such, there may be a theoretical benefit to early direct capsular decompression in proximal femur fractures to mitigate not only avascular osteonecrosis but also articular pressure necrosis. However, the general evidence-based consensus is equivocal regarding the utility of this surgical option in the prevention of osteonecrosis [6].

Perhaps the most acute causative factor in PTOA is the direct chondral damage resulting at the time of injury (Fig. 9.1). This is particularly true in high-energy proximal femur fractures, which are usually seen in younger patients [6]. These cells are subject to matrix damage, disruption of the collagen fibrils, and potentially full thickness articular damage depending on the loading rate and force [7]. Factors predicting worse instantaneous cartilage injury include fracture mechanisms that have simultaneous compression and shear forces such as Pipkin IV fracture dislocations (Table 9.1), and prolonged increases in both load borne by the articular surface and duration of the increased load [7].

With repetitive loading, joint instability and incongruity exacerbate the acute chondral compromise in the form of increasingly symptomatic PTOA. Within the proximal femur, the factors particularly involved include vascular insufficiency, which commonly precedes joint incongruity, while abnormal joint reactive forces via planar malalignment increase instability and contact pressures. The resultant lack of bony subchondral support diminishes the stress-sharing capacity of underlying trabeculae. As such, increased stresses are seen by the overlying articular surface making it prone to thinning and early arthrosis [7].

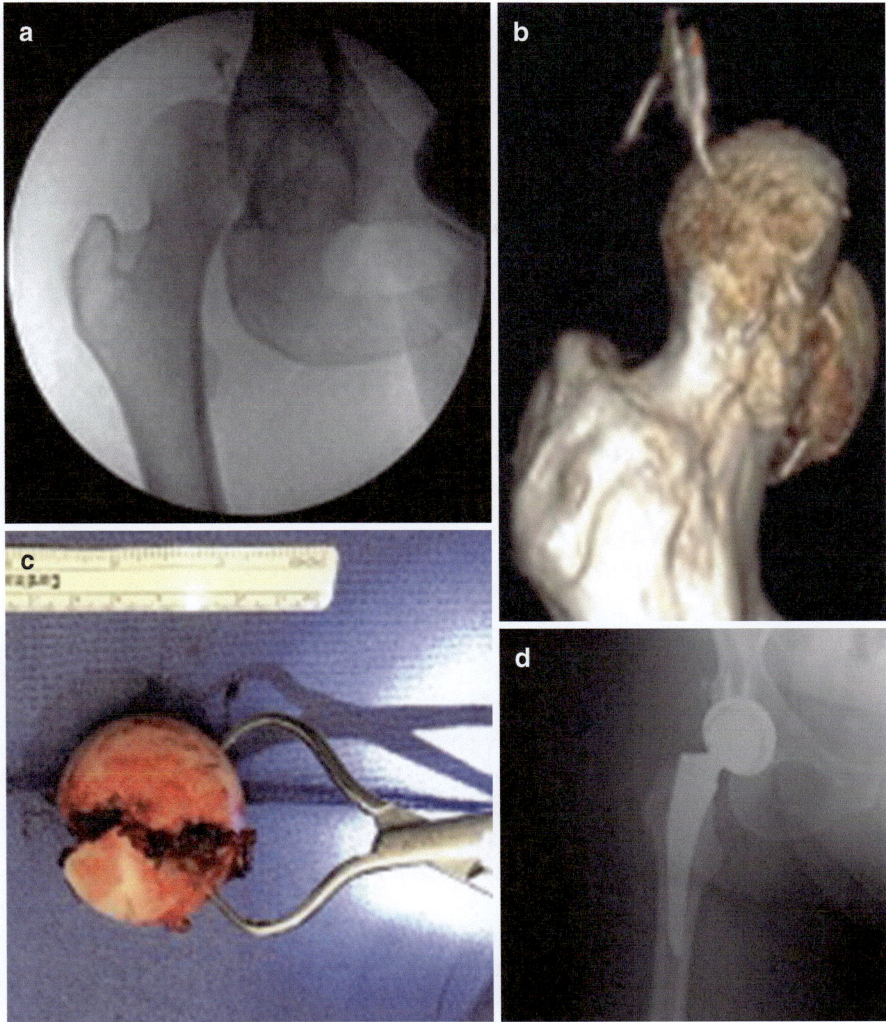

Fig. 9.1 (**a**) Radiograph demonstrating Pipkin IV fracture dislocation in a 48-year-old patient. (**b**) 3-D reconstruction CT image depicting substantial femoral head collapse. (**c**) Intraoperative image of excised femoral head with split-depression fracture. (**d**) Treatment with index total hip arthroplasty (THA)

Table 9.1 Pipkin classification

Type	Fracture pattern
I	Infrafoveal
II	Suprafoveal extension
III	Type I or II with associated femoral neck fracture
IV	Type I or II with associated acetabular fracture

Fracture Specifics

Hip Dislocation

Though the articular surface in isolated femoral head fractures experiences substantial shear forces, prompt reduction generally results in minimal long-term consequences. In isolated dislocations without hip fracture, prompt reduction results in excellent long-term clinical outcomes [8]. At 11-year follow-up, six of seven patients with isolated dislocations had good to excellent Thompson and Epstein objective outcome scores and only one patient had mild pain with cystic changes on radiograph. Therefore, the poor functional outcome in 53% of posterior dislocations and 25% of anterior dislocations seen in this study were attributed to other injuries associated with the dislocation as rates of good to excellent subjective clinical outcomes are 85–100% in isolated hip dislocations [8].

Femoral Head Fracture

PTOA following femoral head fracture results primarily from direct chondral injury. In the long term, failure following femoral head fractures results from avascular necrosis, which is apparent in 10% of patients at 12 months postinjury [9]. Additionally at a mean of 12 months postoperatively, Scolaro et al. demonstrated 12% early fixation failure rate in a population primarily treated with open reduction internal fixation (53%), fragment excision (25%), and hemiarthroplasty (2%) [9]. At a mean of 5 years postinjury, PTOA is present in nearly 20% of patients [1]. Factors predicting worse outcome include nonsurgical management and increasing Pipkin type (Table 9.1) [1, 9, 10].

Fractures of the femoral head present a relatively difficult treatment challenge as both exposure and fixation options are limited. Pipkin I fractures may be treated nonoperatively with open fragment excision or internal fixation [11]. Recently, internal fixation has been described using an arthroscopic approach though long-term outcomes are pending [12]. In large Pipkin I fracture fragments, open reduction with internal fixation (ORIF) has demonstrated better clinical and radiographic outcomes as compared to fragment excision [13, 14].

In Pipkin III fractures, Scolaro et al. recommend strong consideration of arthroplasty based on 100% failure of ORIF in their study [9]. However, AVN-related failures have been markedly reduced with the vascular preserving surgical hip dislocation popularized by Gans [15]. This is particularly true in Pipkin I and II fractures treated with early (<6 hour) surgical hip dislocation – one study with a mean of 36-month follow-up found 0% rate of osteonecrosis, and 100% union rate [11]. Another study demonstrated 85% excellent clinical outcomes (HHS score >80) utilizing a surgical hip dislocation in all operatively managed Pipkin fractures and 8% avascular necrosis rate [16].

While traditionally reserved for Pipkin I and II fractures, a limited series of patients with Pipkin IV fractures demonstrated 88% success (no PTOA) with a modified Gibson approach. This posterior approach allows for increased anterior acetabular exposure through a modification of the proximal exposure via development of the plane between the gluteus maximus and tensor fascia lata rather than the gluteal splitting seen in the Kocher-Langenbeck approach. However, longer-term and larger-scale studies are needed to substantiate this approach for all Pipkin IV fractures [17]. We routinely use a modified Smith-Peterson approach for fixation for infrafoveal fractures while reserving the surgical hip dislocation of Ganz for suprafoveal and Pipkin type IV fractures.

Femoral Neck

PTOA in femoral neck fractures is primarily a failure of fixation and vascularity. The latter complication is particularly elevated in femoral neck fractures given the intracapsular location and tenuous blood supply to the femoral head. This may be compromised during the initial fracture or iatrogenically during fixation. As such, proximal femur fractures with higher displacement are at greatest risk of vascular injury and resultant long-term avascular necrosis (Fig. 9.2). At 5 years postinjury, 20% of femoral neck fractures repaired with internal fixation will undergo revision arthroplasty primarily due to avascular necrosis [18].

In elderly patients, fixation failure in the form of nonunion occurs in approximately 4–5% of stable femoral neck fractures (Garden 1 and 2, Table 9.3) patients [19, 20]. However, all-cause fixation failure is nearly 12–34.6% in this population due to avascular necrosis, nonunion, and fixation failure [21–24]. In younger patients with femoral neck fractures (<60 years old), Slobogean reported a substantially elevated rate of both malunion and nonunion at 7.1 and 9.3%, respectively [25]. Factors predicting a high likelihood of osteosynthesis failure include subcapital fracture location, Pauwel type 3 fractures (Table 9.2), Garden III or IV fractures (Table 9.3), and apex anterior tilt of the femoral head when treated with cancellous screws [26–28].

Pauwel III fractures provide a particularly difficult treatment challenge. Initial treatment with cannulated screws demonstrated significantly higher nonunion rates [29]. Moreover, treatment of this fracture pattern with cancellous screw fixation has also demonstrated significantly lower cycles to 15 mm shortening compared to dynamic hip screw or blade plate fixation [30]. This is substantial as recent data demonstrate femoral neck shortening of ≥ 10 mm has been implicated in worse functional outcomes including statistically lower Harris Hip Scores and SF-36 physical component scores [31]. Given the higher shear forces experienced in Pauwel III fractures, the use of autologous bone grafting at the time of the index procedure has been tried with good short-term success. In a study of 17 patients with Pauwel III fractures, 100% healed at a mean of 14.1 weeks, and less than 6% required arthroplasty at 27-month follow-up [32].

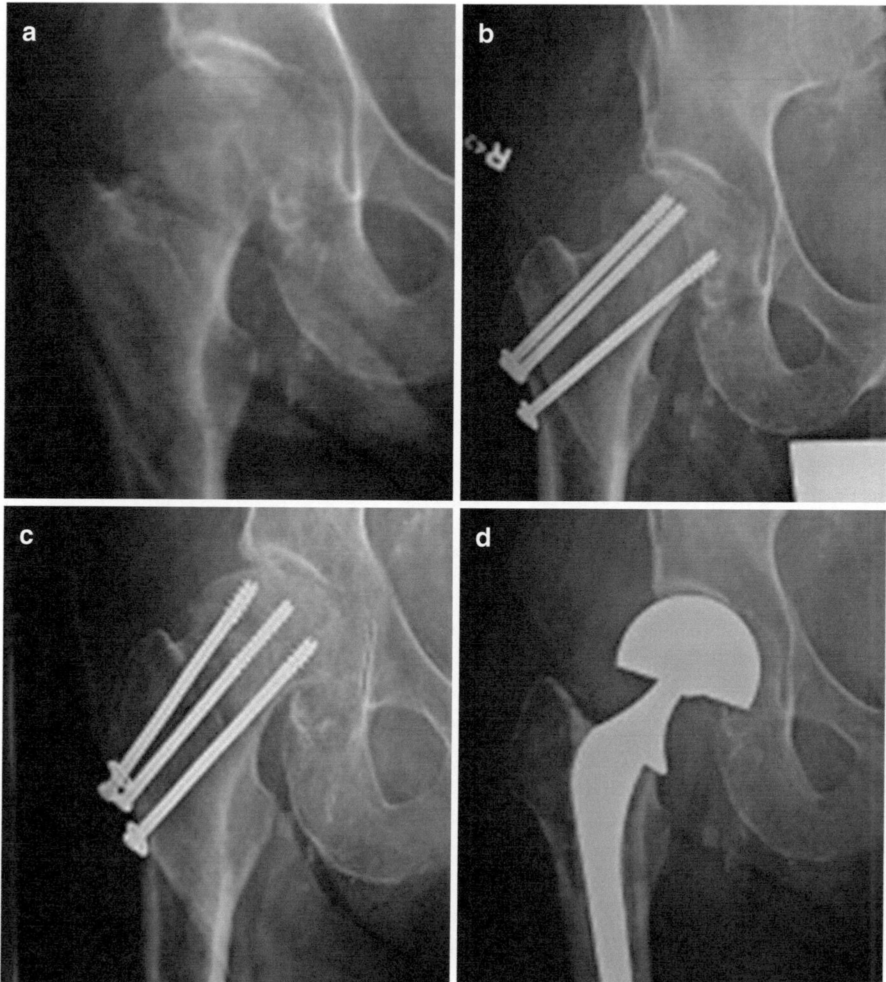

Fig. 9.2 (**a**) Nondisplaced femoral neck fracture. (**b**) Immediate postoperative imaging. (**c**) Femoral head collapse 6 months following index procedure. (**d**) Conversion to hemiarthroplasty

Table 9.2 Pauwel classification

Type	Fracture angle (degrees)
I	<30
II	30–50
III	>50

Table 9.3 Garden classification

Type	Fracture pattern
I	Incomplete
II	Complete, nondisplaced
III	Complete, partially displaced
IV	Complete, highly displaced

Intertrochanteric

PTOA following intertrochanteric fractures primarily occurs due to fixation failure (Fig. 9.3). Fortunately, due to substantial vascular supply, soft tissue preservation with closed reduction techniques, and robust cancellous bone, fixation failure occurs in only 1–2% of trochanteric fractures treated with intramedullary nailing [33, 34]. Factors predicting increased nonunion rate are the essential components of "unstable" trochanteric fractures including reverse obliquity, subtrochanteric extension, lateral wall comminution, and loss of medial calcar support [35–37]. However, the most important factor predicting PTOA via uneven joint force distribution is malreduction [33, 38]. Alteration of greater than 5 degrees of varus in the coronal plane,

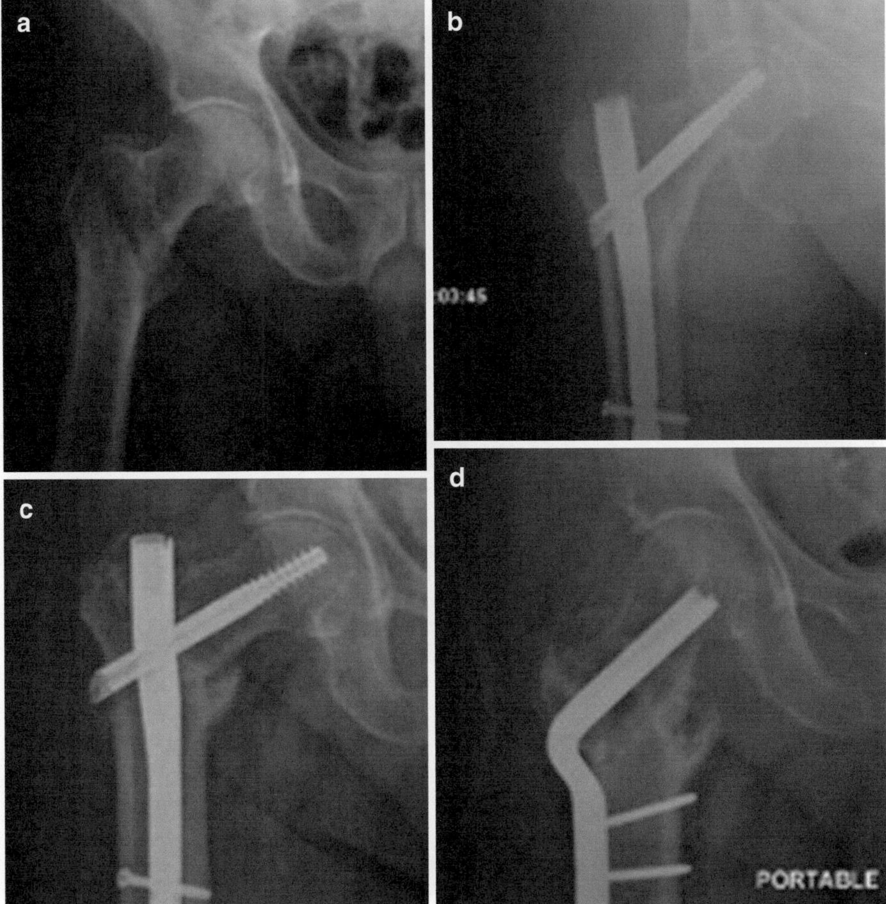

Fig. 9.3 (**a**) Minimally displaced intertrochanteric fracture. (**b**) Immediate postoperative radiographs. (**c**) Varus failure 6 months after index procedure. (**d**) Valgus intertrochanteric osteotomy with revision open reduction internal fixation

10 degrees in the sagittal plane, and 15 degrees in the axial plane focuses load on the superior femoral head, leading to arthrosis [33, 38].

Additionally, cut-out is of particular concern in trochanteric fractures (Fig. 9.4). It is estimated to occur in approximately 2% of patients treated with intramedullary nailing [39, 40]. Factors predicting cut-out including nonanatomic reduction, suboptimal bone quality, and tip-apex distance greater than 25 mm [39–41].

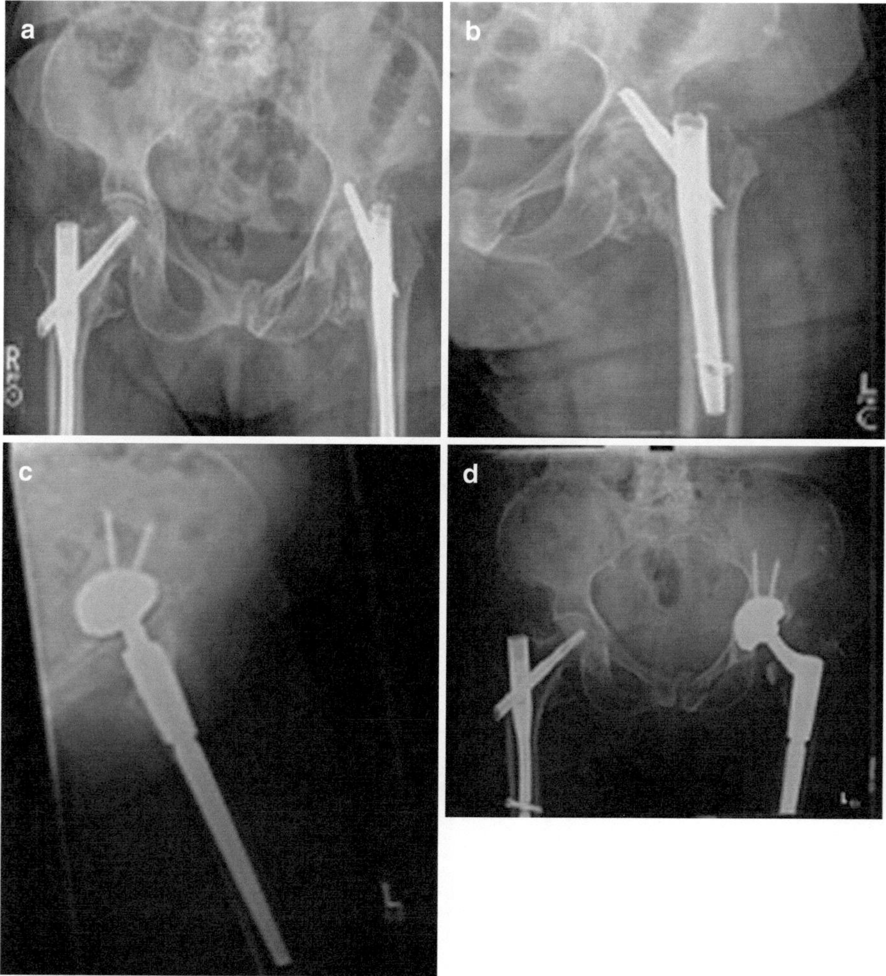

Fig. 9.4 (**a, b**) AP and lateral radiographs of left hip demonstrating cut out of cephalomedullary device. (**c, d**) One year following removal of hardware and conversion to THA

Management

The most definitive management for PTOA of the femoral head is hemi-, or total (THA), hip arthroplasty. These surgeries are supported by strong data demonstrating excellent outcomes, which have led some to opine that prevention of PTOA in patients with prefracture arthrosis should be accomplished with arthroplasty in amenable proximal femur fractures (7). However, arthroplasty in the setting of fracture is still associated with inherent risk over internal fixation including higher rates of wound infection, transfusion, and in-hospital morbidity. Additionally, due to limitations in prosthetic longevity, physiologically younger patients may be better served with osteosynthesis of native bone which may delay arthroplasty on average by 74 months [42]. Also, consideration of nonoperative and less invasive operative options are necessary in femoral head PTOA.

Nonoperative

There is a limited role for nonoperative management at the index injury time. This is usually reserved for critically ill patients. However, some Pipkin I fractures are amenable to initial nonoperative management but this option is usually not recommended as the rate of PTOA in nonoperatively managed Pipkin 1 fractures is 10% higher compared to operatively treated patients [10].

In the long-term, given that posttraumatic arthritis is a subset of osteoarthritis, it responds to the same conservative treatment that is well defined for the more common degenerative osteoarthritis. Antiinflammatory medications of varying potency and physical therapy are first-line, and often permanent, solutions to arthritic pain. Targeted intracapsular corticosteroid injections may also be of benefit from both a diagnostic and therapeutic perspective.

Operative

Arthroscopy

Hip arthroscopy for joint preservation is an increasingly common procedure. However, as with other joint arthroscopies, there is limited evidence to suggest that arthroscopic surgery of hip arthrosis provides improved clinical outcomes [43]. Chondral pathology at the time of hip arthroscopy for all indications is associated with 58-times greater risk for conversion to arthroplasty compared to patients without evidence of chondral damage [44]. Moreover several studies found that 16–44% of patients with arthrosis at the time of hip arthroscopy progress to THA within a maximum of 7 years [44–47].

Table 9.4 Tönnis classification

Grade	Radiographic changes
0	No evidence of OA
I	Sclerosis with minimal joint space narrowing or osteophytes
II	Moderate joint space narrowing with subchondral cyst formation
III	Severe joint space narrowing, subchondral cysts, deformation of femoral head

In the trauma population hip arthroscopy has more sparse literature. A study of 36 patients undergoing arthroscopy following closed reduction of hip dislocation found a 92% rate of loose bodies, and 78% rate of loose bodies in patients with imaging identifying concentric reduction and no loose bodies [48]. However, no outcome measures were reported in this study [48]. In a recent 2015 study of 13 patients undergoing hip arthroscopy following femoral head dislocation or acetabular fracture, 3.5-year follow-up demonstrated significant improvement in VAS scores and Modified Harris Hip Scores [49]. However, only Tönnis grade 0 or 1 (Table 9.4) patients were included in the study, and only 7 of 13 patients were femoral head dislocation patients. It is unknown how many of these patients had a concomitant acetabular fracture, which limits application to the proximal femur PTOA population. In another early study of hip arthroscopy in 38 patients, the diagnosis of arthritis resulted in an average Harris Hip Score increase of 18 and 14 points in patients with chondral injury, and arthritis, respectively, over a 10-month period [50]. However, the Harris Hip Score in those patients with a diagnosis of avascular necrosis decreased by 11 over the same time [50]. As previously mentioned, the etiology of PTOA in proximal femur fractures is strongly related to avascular necrosis. As such current data is inconclusive and further study is necessary to determine whether arthroscopy has a role in the treatment of young patients with severe PTOA following proximal femur fractures.

Hip Preservation

Management of femoral head chondral defects includes open and arthroscopic approaches. A number of treatments including chondroplasty, microfracture, fibrin adhesives, autologous chondrocyte transplantation, and osteochondral autologous transplants have been described [51, 52]. Microfracture has demonstrated positive clinical outcomes at 2-years postsurgery in Tönnis grade 0 or 1 patients [53]. However, there is a high rate of conversion to arthroplasty in patients with greater than Tönnis 1 radiographic changes. Additionally, other data suggests that microfracture does not improve patient reported outcomes at 2 years [54]. Other techniques including periacetabular osteotomy may have a role in the treatment of PTOA though this is yet to be described in the literature.

Osteotomy

Varus malunion is a common mode of failure following treatment of femoral neck fractures. If left uncorrected, PTOA occurs usually within 1 year of onset. In younger patients, and those where arthroplasty is relatively contraindicated, a valgus-producing osteotomy is a popular method of deformity correction to allow more even joint force distribution. This osteotomy may be inter- or subtrochanteric with success rates ranging between 85% and 100% [55]. One study of 60 patients with nonunited Garden III/IV, and Pauwel II/III, femoral neck fractures demonstrated 93% radiographic union rates and 90% good or excellent clinical outcomes after valgus subtrochanteric osteotomy and dynamic hip screw fixation [56]. However, postosteotomy AVN ranges from 10% and 40% although less than 10% of these patients are eventually converted to THA [55].

Core Decompression

In early-stage osteonecrosis, core decompression is a validated method of improving patient function and symptoms [57, 58]. In Fairbank's original study, 88% of Ficat stage I patients (mild osteopenia on radiograph and focal edema on MRI) required no further surgery at 11-year follow-up [58]. However, core decompression does carry the risk of postsurgical fracture and as such should be used with caution in those who are high fall risk. While the literature regarding core decompression is robust, there remains limited external applicability to the trauma patient at the present time. Most studies are based on level IV evidence and primarily evaluate for nontraumatic etiologies of femoral head osteonecrosis [58, 59].

Arthroplasty

Arthroplasty for proximal femur fractures is increasingly indicated during the index fracture. Elderly patients with displaced femoral neck fractures treated with arthroplasty have significantly lower complications, reoperation rates, less postoperative pain, and better overall function when compared to internal fixation [60]. Options for arthroplasty include THA and hemiarthroplasty. Hemiarthroplasty is commonly performed in those patients with relatively poorer health status, and risk factors for recurrent dislocation as the risk of dislocation for THA following fractures is four times higher than for THA performed due to arthritic indications [61–63] However prosthetic-induced acetabular wear causes substantial pain, and at 14 months postoperatively the clinical outcomes for THA are significantly better than hemiarthroplasty in properly selected patients [61, 62, 64]. Additionally, hemiarthroplasty confers no mortality or infection benefit at 4 years postoperatively when compared to THA, and uncemented prosthesis carries 720% higher chance of 5 year periprosthetic fracture when compared to cemented implants [61, 63, 65]. Therefore, the decision to perform hemiarthroplasty as the index procedure should primarily factor in poor projected patient longevity and household ambulation status as large database outcomes trend toward no difference in short-term complications or mortality in hemi- versus total hip arthroplasty [61, 63]. In younger patients aged 40–65, recent data indicate these patients may have greater clinical benefit and overall more cost-effective care with index THA (Fig. 9.1) [66].

With respect to painful PTOA, arthroplasty is the most definitive treatment option. Nearly 50% of patients with femoral head injury or acetabular impaction will require future arthroplasty [67]. The results of THA in patients with PTOA of the hip following acetabular or proximal femur fractures are inferior compared to primary degenerative OA. In one study of 1199 patients, 63 had THA for PTOA. They fared worse with respect to perioperative complications and demonstrated 13% revision rate due to persistent dislocation or infection at an average of 3.5 years postoperatively [42]. When compared to primary THA, patients undergoing THA conversion due to failed fixation of femoral neck fractures also have greater complications including deep infection, dislocation, and periprosthetic fracture [68]. However, 1 year functional outcomes were not substantially different [68].

As mentioned above, failure of fixation in intertrochanteric fractures increases superior femoral head arthrosis via coxa vara. Arthroplasty is a salvage option for the treatment of PTOA in this population as well. Compared to intertrochanteric fractures undergoing primary arthroplasty due to fracture complexity or poor bone quality, conversion arthroplasty resulted in significantly higher blood loss, operative time, and risk of postoperative periprosthetic fracture. However, 1 year mortality rates were not significantly different [69].

Hip Arthrodesis

Due to the above failure rate, and prospect of multiple revisions in young patients, alternatives to arthroplasty including arthrodesis have been employed. Patients considered for this procedure include those with monoarticular disease, high functional demand, and absence of lumbar or ipsilateral knee pathology [70]. Arthrodesis allows for preservation of bone stock and gluteal musculature and affords the patient satisfactory clinical outcomes while awaiting arthroplasty at a more age-appropriate time [70]. While no studies are available specifically addressing postfracture arthrodesis conversion to arthroplasty, one recent study evaluated 18 patients undergoing the aforementioned procedure. Eight of the 18 patients initially had arthrodesis for fracture. Patients undergoing conversion of previous arthrodesis to THA have substantial clinical improvement but also have increased incidence of neurologic injury and heterotopic ossification and tend to require use of ambulatory aids over long distances [71].

Conclusion

PTOA is a common sequelae following proximal femur injury. Initial forces result in chondral injury that is exacerbated by chronic changes in underlying bony support, which increases chondral contact pressures. Fortunately, advances in vascular-preserving approaches and an emphasis on prompt treatment of proximal femur fractures have improved long-term outcomes following these injuries. Given the number of treatment options with strong outcomes in the literature, the optimal treatment of symptomatic proximal femur PTOA is patient specific and ranges from osteotomy to arthroplasty to arthrodesis. With data demonstrating increasingly robust outcomes in PTOA hip arthroscopy, this surgical technique remains on the forefront of new treatment options and will continue to have an expanding role in the diagnosis and treatment of proximal femur PTOA.

References

 1. Giannoudis PV, Kontakis G, Christoforakis Z, Akula M, Tosounidis T, Koutras C. Management, complications and clinical results of femoral head fractures. Injury. 2009;40(12):1245–51. https://doi.org/10.1016/j.injury.2009.10.024.
 2. Oransky M, Martinelli N, Sanzarello I, Papapietro N. Fractures of the femoral head: a long-term follow-up study. Musculoskelet Surg. 2012;96(2):95–9. https://doi.org/10.1007/s12306-012-0182-7.
 3. Brown TD, Johnston RC, Saltzman CL, Marsh JL, Buckwalter JA. Posttraumatic osteoarthritis: a first estimate of incidence , prevalence , and burden of disease. J Orthop Trauma. 2006;20(10):739–44.
 4. Sahyoun NR, Lentzner H, Hoyert D, Robinson KN. Trends in causes of death among the elderly. Aging Trends. 2001;1:1–10.
 5. Furman BD, Mangiapani DS, Zeitler E, et al. Targeting pro-inflammatory cytokines following joint injury: acute intra-articular inhibition of interleukin-1 following knee injury prevents post-traumatic arthritis. Arthritis Res Ther. 2014;16(3):R134. https://doi.org/10.1186/ar4591.
 6. Ly TV, Swiontkowski MF. Treatment of femoral neck fractures in young adults. J Bone Joint Surg Am. 2008;90(10):1–14. https://doi.org/10.1016/0020-1383(82)90049-3.
 7. Olson SA, Guilak F. In: Olson SA, Guilak F, editors. Post-traumatic arthritis: pathogenesis, diagnosis and management: In Vitro Cartilage Explant Injury Models. Boston, MA. Springer. 2015; pp 29–40.
 8. Dreinhöfer KE, Schwarzkopf SR, Haas NP, Tscherne H. Isolated traumatic dislocation of the hip. Long-term results in 50 patients. J Bone Joint Surg Br. 1994;76(1):6–12. http://eutils.ncbi.nlm.nih.gov/entrez/eutils/elink.fcgi?dbfrom=pubmed&id=8300683&retmode=ref&cmd=prlinks%5Cnpapers2://publication/uuid/96679CC9-0424-438D-AE83-F18C6E52CD68.
 9. Scolaro JA, Marecek G, Firoozabadi R, Krieg JC, Routt ML, Chip R. Management and radiographic outcomes of femoral head fractures. J Orthop Traumatol. 2017:1–7. https://doi.org/10.1007/s10195-017-0445-z.
10. Nast-Kolb D, Ruchholtz S, Schweiberer L. Behandlung von Pipkin-Frakturen. Orthopade. 1997;26:360–7.
11. Gavaskar AS, Tummala NC. Ganz surgical dislocation of the hip is a safe technique for operative treatment of Pipkin fractures. Results of a prospective trial. J Orthop Trauma. 2015;29(12):544–8. https://doi.org/10.1097/BOT.0000000000000399.

12. Kekatpure A, Ahn T, Lee SJ, Jeong MY, Chang JS, Yoon PW. Arthroscopic reduction and internal fixation for Pipkin Type I femoral head fracture: technical note. Arthrosc Tech. 2016;5(5):e997–e1000. https://doi.org/10.1016/j.eats.2016.05.001.
13. Kim K, Park S, Kim Y. Disc height and segmental motion as risk factors for recurrent lumbar disc herniation. Spine (Phila Pa 1976). 2009;34(24):2674–8.
14. Park KS, Lee KB, Na BR, Yoon TR. Clinical and radiographic outcomes of femoral head fractures: excision vs. fixation of fragment in Pipkin type I: what is the optimal choice for femoral head fracture? J Orthop Sci. 2015;20(4):702–7. https://doi.org/10.1007/s00776-015-0732-6.
15. Ganz R, Gill TJ, Gautier E, Ganz K, Krügel N, Berlemann U. Surgical dislocation of the adult hip. J Bone Joint Surg [Br]. 2001;83(8):1119–24. https://doi.org/10.1302/0301-620X.83B8.11964.
16. Masse A, Aprato A, Alluto C, Favuto M, Ganz R. Surgical hip dislocation is a reliable approach for treatment of femoral head fractures. Clin Orthop Relat Res. 2015;473:3744–51. https://doi.org/10.1007/s11999-015-4352-4.
17. Yu Y-H, Hsu Y-H, Chou Y-C, Tseng I-C, Su C-Y, Wu C-C. Surgical treatment for Pipkin type IV femoral head fracture: an alternative surgical approach via a modified Gibson approach in nine patients. 2017;25(1):1–6. https://doi.org/10.1177/2309499016684970.
18. Nikolopoulos K, Papadakis S, Kateros K, et al. Long-term outcome of patients with avascular necrosis, after internal fixation of femoral neck fractures. Injury. 2003;34(7):525–8. https://doi.org/10.1016/S0020-1383(02)00367-4.
19. Min B, Lee K, Bae K, Lee S, Lee S, Choi J. Result of internal fixation for stable femoral neck fractures in elderly patients. Hip Pelvis. 2016;28(1):43–8.
20. Chen W-C, Yu S-W, Tseng I-C, Su J-Y, Tu Y-K, Chen W-J. Treatment of undisplaced femoral neck fractures in the elderly. J Trauma. 2005;58(5):1035–1039; discussion 1039. https://doi.org/10.1097/01.TA.0000169292.83048.17.
21. Kain MS, Marcantonio AJ, Iorio R. Revision surgery occurs frequently after percutaneous fixation of stable femoral neck fractures in elderly patients. Clin Orthop Relat Res. 2014;472(12):4010–4. https://doi.org/10.1007/s11999-014-3957-3.
22. Clement ND, Green K, Murray N, Duckworth AD, McQueen MM, Court-Brown CM. Undisplaced intracapsular hip fractures in the elderly: predicting fixation failure and mortality. A prospective study of 162 patients. J Orthop Sci. 2013;18(4):578–85. https://doi.org/10.1007/s00776-013-0400-7.
23. Seo J, Shin S, Jun S, Cho C, Lim BH. The early result of cementless arthroplasty for femur neck fracture in elderly patients with severe osteoporosis. Hip Pelvis. 2014;26(4):256–62.
24. Kim Y, Lee J, Song J, Oh S. The result of in situ pinning for valgus impacted femoral neck fractures of patients over 70 years old. Hip Pelvis. 2014;26(4):263–8.
25. Slobogean GP, Sprague SA, Scott T, Bhandari M. Complications following young femoral neck fractures. Injury. 2015;46(3):484–91. https://doi.org/10.1016/j.injury.2014.10.010.
26. Jo S, Lee SH, Lee HJ. The correlation between the fracture types and the complications after internal fixation of the femoral neck fractures. Hip Pelvis. 2016;28(1):35–42. https://doi.org/10.5371/hp.2016.28.1.35.
27. Kang JS, Moon KH, Shin JS, Shin EH. Clinical results of internal fixation of subcapital femoral neck fractures. Clin Orthop Surg. 2016;8:146–52.
28. Do LND, Marstein T, Foss OA, Basso T. Reoperations and mortality in 383 patients operated with parallel screws for Garden I-II femoral neck fractures with up to ten years. Injury. 2016;47(12):2739–42. https://doi.org/10.1016/j.injury.2016.10.033.
29. Liporace F, Gaines R, Collinge C, Gj H. Results of internal fixation of Pauwels type-3 vertical femoral neck fractures. J Bone Joint Surg. 2008;90:1654–9. https://doi.org/10.2106/JBJS.G.01353.
30. Stoffel K, Zderic I, Gras F, et al. Biomechanical evaluation of the femoral neck system in unstable Pauwels III Femoral neck fractures: a comparison with the dynamic hip screw and cannulated screws. J Orthop Trauma. 2017;31(3):131–7. https://doi.org/10.1097/BOT.0000000000000739.

31. Slobogean GP, Stockton DJ, Zeng B, Wang D, Ma B, Pollak AN. Femoral neck shortening in adult patients under the age of 55 years is associated with worse functional outcomes : analysis of the prospective multi-center study of hip fracture outcomes in China. Injury. 2017; https:// doi.org/10.1016/j.injury.2017.06.013.

32. Luo D, Zou W, He Y, et al. Modi fi ed dynamic hip screw loaded with autologous bone graft for treating Pauwels type-3 vertical femoral neck fractures. Injury. 2017;48(7):1579–83. https:// doi.org/10.1016/j.injury.2017.05.031.

33. Mavrogenis AF, Panagopoulos GN, Megaloikonomos PD, et al. Complications after hip nailing for fractures. Orthopedics. 2016;39(1):e108–16. https://doi.org/10.3928/01477447-20151222-11.

34. Dhammi I, Singh A, Mishra P, Jain A, Rehan-Ul-Haq, Jain S. Primary nonunion of intertrochanteric fractures of femur: analysis of results of valgization and bone grafting. Indian J Orthop. 2011;45(6):514. https://doi.org/10.4103/0019-5413.87122.

35. Lam SW, Teraa M, Leenen LPH, Van Der Heijden GJMG. Systematic review shows lowered risk of nonunion after reamed nailing in patients with closed tibial shaft fractures. Injury. 2010;41(7):671–5. https://doi.org/10.1016/j.injury.2010.02.020.

36. Griffin XL, Costa ML, Parsons N, Smith N. Electromagnetic field stimulation for treating delayed union or non-union of long bone fractures in adults. Cochrane Database Syst Rev. 2011;4:CD008471. https://doi.org/10.1002/14651858.CD008471.pub2.

37. Bhandari M, Guyatt G, Tornetta P, et al. Study to prospectively evaluate reamed intramedullary nails in patients with tibial fractures (S.P.R.I.N.T.): study rationale and design. BMC Musculoskelet Disord. 2008;9:91. https://doi.org/10.1186/1471-2474-9-91.

38. McKellop HA, Sigholm G, Redfern FC, Doyle B, Sarmiento A, Luck JV Sr. The effect of simulated fracture-angulations of the tibia on cartilage pressures in the knee joint. J Bone Joint Surg Am. 1991;73(9):1382–91. http://www.ncbi.nlm.nih.gov/entrez/query.fcgi?cmd=Retrieve &db=PubMed&dopt=Citation&list_uids=1918121.

39. Bojan AJ, Beimel C, Taglang G, Collin D, Ekholm C, Jönsson A. Critical factors in cut-out complication after gamma nail treatment of proximal femoral fractures. BMC Musculoskelet Disord. 2013;14:1. https://doi.org/10.1186/1471-2474-14-1.

40. Bojan AJ, Beimel C, Speitling A, Taglang G, Ekholm C, Jönsson A. 3066 consecutive Gamma Nails. 12 years experience at a single centre. BMC Musculoskelet Disord. 2010;11:133–43. https://doi.org/10.1186/1471-2474-11-133.

41. Baumgaertner MR, Solberg BD. Awareness of tip-apex distance reduces failure of fixation of trochanteric fractures of the hip. J Bone Joint Surg Br. 1997;79(6):969–71. https://doi. org/10.1302/0301-620x.79b6.7949.

42. Khurana S, Nobel TB, Merkow JS, Walsh M, Egol KA. Total hip arthroplasty for posttraumatic osteoarthritis of the hip fares worse than THA for primary osteoarthritis. Am J Orthop. 2015;44:321.

43. Viswanath A, Khanduja V. Can hip arthroscopy in the presence of arthritis delay the need for hip arthroplasty? J Hip Preserv Surg. 2017;4(1):3–8. https://doi.org/10.1093/jhps/hnw050.

44. Kemp JL, MacDonald D, Collins NJ, Hatton AL, Crossley KM. Hip arthroscopy in the setting of hip osteoarthritis: systematic review of outcomes and progression to hip arthroplasty. Clin Orthop Relat Res. 2014;473(3):1055–73. https://doi.org/10.1007/s11999-014-3943-9.

45. Domb BG, Gui C, Lodhia P. How much arthritis is too much for hip arthroscopy: a systematic review. Arthroscopy. 2015;31(3):520–9. https://doi.org/10.1016/j.arthro.2014.11.008.

46. Haviv B, O'Donnell J. The incidence of total hip arthroplasty after hip arthroscopy in osteoarthritic patients. Sport Med Arthrosc Rehabil Ther Technol. 2010;2:18. https://doi. org/10.1186/1758-2555-2-18.

47. Daivajna S, Bajwa A, Villar R. Outcome of arthroscopy in patients with advanced osteoarthritis of the hip. PLoS One. 2015;10(1):1–6. https://doi.org/10.1371/journal.pone.0113970.

48. Mullis BH, Dahners LE. Hip arthroscopy to remove loose bodies after traumatic dislocation. J Orthop Trauma. 2006;20(1):22–6. https://doi.org/10.1097/01.bot.0000188038.66582.ed.

49. Hwang JT, Lee WY, Kang C, Hwang DS, Kim DY, Zheng L. Usefulness of arthroscopic treatment of painful hip after acetabular fracture or hip dislocation. CiOS Clin Orthop Surg. 2015;7(4):443–8. https://doi.org/10.4055/cios.2015.7.4.443.
50. Byrd JWT, Jones KS. Prospective analysis of hip arthroscopy with 2-year follow-up. Arthroscopy. 2000;16(6):578–87. https://doi.org/10.1053/jars.2000.7683.
51. Ahmadpoor P, Reisi S, Makhdoomi K, Ghafari A, Sepehrvand N, Rahimi E. Osteoporosis and related risk factors in renal transplant recipients. Tranplantation Proc. 2009;41(7):2820–2. https://doi.org/10.1016/j.transproceed.2009.07.018.
52. Makhni EC, Stone AV, Ukwuani GC, Zuke W, Garabekyan T, Mei-dan O. A critical review management and surgical options for articular defects in the hip. Clin Sport Med. 2017;36:573–86. https://doi.org/10.1016/j.csm.2017.02.010.
53. Trask DJ, Keene JS. Analysis of the current indications for microfracture of chondral lesions in the hip joint. Am J Sports Med. 2016;44(12):3070–6. https://doi.org/10.1177/0363546516655141.
54. Domb BG, Gupta A, Dunne KF, Gui C, Chandrasekaran S. Microfracture in the hip results of a matched-cohort controlled study with 2-year follow-up. Am J Sports Med. 2015;43(8):1865–74. https://doi.org/10.1177/0363546515588174.
55. Varghese VD, Livingston A, Boopalan PR, Jepegnanam TS. Valgus osteotomy for non-union and neglected neck of femur fractures. World J Orthop. 2016;7(5):301–7. https://doi.org/10.5312/wjo.v7.i5.301.
56. Gupta S, Kukreja S, Singh V. Valgus osteotomy and repositioning and fixation with a dynamic hip screw and a 135° single-angled barrel plate for un-united and neglected femoral neck fractures. J Orthop Surg. 2014;22(1):20–4.
57. Rajagopa M, Samora JB, Ellis TJ. Efficacy of core decompression as treatment for osteonecrosis of the hip: a systematic review. Hip Int. 2012;22(5):489–93. https://doi.org/10.5301/HIP.2012.9748.
58. Fairbank AC, Bhatia D, Jinnah RH, Hungerford DS. Long-term results of core decompression for ischaemic necrosis of the femoral head. J Bone Joint Surg Br. 1995;77(1):42–9. http://www.ncbi.nlm.nih.gov/pubmed/7822394
59. Powell ET, Lanzer WL, Mankey MG. Core decompression for early osteonecrosis of the hip in high risk patients. Clin Orthop Relat Res. 1997;335:181.
60. Ye CY, Liu A, Xu MY, Nonso NS, He RX. Arthroplasty versus internal fixation for displaced intracapsular femoral neck fracture in the elderly: systematic review and meta - analysis of short - and long - term effectiveness. Chin Med J. 2016;129(21) https://doi.org/10.4103/0366-6999.192788.
61. Evidence-based clinical practice guideline: management of hip fracture in the elderly; 2014.
62. Ullmark G. Femoral head fractures: Hemiarthroplasty or total hip arthroplasty? Hip Int. 2014;24(1):S12–4. https://doi.org/10.5301/hipint.5000167.
63. SooHoo NF, Farng E, Chambers L, Znigmond DS, Lieberman JR. Comparison of complication rates between hemiarthroplasty and total hip arthroplasty for intracapsular hip fractures. Orthopedics. 2013;36(4):e384–9. https://doi.org/10.3928/01477447-20130327-09.
64. Roberts KC, Brox WT, Jevsevar DS, Sevarino K. Management of hip fractures in the elderly. J Am Acad Orthop Surg. 2015;23(2):131–7. https://doi.org/10.5435/JAAOS-D-14-00432.
65. Langslet E, Frihagen F, Opland V, Madsen JE, Nordsletten L, Figved W. Cemented versus uncemented hemiarthroplasty for displaced femoral neck fractures: 5-year followup of a randomized trial. Clin Orthop Relat Res. 2014;472(4):1291–9. https://doi.org/10.1007/s11999-013-3308-9.
66. Swart E, Roulette P, Leas D, Bozic KJ, Karunakar M. ORIF or arthroplasty for displaced femoral neck fractures in patients younger than 65 years old: an economic decision analysis. J Bone Joint Surg Am. 2017;99(1):65–75. https://doi.org/10.2106/JBJS.16.00406.
67. Clarke-Jenssen J, Roise O, Storeggen SAO, Madsen JE. Long-term survival and risk factors for failure of the native hip joint after operatively treated displaced acetabular fractures. Bone Joint J. 2017;99(B):834–40. https://doi.org/10.1302/0301-620X.99B6.BJJ-2016-1013.R1.

68. Mahmoud SSS, Pearse EO, Smith TO, Hing CB. Outcomes of total hip arthroplasty , as a salvage procedure , following failed internal fixation of intracapsular fractures of the femoral neck. Bone Joint J. 2016;98(B):452–60. https://doi.org/10.1302/0301-620X.98B4.36922.
69. Lee Y, Kim JT, Alkitaini AA, Kim K, Ha Y, Koo K. Conversion hip arthroplasty in failed fixation of intertrochanteric fracture : a propensity score matching study. J Arthroplast. 2017;32(5):1593–8. https://doi.org/10.1016/j.arth.2016.12.018.
70. Beaulé PE, Matta JM, Mast JW. Hip arthrodesis: current indications and techniques. J Am Acad Orthop Surg. 2002;10(4):249–58.
71. Aderinto J, Lulu OB, Backstein DJ, Safir O, Gross AE. Functional results and complications following conversion of hip fusion to total hip replacement. J Bone Joint Surg Br. 2012;94(11 Suppl A):36–41. https://doi.org/10.1302/0301-620X.94B11.30615.

Chapter 10
Post-traumatic Arthritis of the Distal Femur

Karthikeyan Ponnusamy and Ajit Deshmukh

> **Key Points**
> - Distal femoral fracture nonunions are associated with a high burden of posttraumatic arthritis.
> - Surgical options include osteoarticular autograft and allograft, realignment osteotomies, and unicompartmental or total knee arthroplasty.
> - It is critical to restore the joint line in the treatment of posttraumatic arthritis of the knee.
> - Higher levels of constraint may be necessary in TKA for posttraumatic arthritis.

Epidemiology

Adults sustain distal femur fractures at a rate of 4.5/100,000. Most of these fractures occur in female patients (67% vs. 33% in males) [1]. The two predominant age groups presenting with this injury are young adults who are involved in high-energy mechanisms and elderly who are involved in low-energy falls.

As with any periarticular fracture there are concerns that a combination of initial trauma to the articular cartilage and residual articular step-off or malalignment can accelerate the development of arthritic changes in the joint. One systematic review examined the impact of articular step-off for various joints. When they looked at studies for the distal femur, they only identified rabbit models that demonstrated

K. Ponnusamy
Pinnacle Orthopaedics, Canton, GA, USA

A. Deshmukh (✉)
Department of Orthopaedic Surgery, New York University, New York, NY, USA
e-mail: Kimberly.murillo@NYULangone.org

© Springer Nature Switzerland AG 2021
S. C. Thakkar, E. A. Hasenboehler (eds.), *Post-Traumatic Arthritis*,
https://doi.org/10.1007/978-3-030-50413-7_10

that as long as the step-off was smaller than the thickness of the articular cartilage, there was sufficient remodeling. However, in cases of step-off greater than the thickness of the articular cartilage and knee instability there could be rapid articular degeneration [2]. Another consideration is that residual malalignment from femoral malunion can alter joint loading and lead to degenerative changes. Kettelkamp et al. examined the significance of knee malalignment following fracture malunion and reported that degenerative knee changes developed at a range of 10–60 years after the fracture with an average of 31.7 years [3].

There are only a limited number of trials with sufficient follow-up to ascertain the clinical impact of posttraumatic arthritis from distal femoral fractures. One study by Rademakers et al. reported outcomes at a mean of 14 years (range 5–25 years) and found radiological evidence of moderate to severe osteoarthritis in 36% of patients, but 72% of these patients had good to excellent functional outcome scores [4]. Comparable results were reported by Thomson et al. at an average of 80 months follow-up, where 54% of patients had significant degenerative changes in the knee and 32% had no radiographic arthritic changes. None of these patients had undergone a total knee arthroplasty by the last follow-up [5]. To summarize, patients who have sustained a distal femoral fracture are at risk of developing radiological findings of arthritic changes, but clinical follow-up to 14 years afterward suggests almost three quarters of patients are not impaired by these findings. However, there remain a quarter of patients with radiological findings of posttraumatic arthritis that have more severe symptoms. Further follow-up is needed to determine if and when the previously asymptomatic patients with arthritic changes will become symptomatic.

Natural History of Distal Femur Fracture Healing

Most cases of distal femur fractures are treated surgically with the following implants as possible options: blade plates, locking plates, condylar screws, and retrograde intramedullary nails [6]. Current first-line management usually focuses on locking plates and retrograde intramedullary nails. In patients with significant medical comorbidities and limited ambulatory status, nonoperative options of functional bracing or casting can be considered.

Surgical treatment of distal femur fractures is usually successful, but the nonunion rate is reported to be 10%. Nonunions have been most commonly associated with open fractures, comminution, bone loss, and infection. Monroy et al. compared the results of revision ORIF for distal femur nonunions vs. ORIF for acute distal femur fractures and found that there was statistically no difference in time to union (mean of 7 months for nonunions vs. 5 months for acute fractures) and no statistical difference in range of motion and clinical outcome scores [7]. Ebraheim et al. in their systematic review on the subject of nonunions in distal femur fractures also found that open fractures and bone loss were the most common factors, followed by hardware failure and infection. After revision fixation of nonunions, 97% healed at an average of 9.86 months. They found that metaphyseal comminution was the fracture pattern most associated with nonunion. When the initial fixation utilized dynamic condylar screws and blade plates, there was a higher likelihood of nonunion than with locking plates. The most common fixation used for revisions was fixed angle platting with cancellous bone autograft, and this approach was successful in achieving union for 97.4% of patients at an average time of 7.8 months [6].

Patient Evaluation

Despite the generally successful results of the management of distal femur fractures, there will continue to be a subset of patients who will continue to have knee pain due to nonunion, posttraumatic arthritis, knee instability, or other etiologies. As with any patient, evaluation needs to begin with the history. Key aspects of the history that need to be determined is history regarding the treatment and outcomes from initial distal femur fracture management and time course of symptoms since then. Any aspects suggestive of infection must be highlighted, such as requiring antibiotics in the postoperative period, prolonged wound drainage, and repeat surgeries. Prior operative reports should be obtained if possible to identify the implant and facilitate the removal of the implant if warranted. The physical exam should focus on locating the prior surgical incisions, knee range of motion and ligamentous stability, and patellar tracking. Imaging should begin with standing AP radiograph, PA flexed, lateral, and sunrise views. Advanced cross-sectional imaging can be considered in cases of nonunion with CTs or localized articular injuries or ligamentous damage with MRIs. Prior hardware may affect the quality of the cross-sectional imaging, and specific metal suppression techniques should be considered.

Nonoperative Management of Posttraumatic Arthritis

Nonoperative management for posttraumatic arthritis includes the same treatment modalities as with osteoarthritis. McAlindon et al. conducted a systematic review of 29 treatment modalities to determine whether they should be utilized in nonoperative treatment of knee osteoarthritis. They reported that there was evidence supporting the use of intraarticular steroid injections, physical therapy and exercise, weight loss, acetaminophen, assistive walking devices, and oral or topical NSAIDs [8].

Operative Management of Posttraumatic Arthritis

Surgical options include osteoarticular autograft and allograft, realignment osteotomies, and unicompartmental or total knee arthroplasty (TKA) [9]. In cases of young and active patients with localized articular cartilage defects, osteochondral autograft or allografts can be considered. Gross et al. have published on the use of osteochondral allografts for both the distal femur and proximal tibia [10]. Their distal femur allograft survival rate was 95% at 5 years and 85% at 10 years. With an average of 10-year follow-up, they had 9 of 60 undergo subsequent total knee arthroplasty [10]. As reported by Kettelkamp et al., [3] malalignment after femoral fractures can lead to degenerative arthritic changes in the knee at an average of 30 years after initial injury. Consequently, realignment osteotomies can be a useful tool when managing a young patient with knee pain subsequent to malunited distal femoral fracture. Lustig et al. reported their experience of treating posttraumatic knee arthritis with osteotomy alone (femur, tibia, or both). They found that with an average of 3.8 years of follow-up, two of six patients with an intraarticular malunion went on to a total knee arthroplasty. Whereas, the 22 patients who had an extraarticular malunion did not have an arthroplasty during the time of follow-up. In addition, they found that, in general, patients had improvements in pain scores, but those with extraarticular malunion had the greatest improvement [2, 3].

For end stage posttraumatic arthritis, the treatment of choice would be TKA. However, for patients who undergo TKA for posttraumatic arthritis, it has been reported that they have higher complication rates than primary TKA for osteoarthritis. They have a higher risk for revision surgery with a hazard ratio of 2.23 (CI 95% 1.69–2.88) and postoperative infection of 2.85 (1.97–3.98) [11]. These cases are technically more demanding, but patients can have good outcomes if appropriate limb alignment and implant positioning are achieved [12].

Primary Arthroplasty for Elderly Patients with Acute Comminuted Distal Femur Fractures

In the elderly and frail patient population, the 1-year mortality rate has been reported to be 22% after sustaining a supracondylar femur fracture. This older study went on to further report that 9% of patients needed an above-knee amputation at a later time point due to loss of fracture reduction and/or infection [13]. Due to this suboptimal outcome, over the last couple decades several case series on the use of primary TKA or distal femoral replacement for distal femur fractures have been published. The goal was that an immediate arthroplasty would allow immediate weight bearing and allow patients to regain mobility faster with the theory that they will have fewer complications.

One case series did not demonstrate any improvement in mortality rate and reported a 1-year mortality rate of 30%. They did find a revision rate of 9.5% which is better than reports of complication rates up to 25% for primary TKA for posttraumatic osteoarthritis [14].

Malviya et al. examined the use of acute primary TKA for periarticular distal femur and proximal tibia fractures. They reported that 10 of the 11 distal femur fractures were treated with a rotating hinge, and one was treated with a varus/valgus constrained implant and that they had good clinical outcomes in their case series [15]. Bettin et al. reported on 18 patients who had sustained comminuted intraarticular, osteoporotic, arthritic fractures and were treated with cemented distal femoral replacements. They had two patients who had complications with their implants (one periprosthetic fracture and one deep infection). They reported that the patients in their series were extremely or very satisfied with their outcomes but did not have a comparison arm [16]. Rosen and Strauss reported their use of distal femur replacements in a case series of 24 patients for distal femur fractures and found 71% returned to their preoperative ambulation level [17].

As of now only one retrospective comparative study of ORIF with distal femur replacement has been reported by Hart et al. They found that at 1-year follow-up all the distal femur replacement patients were ambulating while 25% of the ORIF patients were wheelchair bound, but this was not statistically significant. They found comparable reoperation rates of 10% in the distal femur replacement group and 11% in the ORIF group. The ORIF group had fractures healed at an average of 24 weeks but had a nonunion incidence of 18% [18]. Due to the relative rarity of converting a distal femur ORIF to TKA, Bohm et al. suggested that ORIF should be used in most acute fracture cases. However, for specific patient populations with prior arthritis, not compliant with weight-bearing restrictions, and very comminuted fractures, a primary arthroplasty could be considered [19].

One of the surgical considerations for treating acute fractures is that higher levels of constraint such as a rotating hinge prosthesis may be necessary since there is a higher likelihood that the collateral ligaments are compromised by the fracture. In order to determine the joint line in a highly comminuted fracture, one method that can be used in acute fractures is obtaining a temporary reduction with the use of an external fixator or other methods. Alternatively, the joint line can be determined relative to anatomic landmarks such as 1 cm proximal to the fibular head or 2.5 cm distal to the femoral epicondyles (based on their reduced position). Sizing the femur in an acute fracture may be difficult, and estimates based on the trials may be needed. In addition, depending on the level of bone loss/comminution, augments, wedges, sleeves, or cones may be needed [20].

When acute fractures with severe comminution of the condyles are treated with arthroplasty, then a distal femoral replacement may be needed. Some of the technical challenges are to determine the length and rotation of the femur. This can be accomplished by obtaining provisional reduction with traction and from there the rotation can be determined based on the transepicondylar axis. Another consideration is whether to press-fit or cement the stem. Given the likely poor bone quality, the stem will likely need to be cemented [19]. Arthroplasty can be more challenging in these cases but focusing on proper alignment, positioning, and fixation can lead to good patient outcomes.

Surgical Considerations at Arthroplasty for Posttraumatic Arthritis

When comparing posttraumatic arthritis to osteoarthritis for the etiology for TKA, it has been reported that TKA takes about 30 minutes longer in the posttraumatic case [21]. Extensor mechanism issues are a common source of difficulty in performing these procedures. Lateral release was needed in 47% of TKAs reported by Weiss et al. [12] and 46% for Papadopoulos et al. [22]. Other techniques that needed to be used were quadriceps V-Y turndown, vastus medialis advancement, LCL transfer, extensor mechanism realignment, and collateral ligament reconstruction [12, 22].

One of the first considerations for performing a total knee arthroplasty is determining the level of constraint needed. The next step is determining the joint line and component rotation. If the fracture has healed in appropriate alignment and rotation, then standard techniques can be used. However, in cases of deformity or retained hardware that would prevent or severely complicate intramedullary alignment, patient-specific instrumentation, imageless hand-held navigation devices, or computer navigation can be very helpful to establish the alignment.

For larger bony defects, structural allograft or metal augments can be used. Prior hardware and whether it will interfere with the procedure needs to be considered, and the prior hardware can be appropriately removed or retained [12].

Limb alignment needs to be evaluated and malalignment needs to be corrected with intraarticular resections for an arthroplasty or staged/simultaneous osteotomy. If intraarticular resections would compromise the collateral ligaments in order to obtain the necessary alignment correction, a distal femoral osteotomy can be secured with a long-stem femoral component or staged with a plate and screw construct. Bone graft can be placed at osteotomy and nonunion sites [12]. Papadopoulos et al. reported a case series of 48 TKA after distal femoral fractures and found malunions greater than 10 degrees in the coronal plane or 15 degrees in the sagittal plane in 21 knees (44%). Of these with malunions, they were able to correct 15 through intraarticular bony resections and 6 needed osteotomies [22].

Case Example of Staged Osteotomy

A 53-year-old male with a history of a supracondylar left femur fracture treated nonoperatively 35 years ago presented to the clinic with symptomatic left knee pain (Fig. 10.1).

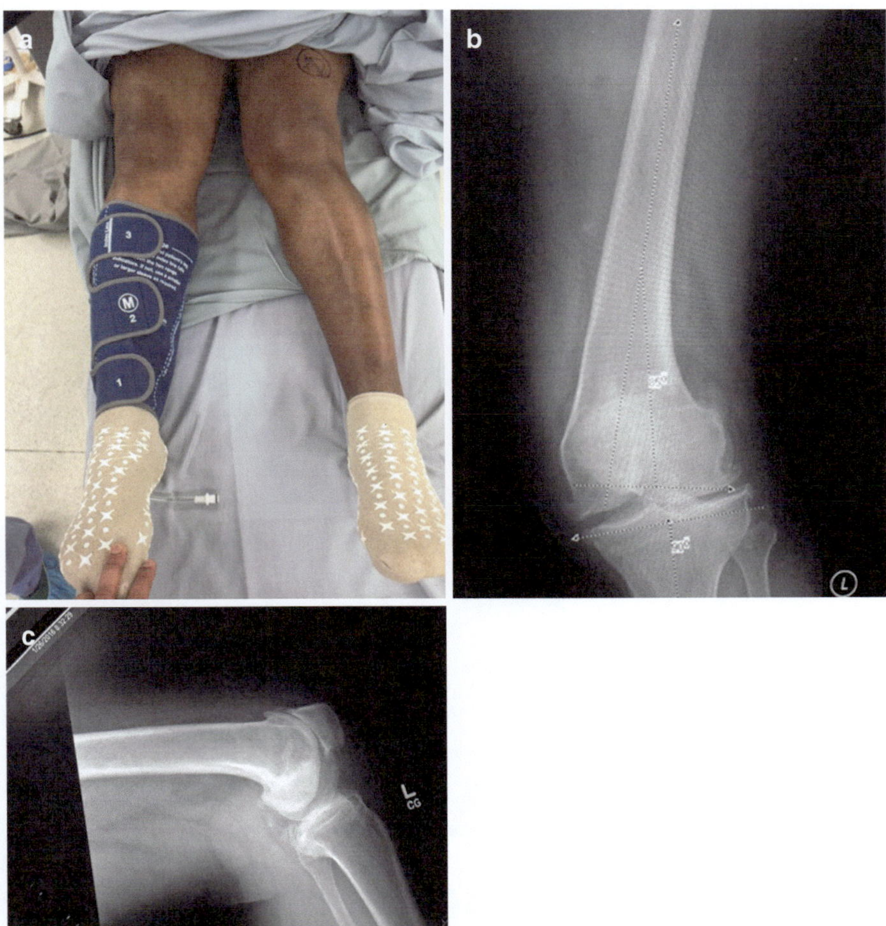

Fig. 10.1 (a–c) Preoperative lower extremity alignment and AP/lateral distal femur

Options to address the deformity would be to perform an intraarticular correction with a TKA or an extraarticular correction with TKA. In the case of the extraarticular correction, the osteotomy could be performed in staged or simultaneous settings. In this case, templating for an intraarticular resection demonstrates that there would be a risk of compromising the MCL origin (Fig. 10.2). Consequently, it was decided to perform an extraarticular correction of the deformity, and it was done in a staged setting.

For this patient a lateral opening wedge osteotomy of the distal femur was planned and performed (Figs. 10.3 and 10.4).

Five months after surgery the osteotomy site had healed (Fig. 10.5).

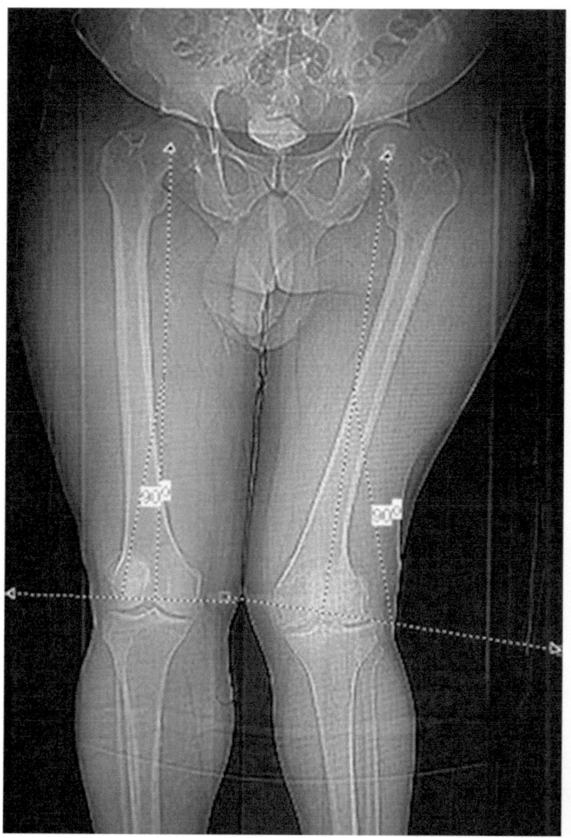

Fig. 10.2 Templating for intraarticular resection

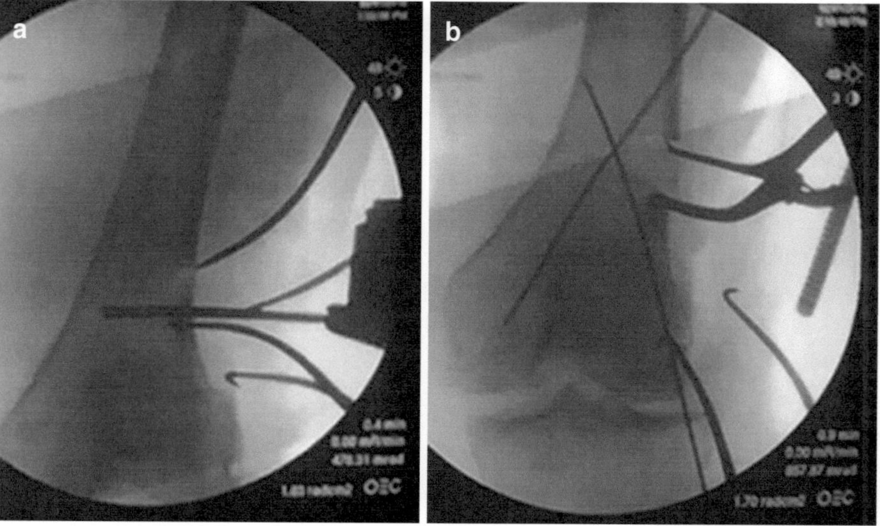

Fig. 10.3 (**a**) Intraoperative fluoroscopy picture after the osteotomy was performed; (**b**) change in alignment after insertion of the bone graft wedge with provisional fixation

Fig. 10.4 Postoperative picture of the patient's lower extremity

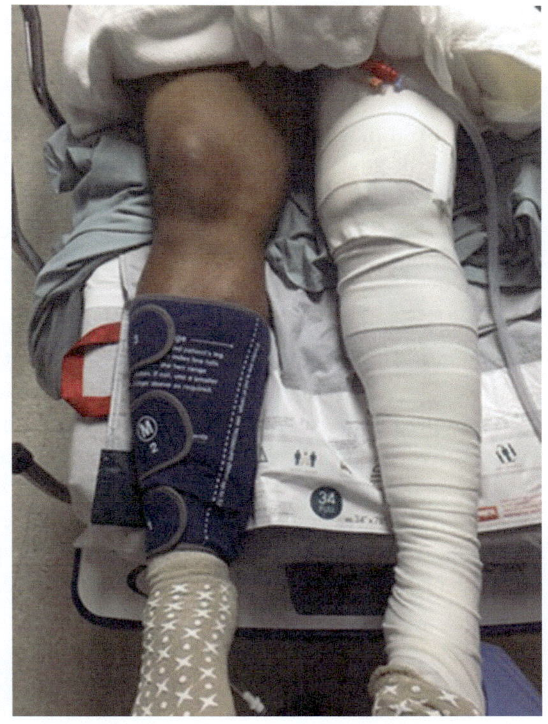

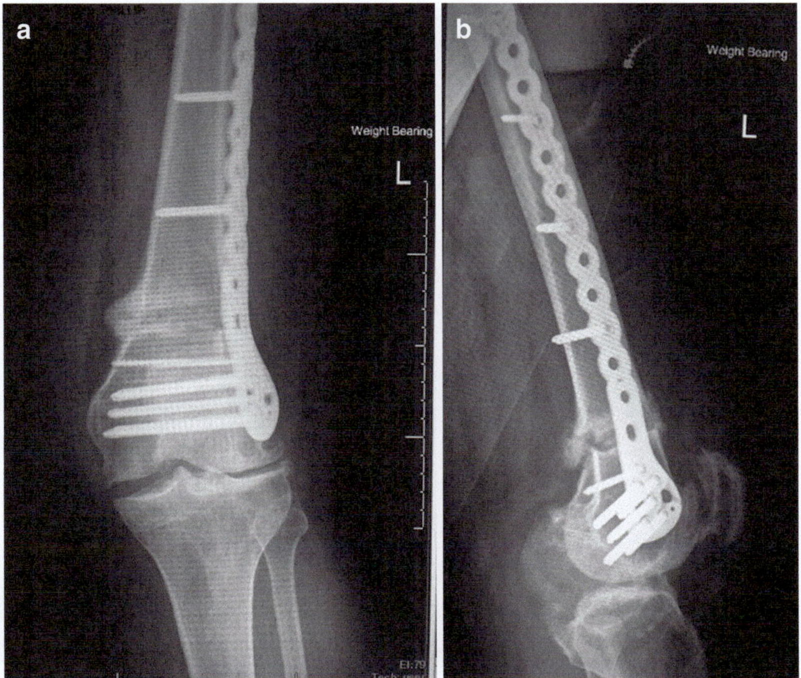

Fig. 10.5 (**a**, **b**) AP and lateral X-rays at 5 months after healing of osteotomy

Case Example of Intraarticular Correction of Deformity and TKA

A 60-year-old male with history of a nonoperatively managed femur 45 years ago presents with advanced arthritic changes of his knee and instability of his knee (Figs. 10.6 and 10.7).

Preoperative templating plans for planned resections demonstrated that the correction could be obtained through intraarticular osteotomies with the TKA (Fig. 10.8).

For this patient, given the malunion in his femur, a long intramedullary femoral alignment rod could not be used and instead a short rod was used. A 3-degree valgus distal femoral cut was performed as templated. Next the tibial cut was performed with intramedullary referencing and then extension space balancing was performed. Preoperatively there was concern that the MCL was incompetent, and the surgeons were prepared to perform a rotating hinge total knee arthroplasty. Intraoperative evaluation determined that the MCL was still intact and as a result extension space balancing was performed. After release of the posterolateral capsule and pie-crusting of the IT band and LCL, the gaps were within 3–4 mm of each other.

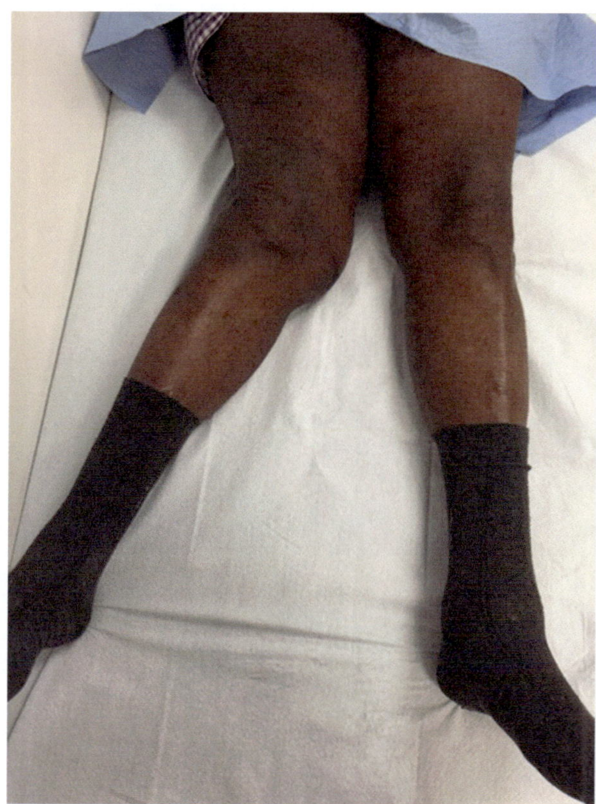

Fig. 10.6 Clinical picture of the deformity

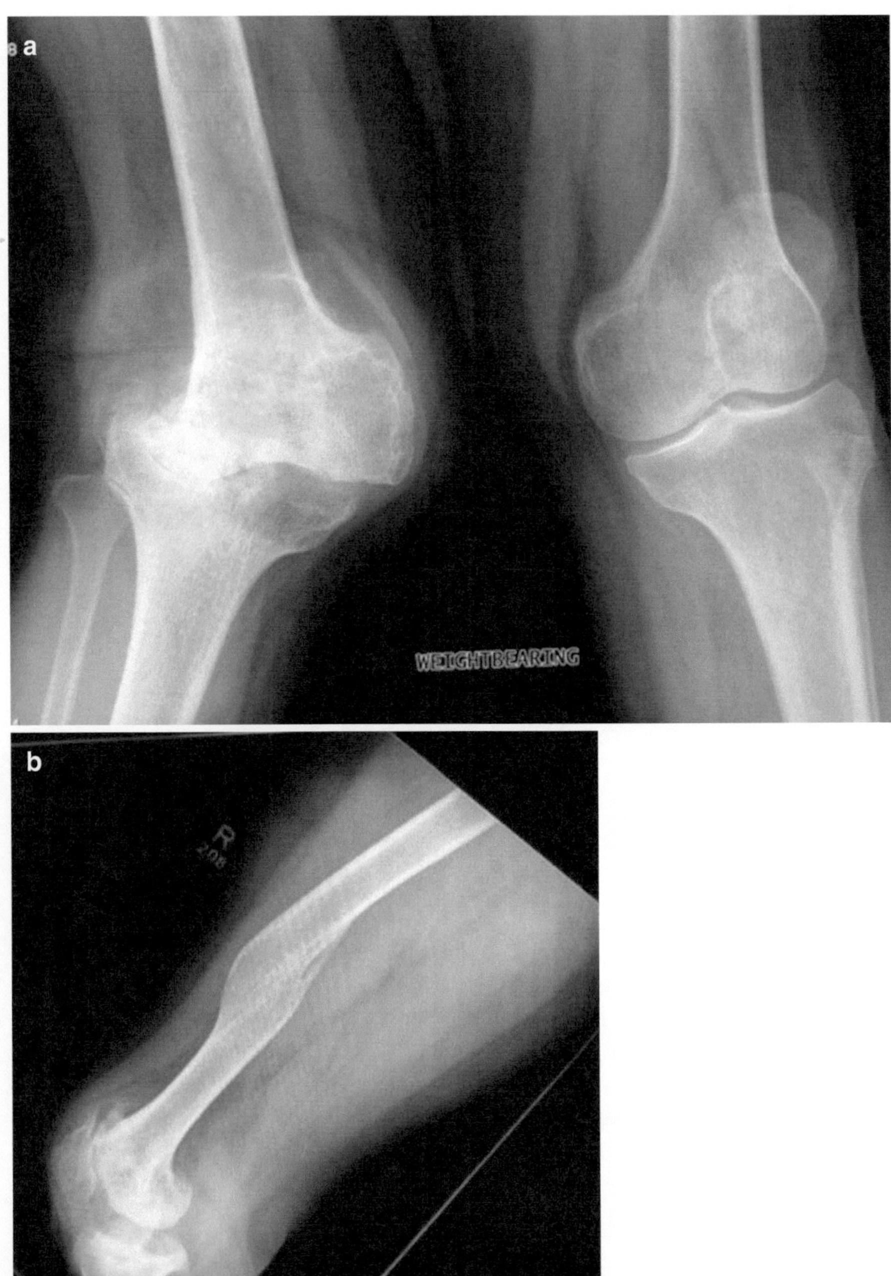

Fig. 10.7 (**a**, **b**) AP and lateral of his knee demonstrating the extraarticular deformity with advanced osteoarthritis and significant coronal plane malunion

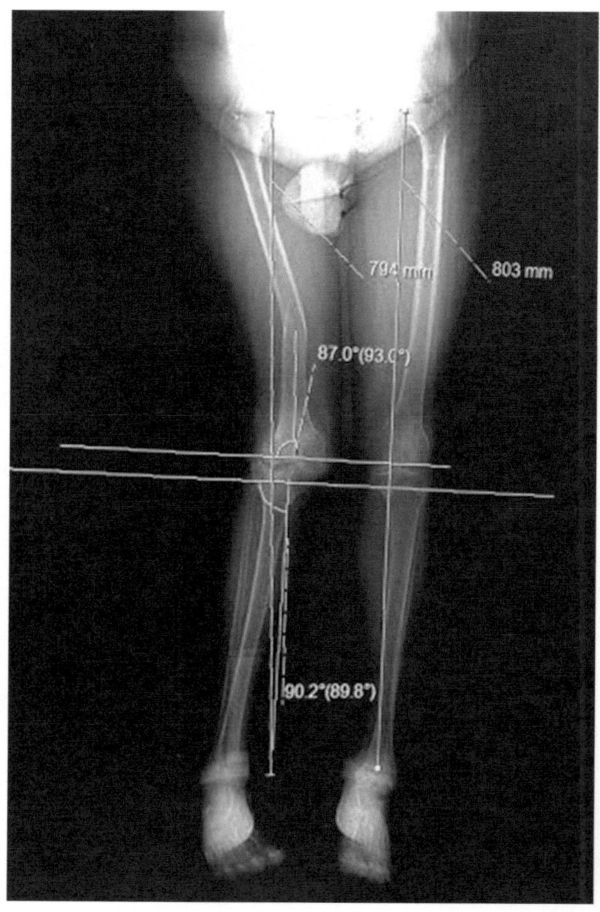

Fig. 10.8 Preoperative templating for intraarticular correction of deformity

Femoral rotation was determined by flexing the knee to 90 degrees and aligning the femoral cutting block with the tibial cut. Preoperative templating determined that a 100 mm sleeve-stem length could be used on the femoral side without reaching the site of malunion. A varus-valgus constrained implant was used, and a stable knee was achieved with good patellar tracking (Figs. 10.9 and 10.10).

Fig. 10.9 Clinical picture
of leg after surgery

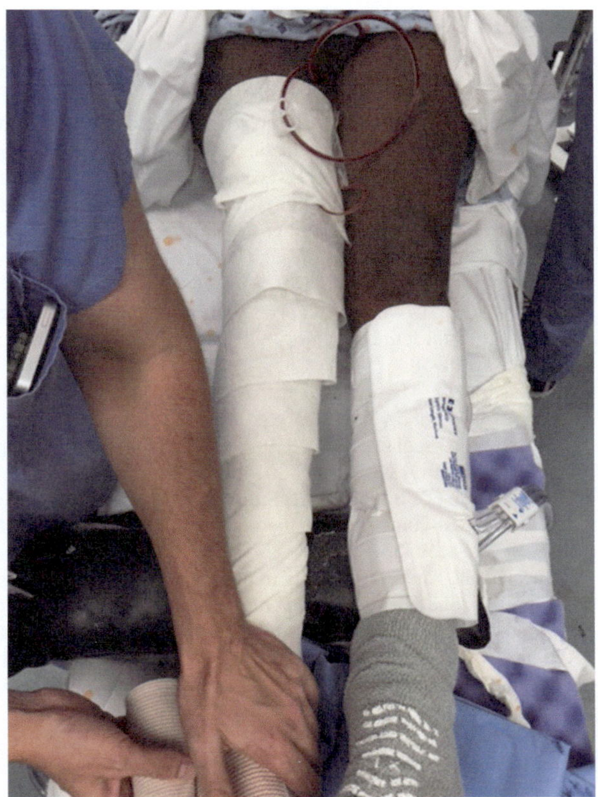

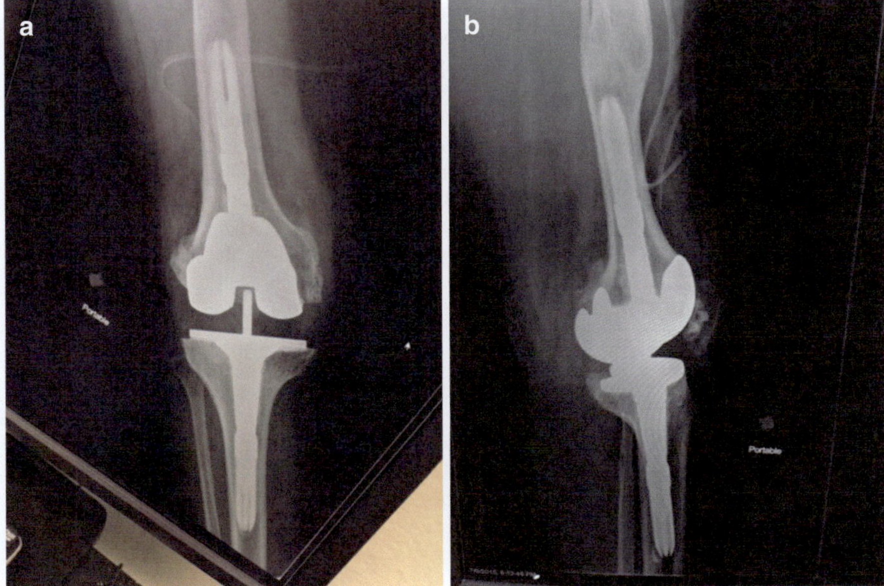

Fig. 10.10 Postoperative AP and lateral X-rays

References

1. Court-Brown CM, Caesar B. Epidemiology of adult fractures: a review. Injury. 2006;37:691–7.
2. Giannoudis PV, Tzioupis C, Papathanassopoulos A, Obakponovwe O, Roberts C. Articular step-off and risk of post-traumatic osteoarthritis. Evidence Today. Injury. 2010;41:986–95.
3. Kettelkamp DB, Hillberry BM, Murrish DE, Heck DA. Degenerative arthritis of the knee secondary to fracture malunion. Clin Orthop Relat Res. 1988;234:159–69.
4. Rademakers MV, Kerkhoffs GMMJ, Sierevelt IN, Raaymakers ELFB, Marti RK. Intra-articular fractures of the distal femur: a long-term follow-up study of surgically treated patients. J Orthop Trauma. 2004;18:213–9.
5. Thomson AB, Driver R, Kregor PJ, Obremskey WT. Long-term functional outcomes after intra-articular distal femur fractures: ORIF versus retrograde intramedullary nailing. Orthopedics. 2008;31:748–50.
6. Ebraheim NA, Martin A, Sochacki KR, Liu J. Nonunion of distal femoral fractures: a systematic review. Orthop Surg. 2013;5:46–50.
7. Monroy A, Urruela A, Singh P, Tornetta P, Egol KA. Distal femur nonunion patients can expect good outcomes. J Knee Surg. 2014;27:83–7.
8. McAlindon TE, Bannuru RR, Sullivan MC, Arden NK, Berenbaum F, Bierma-Zeinstra SM, et al. OARSI guidelines for the non-surgical management of knee osteoarthritis. Osteoarthr Cartil. 2014;22:363–88.
9. Buechel FF. Knee arthroplasty in post-traumatic arthritis. J Arthroplast. 2002;17:63–8.
10. Gross AE, Shasha N, Aubin P. Long-term followup of the use of fresh osteochondral allografts for posttraumatic knee defects. Clin Orthop Relat Res. 2005;435:79–87.
11. Houdek MT, Watts CD, Shannon SF, Wagner ER, Sems SA, Sierra RJ. Posttraumatic total knee arthroplasty continues to have worse outcome than total knee arthroplasty for osteoarthritis. J Arthroplast. 2016;31:118–23.
12. Weiss NG, Parvizi J, Hanssen AD, Trousdale RT, Lewallen DG. Total knee arthroplasty in post-traumatic arthrosis of the knee. J Arthroplast. 2003;18:23–6.
13. Karpman RR, Del Mar NB. Supracondylar femoral fractures in the frail elderly. Fractures in need of treatment. Clin Orthop Relat Res. 1995;316:21–4.
14. Boureau F, Benad K, Putman S, Dereudre G, Kern G, Chantelot C. Does primary total knee arthroplasty for acute knee joint fracture maintain autonomy in the elderly? A retrospective study of 21 cases. Orthop Traumatol Surg Res. 2015;101:947–51.
15. Malviya A, Reed MR, Partington PF. Acute primary total knee arthroplasty for peri-articular knee fractures in patients over 65 years of age. Injury. 2011;42:1368–71.
16. Bettin CC, Weinlein JC, Toy PC, Heck RK. Distal femoral replacement for acute distal femoral fractures in elderly patients. J Orthop Trauma. 2016;30:503–9.
17. Rosen AL, Strauss E. Primary total knee arthroplasty for complex distal femur fractures in elderly patients. Clin Orthop Relat Res. 2004;425:101–5.
18. Hart GP, Kneisl JS, Springer BD, Patt JC, Karunakar MA. Open reduction vs distal femoral replacement arthroplasty for comminuted distal femur fractures in the patients 70 years and older. J Arthroplast. 2017;32:202–6.
19. Bohm ER, Tufescu TV, Marsh JP. The operative management of osteoporotic fractures of the knee: to fix or replace? J Bone Joint Surg Br. 2012;94:1160–9.
20. Parratte S, Bonnevialle P, Pietu G, Saragaglia D, Cherrier B, Lafosse JM. Primary total knee arthroplasty in the management of epiphyseal fracture around the knee. Orthop Traumatol Surg Res. 2011;97:S87–94.
21. Kester BS, Minhas SV, Vigdorchik JM, Schwarzkopf R. Total knee arthroplasty for posttraumatic osteoarthritis: is it time for a new classification? J Arthroplast. 2016;31:1649–1653.e1.
22. Papadopoulos EC, Parvizi J, Lai CH, Lewallen DG. Total knee arthroplasty following prior distal femoral fracture. Knee. 2002;9:267–74.

Chapter 11
Post-traumatic Arthritis of the Proximal Tibia

Stefanie Hirsiger, Lukas Clerc, and Hermes H. Miozzari

> **Key Points**
> - Although tibial plateau fractures are not rare, symptomatic posttraumatic osteoarthritis is rather infrequent.
> - Stepwise treatment algorithms should be followed, starting with activity modification, weight loss and physiotherapy, followed by analgesic medication.
> - Existing literature concerning operative treatment options for posttraumatic osteoarthritis is mainly limited to small case series with little evidence.
> - Corrective osteotomies should be evaluated; if degenerative lesions are too advanced, unicondylar or total knee replacement can ameliorate function.

Introduction

Posttraumatic osteoarthritis (OA) occurring after tibial plateau fractures is more rarely encountered than primary OA. The overall disease burden of posttraumatic OA is estimated to be 12% of all symptomatic OA of the hip, knee, and ankle [1] with 1.2% incidence in the proximal tibia [2]. The last is mostly seen during the fifth decade and secondary to fall from heights or motor vehicle accidents [3]. The complexity of the fracture correlates to the bone quality and the mechanism of injury.

S. Hirsiger · L. Clerc · H. H. Miozzari (✉)
Division of Orthopaedic and Traumatology, Department of Surgery, Geneva University Hospitals, Faculty of Medicine, University of Geneva, Geneva, Switzerland
e-mail: lukas.clerc@hcuge.ch; hermes.miozzari@hcuge.ch

© Springer Nature Switzerland AG 2021
S. C. Thakkar, E. A. Hasenboehler (eds.), *Post-Traumatic Arthritis*,
https://doi.org/10.1007/978-3-030-50413-7_11

Despite several classification systems being available, such as Schatzker [4] or the AO [5], which are based on bony and intraarticular landmarks, none of them are complete or have a direct implication on the surgical treatment. Most tibial plateau fractures are treated operatively. There is only sparse literature defining clear criteria for the indication of surgical treatment. According to older literature, every medial unicondylar fracture (with any displacement) and every medially tilted bicondylar fracture should be operated as well as lateral plateau fractures with a lateral tilt or valgus malalignment exceeding 5°, a displacement with condylar widening of more than 5 mm, and step-offs greater than 3 mm [6]. A recent review found no consensus about the acceptance for any residual articular step-offs after reduction, but in comparison to other joints they seem relatively well tolerated [7]. Posterior fractures, present in about 29% of all Schatzker fracture types [8], are often missed with conventional radiographs; thus CT imaging is recommended for surgical planning [9]. More recently, a three-column concept for classification and fixation has been proposed [10]. The medial, lateral, and posterior columns are evaluated for intra- and extraarticular cortical disruption on 2D and 3D reconstructed CT images. In this updated concept the mechanism of injury is considered and evaluated by analyzing the position of the knee and the direction of the deforming forces at the time of injury: by defining the key articular surface, both the articular approach and hardware to be used can be planned before surgery [11]. The incidence of concomitant soft-tissue injuries has been found to be almost 100% when interpreting acute knee MRI [12]. Meniscal injuries are seen most frequently, followed closely by cruciate- or collateral ligament ruptures but also predating injuries such as asymptomatic meniscal changes with diffuse edema [12]. Unrecognized, chronic ligamentous instability without associate fracture is a major issue that can lead to symptomatic knee OA (Fig. 11.1) [13]. Further, untreated anterior ligament rupture shows associated secondary meniscal ruptures of up to 100% at 10 years [14]. Although there is no hard evidence that the surgical treatment of ligamentous instability can prevent developing symptomatic OA [15], meniscal and ligamentous injuries can lead to instability and persisting pain [16]. They should, therefore, be diagnosed and addressed during osteosynthesis, and an arthroscopically assisted approach might be helpful in these cases [17].

Injured soft tissues along with open wounds can lead to discontinuity of the cutaneous barrier, resulting in soft tissue infections and/or compartment syndrome. Thus, not only the bony and intraarticular damage but also the surrounding soft tissue status should be considered for surgical planning [18]. The optimal treatment of such complex injuries must be individualized, taking into account patients' factors, such as comorbidities, activity level, bone quality, and the presence of predating OA. Surgical options range from conservative treatment to closed/open fracture reduction with either internal or external fixation, or even primary prosthetic replacement in selected cases [19, 20].

Long-term outcomes after tibial plateau fractures are associated with the development of secondary OA. The initial injury and the extent of bony, cartilaginous and soft tissue destruction are crucial to determine the risk of future OA [21]. Indeed, the incidence of OA rises with the complexity of the fracture [22] and is further increased by secondary posttraumatic changes such as an altered limb axis, axis load distribution, or ligamentous instability [23, 24]. Smoking is an independent risk factor for a secondary conversion to a joint replacement procedure [25]. As of today, there is still no consensus in the literature of what is considered an acceptable residual postoperative deformity. However, a persistent postoperative valgus malalignment >5° and articular step-off of more than 2 mm have been shown to be risk factors for early OA and poor outcomes in older patients [23, 26] with degenerative changes appearing between 2 and 11 years after trauma (mean 7 years) and an incidence of posttraumatic OA, based on radiographies, reported between 25% and 45% [27]. Nevertheless, in retrospective analyses, the rate of symptomatic OA ranges only from 2% to 7.5% [24, 25, 28] with major reconstructive surgery needed in 4–7% at 10 years follow-up [27].

Recent developments in imaging allow the quantitative and qualitative evaluation of posttraumatic cartilage defects [29]. Genetic and environmental factors also play an important role in the development of posttraumatic OA [13].

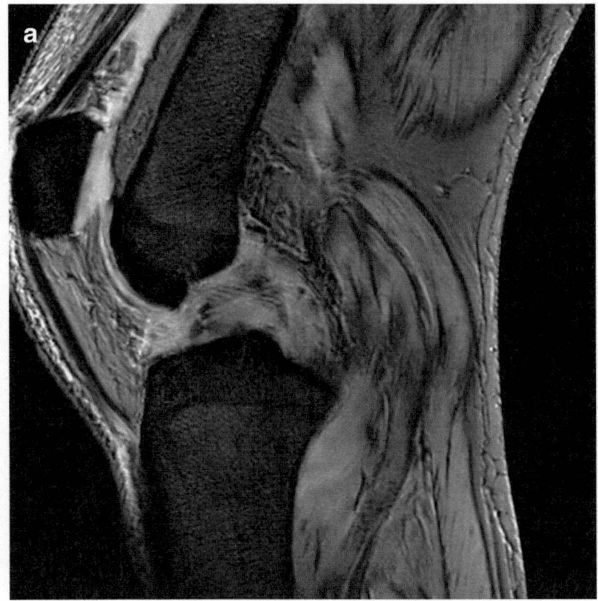

Fig. 11.1 60-year-old patient who sustained a stairway fall with concomitant ACL/PCL/MCL rupture and a nondisplaced fracture of the medial compartment (tibia and femur condyle). The patient presented after 5 months at our office; standard X-rays show a secondary OA mostly involving the medial compartment with joint space narrowing and bone loss, along with ACL and PCL laxity. (**a**) Initial MRI sagittal image: anterior and posterior cruciate rupture visible. (**b**) Long axes (**b**1) and knee anterior-posterior (**b**2) after 5 months showing subluxation and OA of the medial compartment with beginning tibial bone loss. (**c**) Stress X-rays: (**c**1) anterior and posterior drawer and (**c**2) varus and valgus stress. (**d**) Postop X-rays after a primary PS TKA anteroposterior (**d**1) and lateral (**d**2). The MCL and LCL were intact

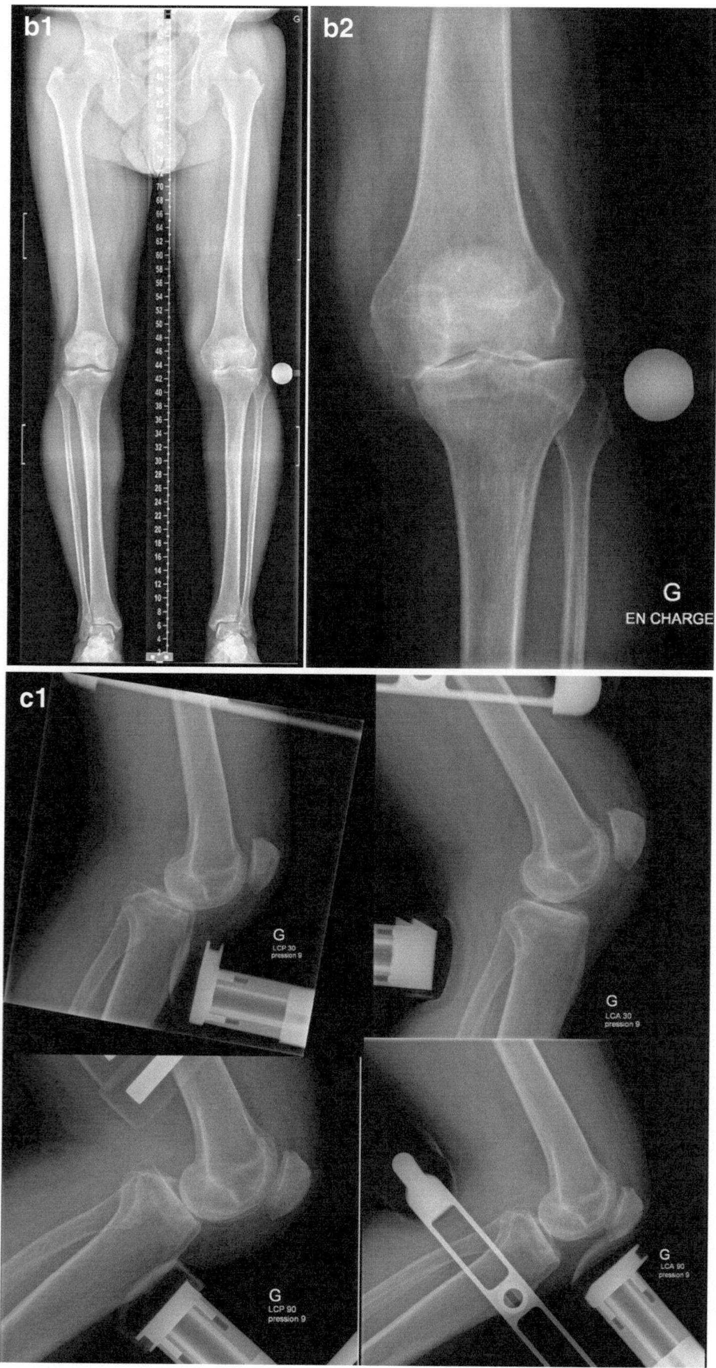

Fig. 11.1 (continued)

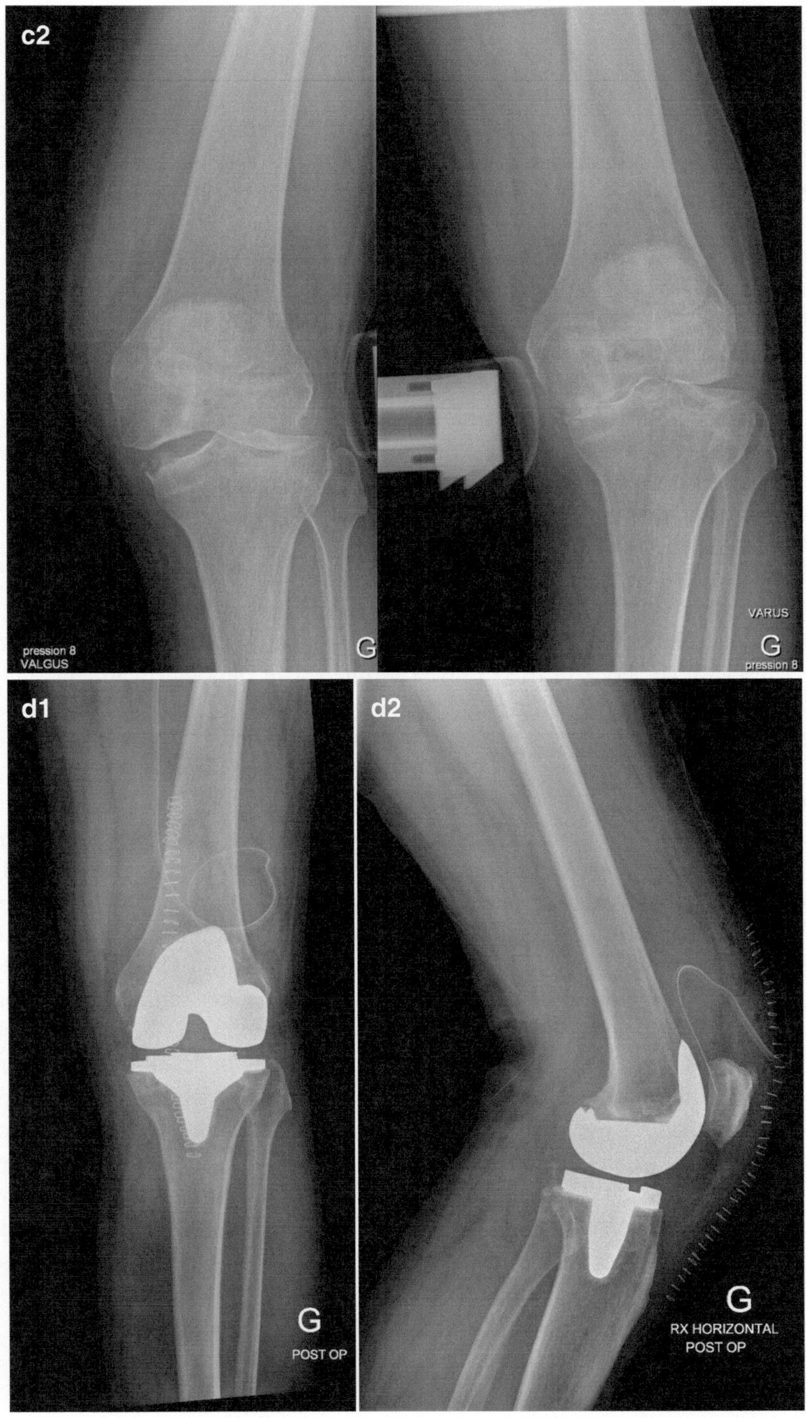

Fig. 11.1 (continued)

Conservative Treatment for Posttraumatic OA

A stepwise medical treatment is paramount in symptomatic knee OA, regardless of its origin. Recently, a consensus statement on the algorithm of the European Society for Clinical and Economic Aspects of Osteoporosis and Osteoarthritis (ESCEO) has been published [30]. Paracetamol (Acetaminophen), despite its minimal efficacy for OA symptoms, is still largely used due to its low cost and presumed safety, but, with higher dosage (>3 g/day), there is evidence of increased risk of upper gastrointestinal events, severe liver damage, loss of renal function, and increase in hypertension [30]. NSAIDs appear to be more effective, but comorbidities and risk of adverse effects have to be taken into account [31]. Topical NSAIDs seem to have an equivalent effect to oral NSAIDs for knee pain with fewer adverse events and 40% less need for concomitant oral administration. Therefore, they may be preferred for geriatric patients, patients at increased risk for gastrointestinal bleed, and those with cardiovascular or renal problems [30]. If NSAIDs are contraindicated, tramadol can be used to provide pain relief [32]. Despite weak evidence, chondroitin sulfate can lead to clinical improvement [33], and short-time beneficial effects of several weeks to months can be obtained with intraarticular infiltrations with corticosteroids [34]. Though widely used, intraarticular viscosupplementation does not provide sufficient evidence for benefit, and it is not recommended by the international osteoarthritis research society (IOARS) [35]. The interest in biologic treatment such as intraarticular platelet-rich plasma and mesenchymal stem cells (bone marrow-, adipose-, and amnion-derived) is growing, but a recent review of the published literature highlights the necessity for larger studies with a higher level of evidence and more standardized protocols [36]. The role of physiotherapy is still debated [37, 38] but seems to be moderately effective for improved function and, with some reservation, for pain [39]. Aquatic exercises may as well have small, short-term and clinically relevant effects on pain, disability and quality of life, though with moderate quality evidence [40]. Adapting activities is important, and there are a number of recreational activities of moderate intensity recommended for OA patients such as swimming, cycling, yoga, tai-chi, and walking. The latter, one of the simplest forms of exercise, has a positive effect on symptomatic knee OA [41], especially when associated with an intensive diet [42]. The role of running in developing knee OA is not clear [43], and some authors advocate a potential protective effect [44]. A prospective control study over two decades in middle- to older-aged long-distance runners could not show any evidence of accelerated OA [45]. In patients with painful OA, on the other hand, high intensity activities such as running, football, Nordic skiing, water skiing, handball, and basketball should be avoided [44]. Weight reduction can have a positive effect on pain and reduce disability in obese patients [46]. A recent study showed that high levels of synovial joint leptine may affect joint pain and might explain the association of pain with female gender and obesity, but the mechanism is not obvious and the causal relationship has yet to be proven [47].

Surgical Treatment for Posttraumatic OA

If conservative treatment proves insufficient to obtain an acceptable function and quality of life for the patient, the evaluation of a surgical treatment deems necessary.

No evidence for a beneficial effect was found for arthroscopic procedures and are, thus, not recommended [48]. Osteotomies can be used in order to diminish load on the degenerative compartment. Other options include osteochondral allografts and, as a last resort, partial or total knee arthroplasty (TKA) [25]. Surgery should be individually adapted; the options will be discussed subsequently.

Osteotomies

Correction osteotomies are a widely used treatment method to address early OA related to deformities of the leg axis and/or ligamentous instability [49]. This conservative technique allows good middle-term outcomes in a majority of patients delaying the time to total knee arthroplasty but is correlated to a relatively high rate of complications of up to 31% [50]. Preliminary results and operative technique of correction of intra- and extraarticular malunion after tibial plateau fractures have been described in case series [51–53]. The proposed intraarticular osteotomies aim at restoring joint anatomy and therefore stability, thus potentially slowing OA development. Knee OA combined with complex extraarticular deformities can be addressed by osteotomy and gradual computer-guided correction with a multiplanar external fixator such as the hexapod [54] (Fig. 11.2).

Osteochondral Allografts

Osteochondral allografts (OCA) could be a valuable alternative to prolong the prosthesis-free lifetime by preserving the joint. The survival of TKA is limited, indeed, especially in young and active patients, with a significantly higher failure within the first 2 years after implantation in the posttraumatic setting [55]. Still, reports about OCA to treat posttraumatic tibial OA remain sparse, showing good outcomes in active patients [56] and a clear improvement of postoperative function, which is also superior to microfracturing [57]. Kaplan-Meier survivorship analysis showed that the survival rate was 95% at 5 years, 80% at 10 years, 65% at 15 years, and 46% at 20 years [58]. Although almost half of the patient needed a conversion to TKA eventually, the mean time to conversion was 12 years [58].

Unicompartmental Knee Arthroplasty

Posttraumatic OA after tibial plateau fractures can be limited to one compartment. If symptomatic and in the absence of metaphyseal deformity, a correction osteotomy should not be considered, unless for a young patient, as it would add to the existing intraarticular pathology an extra axis deformity between the knee and the ankle joint line [59]. In this situation, a unicompartmental knee arthroplasty (UKA) might be considered. Although long-term-survival is lower and, thus, revision rates are potentially higher in UKA compared with total knee prosthesis (TKA) [60], faster rehabilitation, better knee kinematics, and lower complication rate [61] can be advantageous for both relatively young, active patients [62] and the elderly [63]. Since patients with posttraumatic OA needing surgery tend to be younger than for primary OA, this point is relevant [64]. The literature addressing the outcome in posttraumatic OA is sparse. In primary OA, 10 years survival of 95% has been reported for medial UKA [65, 66] and 92% for lateral, diminishing to 84% at 16 years [67]. Sah and Scott compared the results in a small series for lateral UKA used in posttraumatic (10 patients) versus primary OA (38 patients) [64, 68]. The Knee Society knee and function scores (KSS) were significantly lower in the posttraumatic group, with 74 and 65, respectively, versus 95 and 86 in the group for primary OA. More recently, Lustig et al. showed better results for a retrospective series of 13 lateral UKA in the posttraumatic setting, with implant survivorship of 100% at 5 and 10 years and 80% at 15 years along with function and pain relief comparable to primary OA with a KSS score of 89 and 87 for function [64]. We are not aware of studies comparing outcomes of UKA versus TKA for posttraumatic OA. Intraoperative conversion from a scheduled lateral UKA to TKA after evaluation of the neighbor compartments was reported in 52% of the patients [68]. For this reason, the authors advise the use of a medial parapatellar approach, and patients should be informed of a potential conversion to TKA for consent. Alternatively, a lateral parapatellar approach can be used and would easily allow a conversion to TKA.

Total Knee Arthroplasty

In advanced tricompartmental OA, when impairment of knee function and quality of life are important and conservative measures have failed, TKA can be indicated. Compared to a normal population, 10 years after tibial plateau fracture, patients are 5.3 times more likely to need a TKA [24]. The need increases with increasing age (per year over 48), bicondylar fracture pattern, and greater comorbidities [24]. Patients with instability or nonunion of the proximal tibia need TKA earlier than those with malunions (13.3 and 14 vs. 50 months), with a higher incidence of complications [69], such as wound problems, deep infection, patellar tendon avulsion, and reduced range of motion [1, 27]. Outcomes are further diminished in the

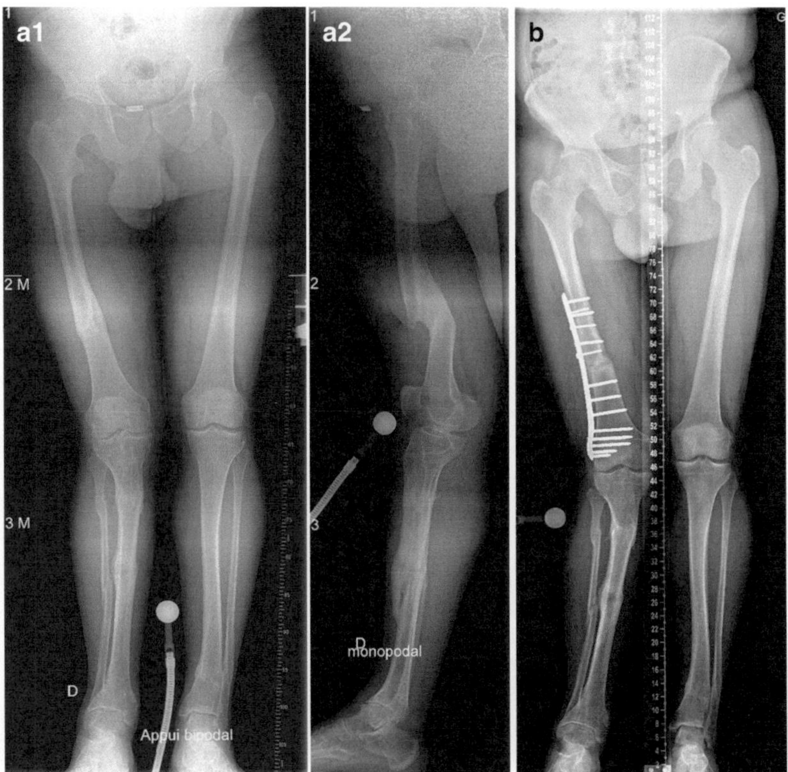

Fig. 11.2 46-year-old patient with a status post three motor vehicle accidents. At age 17 he sustained an open fracture (unknown open grade) of the right femoral diaphysis, treated with transtibial traction. At 18 he had an open fracture of the right tibia and fibula (unknown open grade) also treated nonoperatively. At the age of 43 he sustained a new open fracture Gustilo II of the right tibia and fibula, treated with intramedullary nail fixation despite the preexisting malunion. The fracture healed uneventfully, and the nail was removed after 2 years. The patient presented with worsening right knee pain 1 year later, corresponding to a symptomatic lateral OA with gait disturbance due to a complex valgus deformity of the lower right leg (shortening 5 cm, recurvatum 17°, valgus 11°, tibial slope 15°, external rotation 38°). Decision was made to perform a dual femoral and tibiofibula distraction osteotomy with computer-guided correction using multiplanar external fixator for the tibia and distraction nail for the femur. (**a**) Long leg axis showing the different deformities of the right side ap (**a1**) and sagittal plane (**a2**). (**b**) Long leg axis after corrective femoral osteotomy for a preexisting recurvatum malunion of 17°. A tibial osteotomy was made thereafter without complete correction of the deformity. (**c**) Status post removal of hardware, femur ap (**c1**) and lateral views (**c2**), tibia ap (**c3**), and lateral (**c4**) (**d**) Long leg axis (EOS) at 4 weeks after femoral osteotomy (deflexion, slight varisation, and lengthening) with retrograde expandable nail, and tibia/fibula osteotomy (varisation and translation and slight lengthening) and fixation with hexapod. (**e**) Long leg axis (EOS) after removal of the hexapod at 3.5 months, ap (**e1**) and lateral (**e2**) views. The whole axis has a slight residual valgus, the tibia has healed, and the callotaxis after femoral osteotomy is partially consolidated. (**f**) Long leg axis after healing of the femoral callotaxis before nail removal. The patient is still suffering from lateral OA but correction of the axis did improve the situation and arthroplasty has been delayed

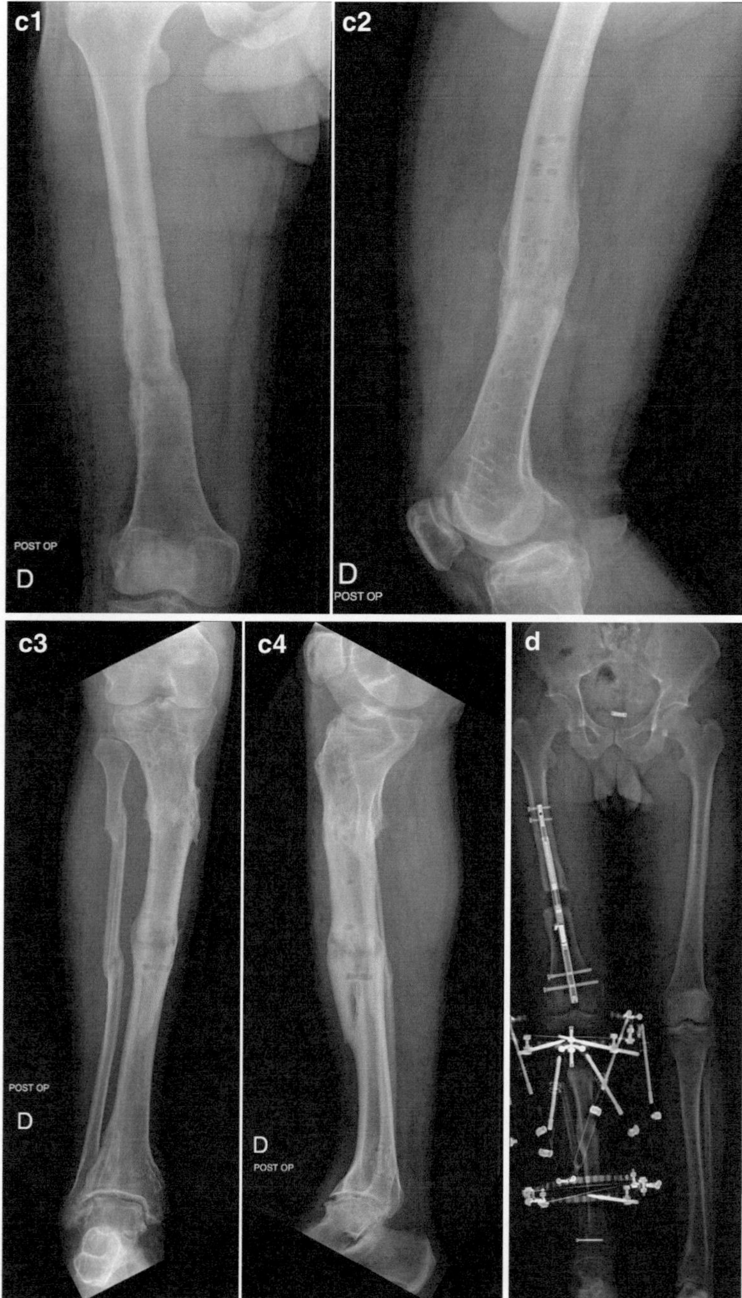

Fig. 11.2 (continued)

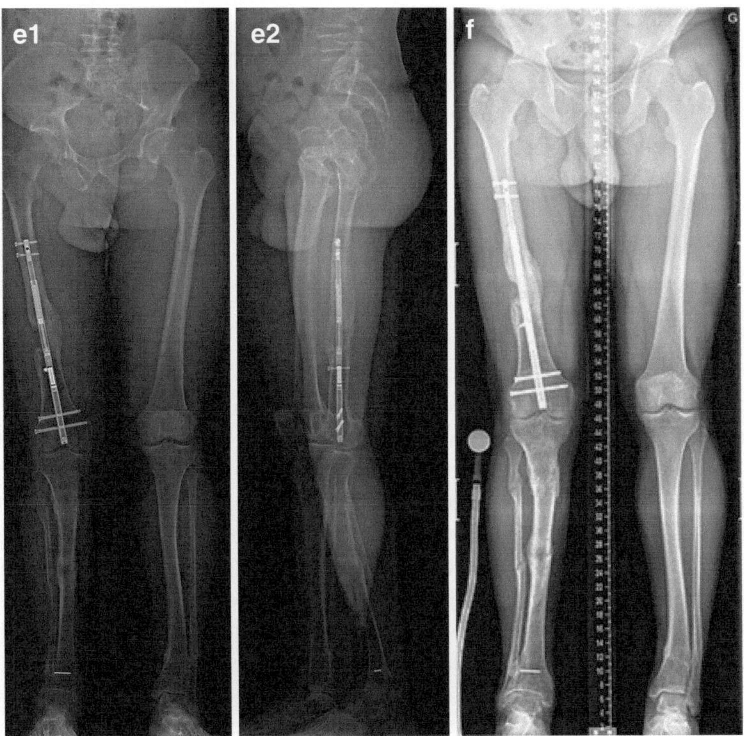

Fig. 11.2 (continued)

presence of combined secondary tibial and femoral deformities or soft tissue compromise [70], resulting in technically more demanding surgeries with extended operative time [71], increased length of stay, and 30-day readmission [72]. Abdel et al. reported a high rate of complications in TKA for posttraumatic OA (34%) compared to primary OA, 90% occurring within the first 2 years [73]. Houdek et al., in a larger retrospective cohort from the same institution, reported an overall revision-free survival of 78% at 15 and 20 years of follow-up with a significant risk for revision in patient aged 60 or less as well as patients with an infection, hematoma, deep vein thrombosis, or pulmonary embolism following arthroplasty [74]. Objective and subjective outcomes rely on sparse literature on (obviously) relatively small series, showing comparable KSS [73], Patient-Reported Outcome Measurements (PROMs), and satisfaction [69, 75]. In the existing studies, implants with different degrees of constraint have been used, from cruciate-retaining to hinge models with or without tibial augments and a long stem [20, 75–77]. Indeed, the type of prosthesis should be adapted to ligamentous stability, bone stock, and bone quality [78].

Primary TKA in the acute setting has been proposed in selected cases of complex fractures in osteoporotic bones of elderly patients; experiences are limited to small case series, but the results are promising [77, 79–82]. Of importance, autonomy in the elderly population is reduced after tibial plateau fractures even when TKA is done in first intention [83]. Additionally, age is an independent risk factor for mortality within 30 days after TKA [84].

Summary

In everyday practice, symptomatic knee OA secondary to tibial plateau fractures is relatively rare. Radiologic incidences varies between 25% and 45% with major reconstructive surgery reported to be needed in only 4–7% at 10 years follow-up [24, 27, 28]. Risk factors for the development of symptomatic OA are complexity of the fracture [22], concomitant intra- and extraarticular soft tissue injury [18], the age of the patient at the time of injury [23], persistent postoperative valgus malalignment >5°, and a persistent articular depression >2 mm [23] or ligamentous instability [24] as well as smoking [25]. When OA becomes symptomatic, a stepwise medical treatment is paramount [30] and activity modification should be addressed at first: moderate activities such as walking have a positive effect on symptomatic knee OA [41], whereas high-level activities should be avoided [44]. Weight reduction can reduce pain and thus improve disability in obese patients [46]. The role of physiotherapy and aquatic exercise is still debated, but given the few side effects, it is recommended [37–40]. Paracetamol (acetaminophen) is still widely used, even though symptom relief is minimal and side effects not infrequent [30], and NSAIDs appear to be more effective [31]. Given the equivalent effect of oral and topical NSAIDs applications, the latter should be preferred to reduce adverse events [30]. Intraarticular infiltrations with corticosteroids can temporarily reduce symptoms [34]. Chondroitin and tramadol can provide some pain relief [30, 32, 33]. When conservative treatment becomes insufficient, surgical treatment must be considered. Especially in young patients, a conservative, joint-preserving surgery should be prioritized whenever possible. Osteotomies have been described for the correction of intra- and extraarticular posttraumatic deformities [51–53]. If OA is too advanced and without extraarticular deformities, unilateral knee arthroplasty (UKA) can be an option. The revision rate is higher in UKA than in TKA [60], but faster rehabilitation, a better knee kinematics, and lower complication rates [61] can be advantageous especially for young, active patients [62]. Good results with implant survivorship of 100% at 5 and 10 years and 80% at 15 years, and good knee function are described [64, 68]. Fifty-two percent of conversions during surgery, from UKA to TKA, after evaluation of the neighbor compartments have been reported [68]. For severe, generalized OA, TKA is preferred. The type of implant constraint can range from cruciate-retaining to posterior-stabilized and up to hinge models with or without augments and a long stem, depending on ligamentous stability, bone stock, and bone quality [20, 75–78]. Compared to TKA for primary OA, the risk for complications is higher in the posttraumatic setting, and surgery is likely to be more complex [1, 27, 70, 71, 73]. Still, even if revision rates are higher [74], PROMs and patient satisfaction are comparable [69, 75]. Primary TKA in the acute fracture setting has been proposed in selected cases of complex fractures in osteoporotic bone of elderly patients, but experiences are limited to small case series [77, 79].

Despite injury prevention, future research should aim at reducing the development of postoperative OA. Sclerostin has been found to play a role in cartilage degeneration in mice [85, 86]. When applied intraarticularly or if upregulated transgenically, it plays a protective role, maintaining cartilage integrity, while its loss promotes osteoarthritis [85, 86]. If such approaches would prove to be safe and effective in humans, pain and functional impairment and, consequently, the need for arthroplasties could eventually be prevented by modification of the degenerative cascade.

Conflict of Interest All authors declare that they have no conflict of interest to disclose and have not received external funding.

Bibliography

1. Bala A, Penrose CT, Seyler TM, Mather RC 3rd, Wellman SS, Bolognesi MP. Outcomes after total knee arthroplasty for post-traumatic arthritis. Knee. 2015;22(6):630–9.
2. Court-Brown CM, Caesar B. Epidemiology of adult fractures: a review. Injury. 2006;37(8):691–7.
3. Albuquerque RP, Hara R, Prado J, Schiavo L, Giordano V, do Amaral NP. Epidemiological study on tibial plateau fractures at a level I trauma center. Acta Ortop Bras. 2013;21(2):109–15.
4. Schatzker J, McBroom R, Bruce D. The tibial plateau fracture. The Toronto experience 1968–1975. Clin Orthop Relat Res. 1979;(138):94–104.
5. Müller ME, Nazarian S, Koch P, Schatzker J. The comprehensive classification of fractures of long bones. Berlin: Springer Science & Business Media; 2012.
6. Honkonen SE. Indications for surgical treatment of tibial condyle fractures. Clin Orthop Relat Res. 1994;302:199–205.
7. Giannoudis PV, Tzioupis C, Papathanassopoulos A, Obakponovwe O, Roberts C. Articular step-off and risk of post-traumatic osteoarthritis. Evidence today. Injury. 2010;41(10):986–95.
8. Yang G, Zhai Q, Zhu Y, Sun H, Putnis S, Luo C. The incidence of posterior tibial plateau fracture: an investigation of 525 fractures by using a CT-based classification system. Arch Orthop Trauma Surg. 2013;133(7):929–34.
9. Chen HW, Chen CQ, Yi XH. Posterior tibial plateau fracture: a new treatment-oriented classification and surgical management. Int J Clin Exp Med. 2015;8(1):472–9.
10. Luo CF, Sun H, Zhang B, Zeng BF. Three-column fixation for complex tibial plateau fractures. J Orthop Trauma. 2010;24(11):683–92.
11. Wang Y, Luo C, Zhu Y, Zhai Q, Zhan Y, Qiu W, et al. Updated three-column concept in surgical treatment for tibial plateau fractures – a prospective cohort study of 287 patients. Injury. 2016;47(7):1488–96.
12. Gardner MJ, Yacoubian S, Geller D, Suk M, Mintz D, Potter H, et al. The incidence of soft tissue injury in operative tibial plateau fractures: a magnetic resonance imaging analysis of 103 patients. J Orthop Trauma. 2005;19(2):79–84.
13. Lohmander LS, Englund PM, Dahl LL, Roos EM. The long-term consequence of anterior cruciate ligament and meniscus injuries: osteoarthritis. Am J Sports Med. 2007;35(10):1756–69.

14. Keene GC, Bickerstaff D, Rae PJ, Paterson RS. The natural history of meniscal tears in anterior cruciate ligament insufficiency. Am J Sports Med. 1993;21(5):672–9.
15. Louboutin H, Debarge R, Richou J, Selmi TA, Donell ST, Neyret P, et al. Osteoarthritis in patients with anterior cruciate ligament rupture: a review of risk factors. Knee. 2009;16(4):239–44.
16. Delamarter RB, Hohl M, Hopp E Jr. Ligament injuries associated with tibial plateau fractures. Clin Orthop Relat Res. 1990;250:226–33.
17. Abdel-Hamid MZ, Chang CH, Chan YS, Lo YP, Huang JW, Hsu KY, et al. Arthroscopic evaluation of soft tissue injuries in tibial plateau fractures: retrospective analysis of 98 cases. Arthroscopy. 2006;22(6):669–75.
18. Borrelli J Jr. Management of soft tissue injuries associated with tibial plateau fractures. J Knee Surg. 2014;27(1):5–9.
19. Pape D, Hoffmann A, Gerich T, Van der Kerkhofe M, Weber M, Pape HC. Fractures of the knee joint in the elderly: osteosynthesis versus joint replacement. Orthopade. 2014;43(4):365–73.
20. Wilkes RA, Thomas WG, Ruddle A. Fracture and nonunion of the proximal tibia below an osteoarthritic knee: treatment by long stemmed total knee replacement. J Trauma. 1994;36(3):356–7.
21. Lotz MK, Kraus VB. New developments in osteoarthritis. Posttraumatic osteoarthritis: pathogenesis and pharmacological treatment options. Arthritis Res Ther. 2010;12(3):211.
22. Manidakis N, Dosani A, Dimitriou R, Stengel D, Matthews S, Giannoudis P. Tibial plateau fractures: functional outcome and incidence of osteoarthritis in 125 cases. Int Orthop. 2010;34(4):565–70.
23. Parkkinen M, Madanat R, Mustonen A, Koskinen SK, Paavola M, Lindahl J. Factors predicting the development of early osteoarthritis following lateral tibial plateau fractures: midterm clinical and radiographic outcomes of 73 operatively treated patients. Scand J Surg. 2014;103(4):256–62.
24. Wasserstein D, Henry P, Paterson JM, Kreder HJ, Jenkinson R. Risk of total knee arthroplasty after operatively treated tibial plateau fracture: a matched-population-based cohort study. J Bone Joint Surg Am. 2014;96(2):144–50.
25. Oladeji LO, Dreger TK, Pratte EL, Baumann CA, Stannard JP, Volgas DA, et al. Total knee arthroplasty versus osteochondral allograft: prevalence and risk factors following Tibial plateau fractures. J Knee Surg. 2019;32(4):380–6.
26. Rademakers MV, Kerkhoffs GM, Sierevelt IN, Raaymakers EL, Marti RK. Operative treatment of 109 tibial plateau fractures: five- to 27-year follow-up results. J Orthop Trauma. 2007;21(1):5–10.
27. Lizaur-Utrilla A, Collados-Maestre I, Miralles-Munoz FA, Lopez-Prats FA. Total knee arthroplasty for osteoarthritis secondary to fracture of the tibial plateau. A prospective matched cohort study. J Arthroplast. 2015;30(8):1328–32.
28. Mehin R, O'Brien P, Broekhuyse H, Blachut P, Guy P. Endstage arthritis following tibia plateau fractures: average 10-year follow-up. Can J Surg. 2012;55(2):87–94.
29. Eagle S, Potter HG, Koff MF. Morphologic and quantitative magnetic resonance imaging of knee articular cartilage for the assessment of post-traumatic osteoarthritis. J Orthop Res. 2017;35(3):412–23.
30. Bruyere O, Cooper C, Pelletier JP, Maheu E, Rannou F, Branco J, et al. A consensus statement on the European Society for Clinical and Economic Aspects of Osteoporosis and Osteoarthritis (ESCEO) algorithm for the management of knee osteoarthritis-from evidence-based medicine to the real-life setting. Semin Arthritis Rheum. 2016;45(4 Suppl):S3–11.
31. Towheed TE, Maxwell L, Judd MG, Catton M, Hochberg MC, Wells G. Acetaminophen for osteoarthritis. Cochrane Database Syst Rev. 2006;1:CD004257.
32. Cepeda MS, Camargo F, Zea C, Valencia L. Tramadol for osteoarthritis: a systematic review and metaanalysis. J Rheumatol. 2007;34(3):543–55.
33. Singh JA, Noorbaloochi S, MacDonald R, Maxwell LJ. Chondroitin for osteoarthritis. Cochrane Database Syst Rev. 2015;1:CD005614.

34. Juni P, Hari R, Rutjes AW, Fischer R, Silletta MG, Reichenbach S, et al. Intra-articular corticosteroid for knee osteoarthritis. Cochrane Database Syst Rev. 2015;10:CD005328.
35. Hunter DJ. Viscosupplementation for osteoarthritis of the knee. N Engl J Med. 2015;372(26):2570.
36. Delanois RE, Etcheson JI, Sodhi N, Henn RF, Gwam CU, George NE, et al. Biologic therapies for the treatment of knee osteoarthritis. J Arthroplast. 2019;34(4):801–13.
37. Bennell KL, Hinman RS, Metcalf BR, Buchbinder R, McConnell J, McColl G, et al. Efficacy of physiotherapy management of knee joint osteoarthritis: a randomised, double blind, placebo controlled trial. Ann Rheum Dis. 2005;64(6):906–12.
38. Fransen M, McConnell S, Harmer AR, Van der Esch M, Simic M, Bennell KL. Exercise for osteoarthritis of the knee: a Cochrane systematic review. Br J Sports Med. 2015;49(24):1554–7.
39. Salamh P, Cook C, Reiman MP, Sheets C. Treatment effectiveness and fidelity of manual therapy to the knee: a systematic review and meta-analysis. Musculoskeletal Care. 2016;15(3):238–48.
40. Bartels EM, Juhl CB, Christensen R, Hagen KB, Danneskiold-Samsoe B, Dagfinrud H, et al. Aquatic exercise for the treatment of knee and hip osteoarthritis. Cochrane Database Syst Rev. 2016;3:CD005523.
41. White DK, Keysor JJ, Neogi T, Felson DT, LaValley M, Gross KD, et al. When it hurts, a positive attitude may help: association of positive affect with daily walking in knee osteoarthritis. Results from a multicenter longitudinal cohort study. Arthritis Care Res (Hoboken). 2012;64(9):1312–9.
42. Messier SP, Mihalko SL, Legault C, Miller GD, Nicklas BJ, DeVita P, et al. Effects of intensive diet and exercise on knee joint loads, inflammation, and clinical outcomes among overweight and obese adults with knee osteoarthritis: the IDEA randomized clinical trial. JAMA. 2013;310(12):1263–73.
43. Timmins KA, Leech RD, Batt ME, Edwards KL. Running and knee osteoarthritis: a systematic review and meta-analysis. Am J Sports Med. 2016;45(6):1447–57.
44. Mobasheri A, Beatt M. An update on the pathophysiology of osteoarthritis. Ann Phys Rehabil Med. 2016;59(5–6):333–9.
45. Chakravarty EF, Hubert HB, Lingala VB, Zatarain E, Fries JF. Long distance running and knee osteoarthritis. A prospective study. Am J Prev Med. 2008;35(2):133–8.
46. Christensen R, Bartels EM, Astrup A, Bliddal H. Effect of weight reduction in obese patients diagnosed with knee osteoarthritis: a systematic review and meta-analysis. Ann Rheum Dis. 2007;66(4):433–9.
47. Lubbeke A, Finckh A, Puskas GJ, Suva D, Ladermann A, Bas S, et al. Do synovial leptin levels correlate with pain in end stage arthritis? Int Orthop. 2013;37(10):2071–9.
48. Thorlund JB, Juhl CB, Roos EM, Lohmander LS. Arthroscopic surgery for degenerative knee: systematic review and meta-analysis of benefits and harms. Br J Sports Med. 2015;49(19):1229–35.
49. Mehl J, Paul J, Feucht MJ, Bode G, Imhoff AB, Sudkamp NP, et al. ACL deficiency and varus osteoarthritis: high tibial osteotomy alone or combined with ACL reconstruction? Arch Orthop Trauma Surg. 2017;137(2):233–40.
50. Woodacre T, Ricketts M, Evans JT, Pavlou G, Schranz P, Hockings M, et al. Complications associated with opening wedge high tibial osteotomy--a review of the literature and of 15 years of experience. Knee. 2016;23(2):276–82.
51. Marti RK, Kerkhoffs GM, Rademakers MV. Correction of lateral tibial plateau depression and valgus malunion of the proximal tibia. Oper Orthop Traumatol. 2007;19(1):101–13.
52. Kerkhoffs GM, Rademakers MV, Altena M, Marti RK. Combined intra-articular and varus opening wedge osteotomy for lateral depression and valgus malunion of the proximal part of the tibia. J Bone Joint Surg Am. 2008;90(6):1252–7.
53. Frosch KH, Krause M, Frings J, Drenck T, Akoto R, Muller G, et al. Posttraumatic deformities of the knee joint : intra-articular osteotomy after malreduction of tibial head fractures. Unfallchirurg. 2016;119(10):859–76.

54. Hughes A, Parry M, Heidari N, Jackson M, Atkins R, Monsell F. Computer hexapod-assisted orthopaedic surgery for the correction of tibial deformities. J Orthop Trauma. 2016;30(7):e256–61.

55. Pitta M, Esposito CI, Li Z, Lee YY, Wright TM, Padgett DE. Failure after modern total knee arthroplasty: a prospective study of 18,065 knees. J Arthroplast. 2018;33(2):407–14.

56. Nuelle CW, Nuelle JA, Cook JL, Stannard JP. Patient factors, donor age, and graft storage duration affect osteochondral allograft outcomes in knees with or without comorbidities. J Knee Surg. 2017;30(2):179–84.

57. Gudas R, Gudaite A, Pocius A, Gudiene A, Cekanauskas E, Monastyreckiene E, et al. Ten-year follow-up of a prospective, randomized clinical study of mosaic osteochondral autologous transplantation versus microfracture for the treatment of osteochondral defects in the knee joint of athletes. Am J Sports Med. 2012;40(11):2499–508.

58. Shasha N, Krywulak S, Backstein D, Pressman A, Gross AE. Long-term follow-up of fresh tibial osteochondral allografts for failed tibial plateau fractures. J Bone Joint Surg Am. 2003;85-A(Suppl 2):33–9.

59. Holschen M, Lobenhoffer P. Complications of corrective osteotomies around the knee. Orthopade. 2016;45(1):13–23.

60. Niinimaki T, Eskelinen A, Makela K, Ohtonen P, Puhto AP, Remes V. Unicompartmental knee arthroplasty survivorship is lower than TKA survivorship: a 27-year Finnish registry study. Clin Orthop Relat Res. 2014;472(5):1496–501.

61. Brown NM, Sheth NP, Davis K, Berend ME, Lombardi AV, Berend KR, et al. Total knee arthroplasty has higher postoperative morbidity than unicompartmental knee arthroplasty: a multicenter analysis. J Arthroplast. 2012;27(8 Suppl):86–90.

62. Hopper GP, Leach WJ. Participation in sporting activities following knee replacement: total versus unicompartmental. Knee Surg Sports Traumatol Arthroscopy. 2008;16(10):973–9.

63. Siman H, Kamath AF, Carrillo N, Harmsen WS, Pagnano MW, Sierra RJ. Unicompartmental knee arthroplasty vs total knee arthroplasty for medial compartment arthritis in patients older than 75 years: comparable reoperation, revision, and complication rates. J Arthroplast. 2017;32(6):1792–7.

64. Lustig S, Parratte S, Magnussen RA, Argenson JN, Neyret P. Lateral unicompartmental knee arthroplasty relieves pain and improves function in posttraumatic osteoarthritis. Clin Orthop Relat Res. 2012;470(1):69–76.

65. Svard UC, Price AJ. Oxford medial unicompartmental knee arthroplasty. A survival analysis of an independent series. J Bone Joint Surg. 2001;83(2):191–4.

66. Berger RA, Meneghini RM, Jacobs JJ, Sheinkop MB, Della Valle CJ, Rosenberg AG, et al. Results of unicompartmental knee arthroplasty at a minimum of ten years of follow-up. J Bone Joint Surg Am. 2005;87(5):999–1006.

67. Argenson JN, Parratte S, Bertani A, Flecher X, Aubaniac JM. Long-term results with a lateral unicondylar replacement. Clin Orthop Relat Res. 2008;466(11):2686–93.

68. Sah AP, Scott RD. Lateral unicompartmental knee arthroplasty through a medial approach. Study with an average five-year follow-up. J Bone Joint Surg Am. 2007;89(9):1948–54.

69. Weiss NG, Parvizi J, Hanssen AD, Trousdale RT, Lewallen DG. Total knee arthroplasty in post-traumatic arthrosis of the knee. J Arthroplast. 2003;18(3 Suppl 1):23–6.

70. Shearer DW, Chow V, Bozic KJ, Liu J, Ries MD. The predictors of outcome in total knee arthroplasty for post-traumatic arthritis. Knee. 2013;20(6):432–6.

71. Dexel J, Beyer F, Lutzner C, Kleber C, Lutzner J. TKA for posttraumatic osteoarthritis is more complex and needs more surgical resources. Orthopedics. 2016;39(3 Suppl):S36–40.

72. Kester BS, Minhas SV, Vigdorchik JM, Schwarzkopf R. Total knee arthroplasty for posttraumatic osteoarthritis: is it time for a new classification? J Arthroplast. 2016;31(8):1649–53.. e1

73. Abdel MP, von Roth P, Cross WW, Berry DJ, Trousdale RT, Lewallen DG. Total knee arthroplasty in patients with a prior tibial plateau fracture: a long-term report at 15 years. J Arthroplast. 2015;30(12):2170–2.

74. Houdek MT, Watts CD, Shannon SF, Wagner ER, Sems SA, Sierra RJ. Posttraumatic total knee arthroplasty continues to have worse outcome than total knee arthroplasty for osteoarthritis. J Arthroplast. 2016;31(1):118–23.
75. Scott CE, Davidson E, MacDonald DJ, White TO, Keating JF. Total knee arthroplasty following tibial plateau fracture: a matched cohort study. Bone Joint J. 2015;97-B(4):532–8.
76. Lonner JH, Pedlow FX, Siliski JM. Total knee arthroplasty for post-traumatic arthrosis. J Arthroplast. 1999;14(8):969–75.
77. Nau T, Pflegerl E, Erhart J, Vecsei V. Primary total knee arthroplasty for periarticular fractures. J Arthroplast. 2003;18(8):968–71.
78. Bedi A, Haidukewych GJ. Management of the posttraumatic arthritic knee. J Am Acad Orthop Surg. 2009;17(2):88–101.
79. Nourissat G, Hoffman E, Hemon C, Rillardon L, Guigui P, Sautet A. Total knee arthroplasty for recent severe fracture of the proximal tibial epiphysis in the elderly subject. Rev Chir Orthop Reparatrice Appar Mot. 2006;92(3):242–7.
80. Parratte S, Bonnevialle P, Pietu G, Saragaglia D, Cherrier B, Lafosse JM. Primary total knee arthroplasty in the management of epiphyseal fracture around the knee. Orthop Traumatol Surg Res. 2011;97(6 Suppl):S87–94.
81. Malviya A, Reed MR, Partington PF. Acute primary total knee arthroplasty for peri-articular knee fractures in patients over 65 years of age. Injury. 2011;42(11):1368–71.
82. Vermeire J, Scheerlinck T. Early primary total knee replacement for complex proximal tibia fractures in elderly and osteoarthritic patients. Acta Orthop Belg. 2010;76(6):785–93.
83. Boureau F, Benad K, Putman S, Dereudre G, Kern G, Chantelot C. Does primary total knee arthroplasty for acute knee joint fracture maintain autonomy in the elderly? A retrospective study of 21 cases. Orthop Traumatol Surg Res. 2015;101(8):947–51.
84. Belmont PJ Jr, Goodman GP, Waterman BR, Bader JO, Schoenfeld AJ. Thirty-day postoperative complications and mortality following total knee arthroplasty: incidence and risk factors among a national sample of 15,321 patients. J Bone Joint Surg Am. 2014;96(1):20–6.
85. Wu J, Ma L, Wu L, Jin Q. Wnt-beta-catenin signaling pathway inhibition by sclerostin may protect against degradation in healthy but not osteoarthritic cartilage. Mol Med Rep. 2017;15(5):2423–32.
86. Bouaziz W, Funck-Brentano T, Lin H, Marty C, Ea HK, Hay E, et al. Loss of sclerostin promotes osteoarthritis in mice via beta-catenin-dependent and -independent Wnt pathways. Arthritis Res Ther. 2015;17:24.

Chapter 12
Post-traumatic Arthritis of the Ankle

Nigel N. Hsu and Lew Schon

> **Key Points**
> - The ankle joint is more susceptible to posttraumatic arthritis than the hip or the knee joint.
> - Ankle biomechanics play a major role in posttraumatic arthritis.
> - Weight-bearing CT scans are new imaging modalities to help with the diagnosis and management of posttraumatic ankle arthritis.
> - The mainstay of surgical treatment is total ankle arthroplasty and ankle arthrodesis.

Introduction

Posttraumatic osteoarthritis accounts for 12% of arthritis across all joints, which represents 5.6 million people, and cost the US health care 3.06 billion dollars annually [1]. For the ankle joint, posttraumatic arthritis is the primary cause of arthritis accounting for 70–79.5% of ankle arthritis [1, 2] compared to 1.6% in the hip and 9.8% in the knee. This variation is due to the mechanical, biochemical, and anatomical factors of the ankle. Although the prevalence of ankle osteoarthritis is about 9 times lower than that of the knee and hip [3], in 2010, approximately 4400 total ankle replacements and 25,000 ankle fusions were performed in the United States [4]. Fifty percent of elderly patients have some form of arthrosis of the foot or ankle [5].

N. N. Hsu (✉)
Department of Orthopaedic Surgery, Johns Hopkins University, Baltimore, MD, USA
e-mail: Nhsu4@jhmi.edu

L. Schon
Department of Orthopaedic Surgery, Mercy Medical Center, Baltimore, MD, USA

© Springer Nature Switzerland AG 2021
S. C. Thakkar, E. A. Hasenboehler (eds.), *Post-Traumatic Arthritis*,
https://doi.org/10.1007/978-3-030-50413-7_12

In this chapter, we will examine the pathophysiology and biomechanics of posttraumatic ankle arthritis and review indications and nonoperative and operative treatment options.

Anatomy

Primary osteoarthritis of the ankle is less common compared to the knee and hip due to its anatomy and biochemical factors. The bony anatomy of the ankle joint confers a high degree of stability and congruence when the joint is loaded [6]. The bony anatomy, ligaments, and joint capsule guide and restrain movement between the talus and the mortise. There is minimal translation of the talus relative to the mortise during normal motion due to the soft tissue around the ankle.

Although the ankle has a smaller area of contact between articular surfaces compared to the hip and knee (350 mm^2 at 500 N of load compared to 1100 mm^2 for the hip and 1120 mm^2 for the knee) [7–9], the tensile fracture stress and tensile stiffness of ankle articular cartilage deteriorate less rapidly with age than those of the hip [10]. The articular cartilage of the ankle is 1–2 mm compared to the articular cartilage in the hip and knee, which is 3–6 mm [11, 12]. The metabolism of cartilage degradation is also different between the ankle and that of the knee. The catabolic cytokine interleukin-1 (IL-1) inhibits proteoglycan synthesis of chondrocytes more in the knee than the ankle, and this is in part due to fewer IL-1 receptors in the ankle articular chondrocyte [3].

The high peak contact stress from smaller contact area, the congruency of the joint, and thinness of ankle articular cartilage make the ankle joint more susceptible to posttraumatic osteoarthritis than the hip and knee. Injuries that damage the joint congruency and articular cartilage lead to joint degeneration within 2 years of injury [6]. Newer studies have found that posttraumatic osteoarthritis can occur after ankle fracture despite anatomic reduction [13], and early inflammatory response could lead to irreversible damage to the cartilage [14]. The synovial fluid analysis showed that after intraarticular ankle fracture, there is a proinflammatory and extracellular matrix degrading environment similar to that described in idiopathic osteoarthritis. Specifically IL-6, IL-8, MMP-1, MMP-2, MMP-3, MMP-9, and MMP-10 were significantly elevated compared to normal synovial fluid [15].

Epidemiology

Trauma and abnormal ankle biomechanics are the most common causes of degenerative changes [16]. Traumatic injuries of the ankle include malleolar fractures, pilon fracture, talus fracture, fracture dislocations, osteochondritis dessicans, ankle sprains, and instability. The most common causes of posttraumatic ankle arthritis are rotational ankle fractures (37%), recurrent ankle instability (14.6%), and single sprain with continued pain (13.7%) [2]. The severity of ankle fractures is correlated to the development of posttraumatic ankle arthritis. Lindsjo reported that the prevalence of ankle arthritis is 14% after ankle fractures and ranges from 4% in Weber A to 33% in Weber C fractures [17]. Pilon fracture of the tibial plafond is a high-energy injury that causes significant morbidity. Posttraumatic osteoarthritis after pilon fracture is 26.6% [18]. Talus fracture is associated with both subtalar and tibiotalar posttraumatic osteoarthritis. The rate of arthritis after talar fracture is 47–97% [19].

Patient Evaluation

History and physical examination are essential in diagnosing posttraumatic osteoarthritis. Determining a history of trauma such as a fracture, ankle sprain, or instability episode can help with diagnosing posttraumatic osteoarthritis of the ankle. Careful examination of the ankle in sitting, standing, and walking is helpful. Examine the range of motion, stability of the soft tissue, and alignment, and deformity of the foot and ankle should be evaluated as well as gait to see the effects of proximal or distal pathology. Plain weight-bearing radiographs of the ankle should be obtained. The hindfoot alignment view is important to evaluate the hindfoot deformity. Computed tomography (CT) can be useful to assess bony issues such as malalignments, cysts, malunions, and nonunions. Magnetic resonance imaging (MRI) is useful for evaluating cartilage, adjacent joint arthritis, ligamentous injuries, and tendon pathology, which may also affect an ankle that is arthritic. Weight-bearing CT is a newer modality that allows us to evaluate the true bone positions in their loaded state to see the effects of cysts, malunions, and nonunions, or to maximize preoperative planning for osteotomies, fusions, or joint replacements.

Conservative Treatment

Nonoperative treatments for posttraumatic ankle arthritis or end-stage arthritis include nonsteroidal antiinflammatory drugs (NSAIDs), injections, use of cane, and orthotics. Injection options include corticosteroids, hyaluronic acid (HA), and platelet-rich plasma (PRP). Steroid injections can provide short-term relief, but repeat injections should be avoided due to catabolic risks to the soft tissue. Low quality studies have shown some improvement in pain and functional scores with hyaluronic acid injections for ankle osteoarthritis [20] although the Cochran review in 2015 states that it is unclear if there is benefit or harm for HA as a treatment for ankle osteoarthritis based on the current evidence [21]. There are a few studies that examined PRP injections for ankle osteoarthritis. Angthong et al. had a series of 5 patients with improvement in functional scores at mean follow-up of 16 months for ankle osteoarthritis [22]. Mei-Dan et al. compared PRP injection to HA in a randomized controlled trial of 30 patients with talar osteochondral lesions and reported improved pain and function in the PRP group [23]. Bone marrow aspirate concentrate (BMAC) injection is also being investigated as an option for ankle arthritis as an isolated treatment or in conjunction with surgical treatment [24]. A cane can unload the joint mechanically. A custom molded ankle-foot orthosis (AFO) that is molded to the calf muscle can unload the ankle. A rigid leather ankle lacer with a solid ankle cushion heel (SACH) and a rocker sole can limit ankle motion and help with pain relief.

Operative Treatment

The goal of surgical management of posttraumatic ankle arthritis is to improve pain, function, and restore alignment. The main surgical options include total ankle arthroplasty (TAA) and ankle arthrodesis (AA). In the last 20 years, we have seen other alternatives that include arthroscopic debridement, allograft transplantation, bipolar fresh total osteochondral allograft, periankle osteotomy, and distraction arthroplasty.

Posttraumatic ankle arthritis is the most common indication for ankle arthrodesis [25]. It is also an option as primary salvage following pilon fracture. It provides reliable pain relief with relatively low reoperation rates. The optimal position for fusion is neutral dorsiflexion, 5 degrees of hindfoot valgus, external rotation comparable to the contralateral side, and the anterior dome of the talus brought to anterior tibia [26]. Fusion can be achieved with open arthrodesis or arthroscopic arthrodesis, and internal fixation with screw or plate vs. external fixation can be used. Figure 12.1 shows preoperative and postoperative radiographs of a patient who underwent ankle arthrodesis for posttraumatic ankle arthritis with valgus deformity. The disadvantages of ankle arthrodesis include loss of ankle motion, decreased gait efficiency, and adjacent joint arthrosis [27]. Coester et al. reported 22-year follow-up in 23 patients who underwent ankle fusion for posttraumatic arthritis and found increased adjacent joint arthritis compared to the contralateral side [28]. Arthroscopic ankle arthrodesis is a good option for patients with limited angular deformities. O'Brien et al. compared arthroscopic to open ankle arthrodesis and found similar fusion rates with significantly less morbidity, shorter operative and tourniquet time, less blood loss, and shorter hospital stay [29]. Winson reported 71% excellent and good outcome in 116 patients who underwent arthroscopic ankle arthrodesis [30].

Total ankle arthroplasty was introduced in the 1970s, and early results were disappointing with a high rate of failure [31]. This was attributed to poor implant design, loosening, and instability [32]. Since then, the development of newer generation of total ankle implants with semiconstrained, cementless design with mobile and fixed bearing has become more popular [33]. The potential benefits of TAA is restoration of ankle kinematics and preventing adjacent joint arthritis. Figure 12.2 shows preoperative and postoperative radiographs of a patient who underwent a total ankle arthroplasty for posttraumatic ankle arthritis. Haddad et al. performed a

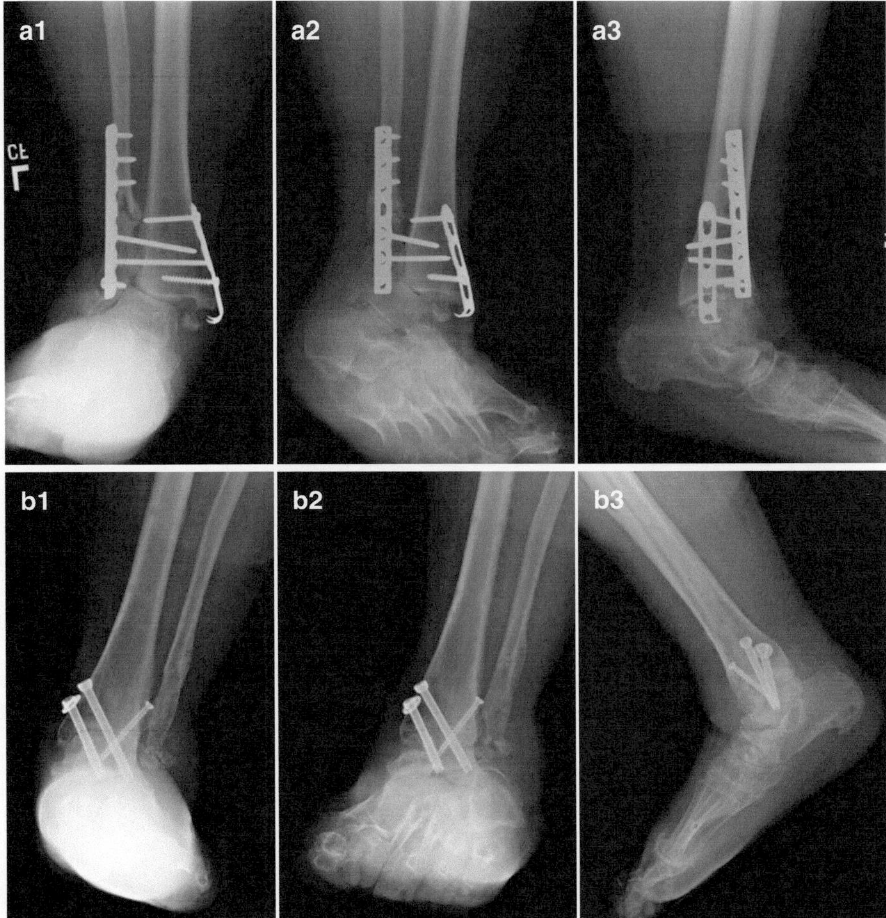

Fig. 12.1 (**a**) Shows the preoperative AP, oblique, and lateral radiographs of a patient with bimalleolar ankle fracture who developed posttraumatic ankle arthritis with collapse of the talus and valgus deformity. (**b**) Shows the postoperative AP, oblique, and lateral radiographs after treatment with removal of hardware and ankle arthrodesis

metaanalysis of the available outcome studies in 2007 that included 852 patients who underwent total ankle arthroplasty with second-generation implants and found 68% of excellent and good results [34]. The 5-year and 10-year implant survival rates were 78% and 77% with 7% revision rate [34]. A multicenter prospective non-randomized trial comparing Scandinavian Total Ankle Replacement (STAR) to ankle fusion in 593 patients showed that by 24 months, TAA had better function and equivalent pain relief as the fusion group [35]. Another multicenter prospective trail in Canada comparing 281 TAA and 107 AA in 5.5 year follow-up reported similar improvement in pain and function, but there was a higher major complication rate (19% vs. 7%) and higher revision rate (17% vs. 7%) in ankles treated with TAA vs.

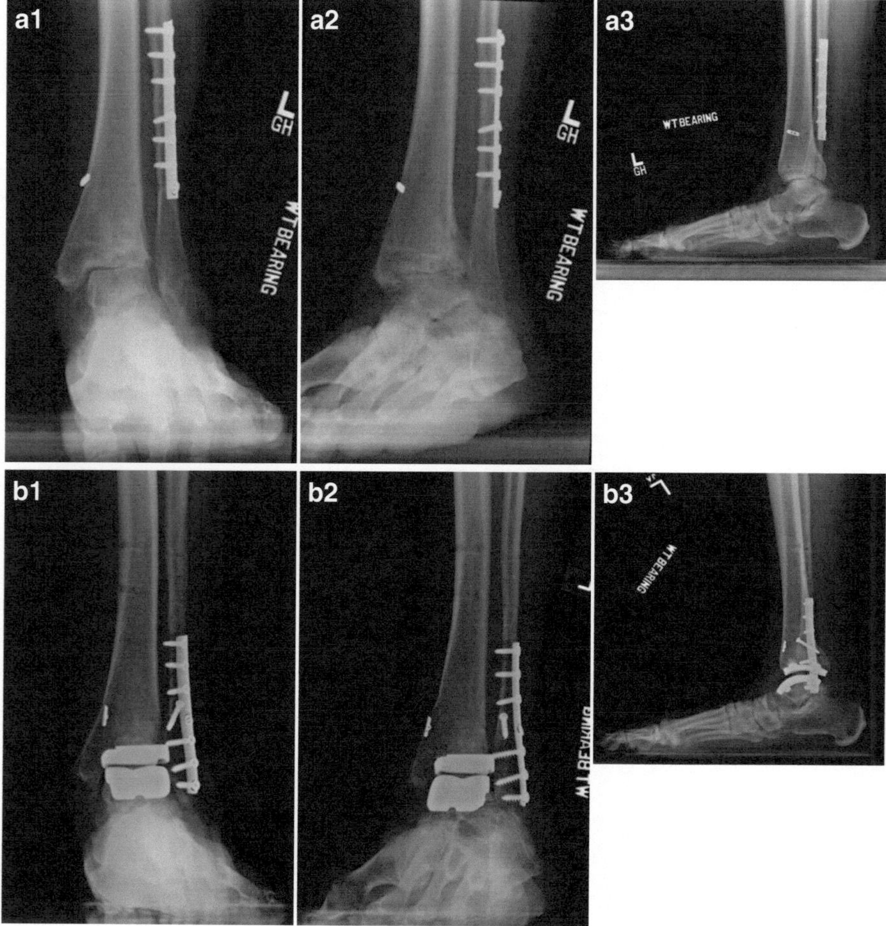

Fig. 12.2 (**a**) Shows the preoperative AP, oblique, and lateral radiographs of a patient with a lateral malleolar ankle fracture with syndesmosis injury status post ORIF and tightrope fixation who developed posttraumatic ankle arthritis. (**b**) Shows the postoperative AP, oblique, and lateral radiographs after treatment with transfibular total ankle arthroplasty

AA [36]. A new total ankle coinvented by the senior author was introduced in the USA 4.5 years ago. The design allows for conservation of bone stock, coronal plane orientation of the rails, porous tantalum surfaces, and highly crosslinked polyethylene. A fibular osteotomy is performed for full joint exposure with preservation of the deep deltoid. This osteotomy allows for correction of sagittal and coronal plane deformities. Of the 105 performed by the senior author, 80% had deformity correction of the tibia, talus, and fibula. Early results are promising with no fibular nonunion, malunion, or implant failure after 12 -months follow-up [37].

In patients with posttraumatic impingement syndrome, ankle arthroscopic debridement can be considered [38]. Arnold reported 81% good or excellent outcome with ankle arthroscopy with resection of hypertrophic synovium, fibrous bands, or tibial spurs after an ankle sprain. The poor outcomes were associated with severe chondral lesions found during arthroscopy. Rasmussen reported 62% pain free 2 years after arthroscopic debridement for impingement, and 27% had pain improvement [39].

In cases of patients with localized articular cartilage defects, allograft transplantation can be considered. It is performed with anatomically matched fresh allograft harvested within 24 hours of death and removal of bacteria, blood, and lipids. Hahn et al. reported significant improvement in pain and functional scores in 18 patients who underwent allograft transplantation for osteochondral lesions of the talar dome [40].

Severe posttraumatic ankle arthritis in young and active patients poses a reconstructive challenge and bipolar fresh total osteochondral allograft (BFTOA) may be an alternative to arthrodesis and total ankle replacement [41]. Figure 12.3 shows intraoperative pictures and postoperative radiographs of a patient who underwent bipolar fresh total osteochondral allograft. Giannini et al. reported improvement in functional scores at 40.9-months follow-up in 26 patients who underwent BFTOA for posttraumatic arthritis. Six out of the 26 patients had failure associated with malalignment of the tibial slope. Bugbee et al. reported 83% improved pain and function in 88 patients who underwent BFTOA at 5.3-year follow-up although 29% required another operation [42].

Supramalleolar osteotomy is an option for patients with varus or valgus ankle arthritis. The goal is to correct the ankle alignment for improved joint loading while preserving the ankle joint [43]. Medial opening wedge osteotomy is used to correct incongruent varus arthritis, and medial closing wedge osteotomy is used for valgus ankle arthritis [43]. Figure 12.4 shows preoperative and postoperative radiographs of a patient who underwent medial opening wedge osteotomy for ankle arthritis with varus deformity. Takakura et al. reported improved pain and function in 9 patients who underwent tibial osteotomy for varus ankle arthritis at 7-year follow-up [44]. Pagenstert et al. reported improved pain and function in 22 patients who underwent osteotomy for valgus ankle arthritis with 4.5-year follow-up [45]. Knupp et al. reported statistical significant improvement in functional scores in 92 patients who underwent osteotomy for varus or valgus ankle arthritis at 43-months follow-up [46].

In young and active patients with posttraumatic ankle osteoarthritis, ankle distraction is another option to preserve the joint. This technique involves external fixator with or without a hinge, and progressive distraction for 3 months while weight bearing. The theory is that by removing the mechanical stress, the cartilage can repair itself [47]. Figure 12.5 shows preoperative and postoperative radiographs of a patient who underwent ankle distraction arthroplasty. Tellisi et al. reported significant pain and functional improvement in 91% of patients who underwent ankle distraction in 25 patients with ankle arthritis at follow-up of 30 months [48]. Nguyen et al. reported intermediate-term follow-up of 36 patients who underwent ankle distraction for end-stage ankle arthritis, and 45% underwent subsequent ankle arthrodesis or total ankle arthroplasty due to pain [49].

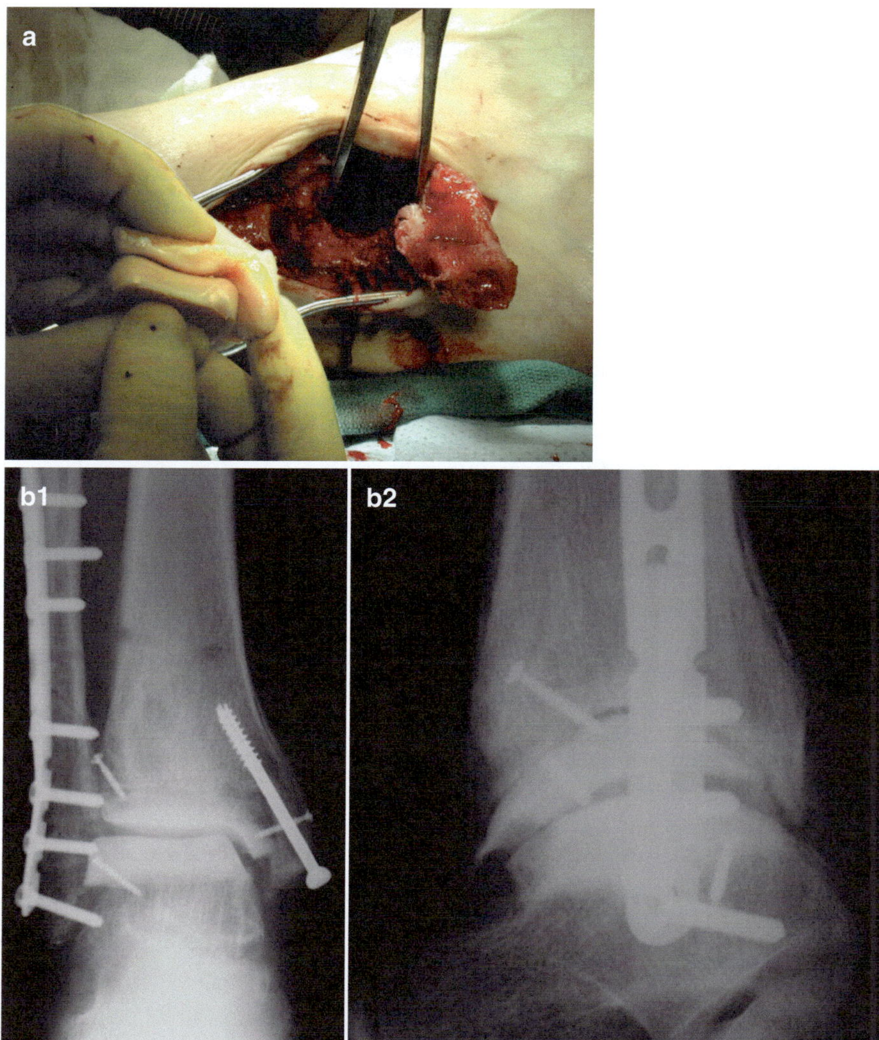

Fig. 12.3 (**a**) Shows an intraoperative photograph of the fresh allograft of the talar dome and tibial plafond prior to implantation. (**b**) Show AP and lateral postoperative radiographs of a patient with posttraumatic ankle osteoarthritis treated with bipolar fresh total osteochondral allograft. Note the small screw fixation in the tibia and talus

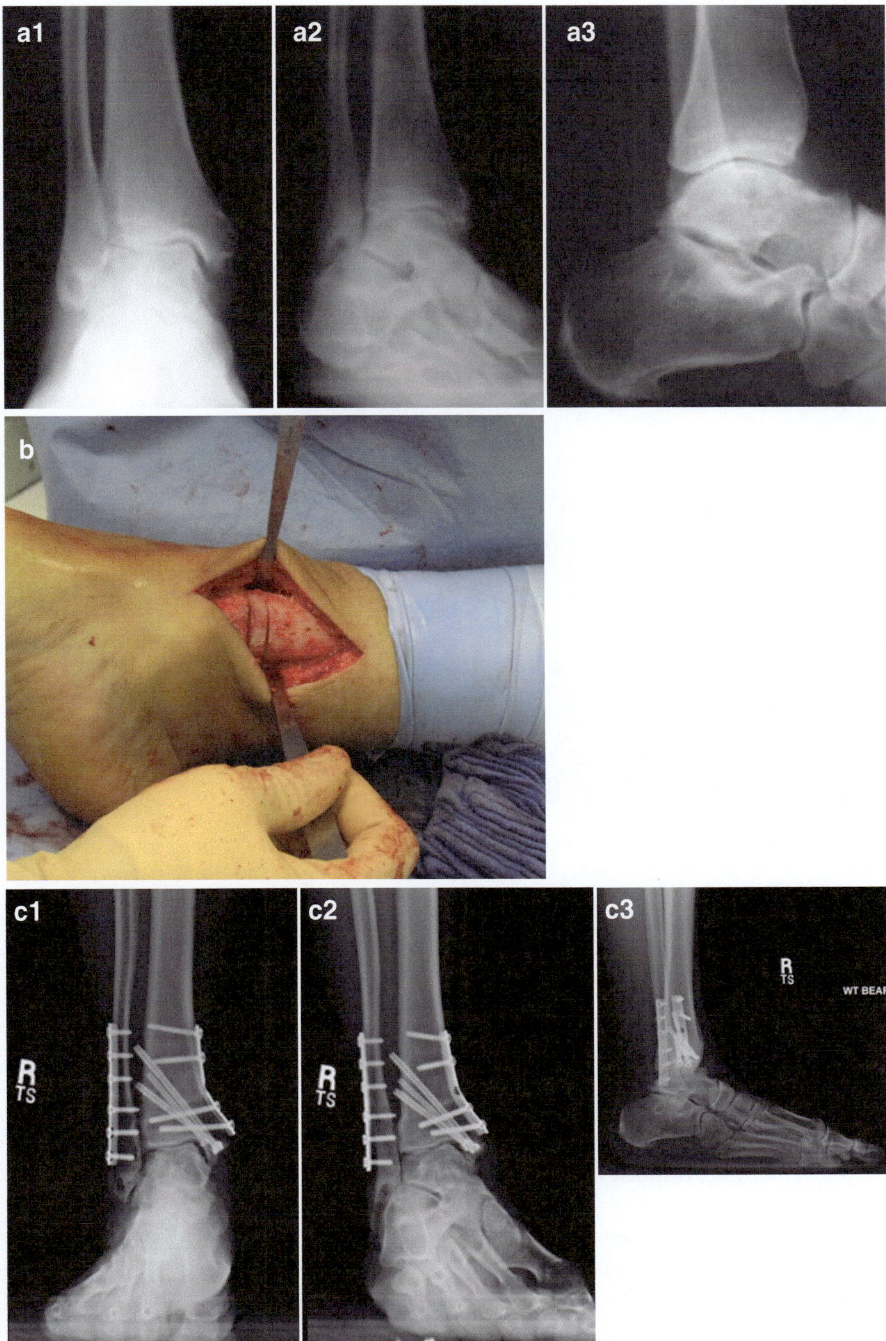

Fig. 12.4 (**a**) Show the preoperative AP, oblique, and lateral radiographs of a patient with varus deformity ankle arthritis treated with medial opening wedge osteotomy. (**b**) Shows the intraoperative image of the medial ankle with an allograft wedge. (**c**) Show the postoperative AP, oblique, and lateral radiographs demonstrating restored alignment

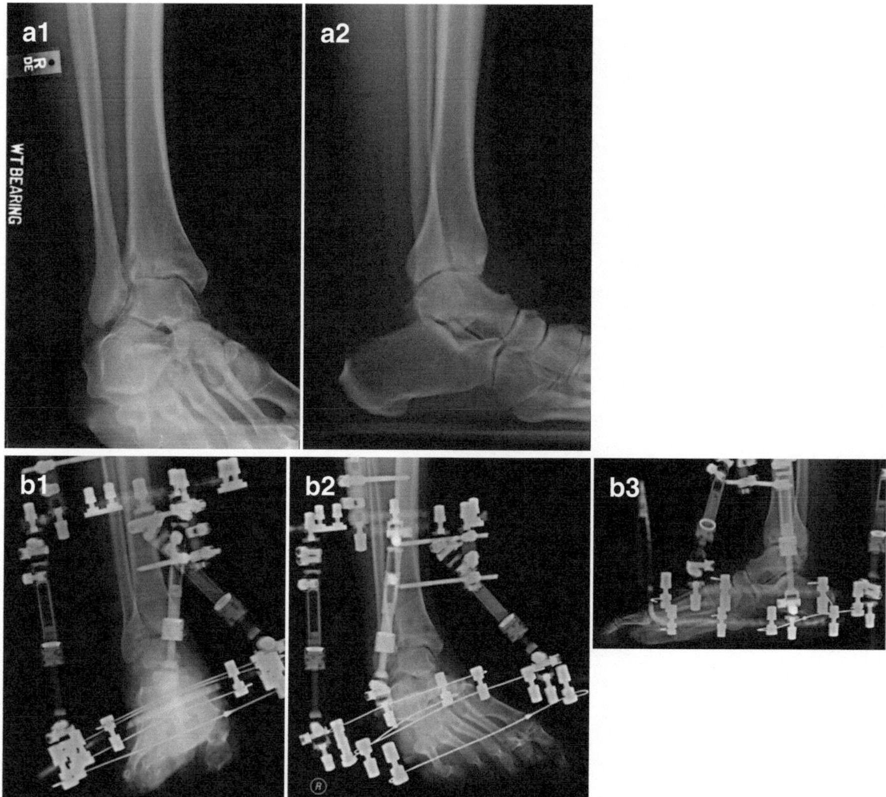

Fig. 12.5 (a) Shows the preoperative oblique and lateral radiographs of a young patient with post-traumatic ankle arthritis. (b) Shows the postoperative AP, oblique, and lateral radiographs after distraction arthroplasty with an external fixator that allows for ankle range of motion

Summary

Post-traumatic arthritis is the primary cause of arthritis in the ankle. It disproportionately affects younger individuals and athletes. Inflammatory events at the time of injury with release of cytokines can lead to irreversible damage to the cartilage. Nonoperative treatments for posttraumatic ankle arthritis include NSAIDs, corticosteroid injections, orthotics and bracing. Surgical treatment is based on the ankle alignment and severity of the arthritis. Primary surgical treatments for end stage ankle arthritis include total ankle arthroplasty and ankle arthrodesis. The literature supports both ankle arthrodesis and total ankle arthroplasty. Other treatment options include arthroscopic debridement, allograft transplantation, bipolar fresh total osteochondral allograft, supramalleolar osteotomy, and distraction arthroplasty. Patient specific factors such as medical comorbidities, malalignment, adjacent joint pathology, age and activity levels are important considerations when selecting the surgical treatment.

References

1. Brown TD, Johnston RC, Saltzman CL, Marsh JL, Buckwalter JA. Posttraumatic osteoarthritis: a first estimate of incidence, prevalence, and burden of disease. J Orthop Trauma. 2006;20(10):739–44.
2. Saltzman CL, Salamon ML, Blanchard GM, et al. Epidemiology of ankle arthritis: report of a consecutive series of 639 patients from a tertiary orthopaedic center. Iowa Orthop J. 2005;25:44–6.
3. Huch K, Kuettner KE, Dieppe P. Osteoarthritis in ankle and knee joints. Semin Arthritis Rheum. 1997;26(4):667–74.
4. Terrell RD, Montgomery SR, Pannell WC, et al. Comparison of practice patterns in total ankle replacement and ankle fusion in the United States. Foot Ankle Int. 2013;34(11):1486–92. LOE: This level IV cross-sectional study examined CPT codes for total ankle replacement and ankle arthrodesis were searched through the PearlDiver Patient Record Database from 2004 to 2009 and found a 57% increase in total ankle replacement from 2004 to 2009.
5. Lawrence RC, Helmick CG, Arnett FC, et al. Estimates of the prevalence of arthritis and selected musculoskeletal disorders in the United States. Arth Rheum. 1998;41(5):778–99.
6. Coughlin MJ, Saltzman CL, Mann RA. Mann's surgery of the foot and ankle: expert consult-online. Philadelphia: Elsevier Health Sciences; 2013.
7. Beaudoin AJ, Fiore SM, Krause WR, Adelaar RS. Effect of isolated talocalcaneal fusion on contact in the ankle and talonavicular joints. Foot Ankle. 1991;12(1):19–25.
8. Brown TD, Shaw DT. In vitro contact stress distributions in the natural human hip. J Biomech. 1983;16:373–84.
9. Ihn JC, Kim SJ, Park IH. In vitro study of contact area and pressure distribution in the human knee after partial and total meniscectomy. Int Orthop. 1993;17(4):214–8.
10. Kempson GE. Age-related changes in the tensile properties of human articular cartilage: a comparative study between the femoral head of the hip joint and the talus of the ankle joint. Biochim Biophys Acta. 1991;1075(3):223–30.
11. Ateshian GA, Soslowsky LJ, Mow VC. Quantitation of articular surface topography and cartilage thickness in knee joints using stereophotogrammetry. J Biomech. 1991;24(8):761–76.
12. Athanasiou KA, Niederauer GG, Schenck RC Jr. Biomechanical topography of human ankle cartilage. Ann Biomed Eng. 1995;23(5):697–704.
13. Dirschl DR, Marsh JL, Buckwalter JA, et al. Articular fractures. J Am Acad Orthop Surg. 2004;12(6):416–23.
14. Catterall JB, Stabler TV, Flannery CR, Kraus VB. Changes in serum and synovial fluid biomarkers after acute injury (NCT00332254). Arthritis Res Ther. 2010;12(6):R229.
15. Adams SB, Setton LA, Bell RD, et al. Inflammatory cytokines and matrix metalloproteinases in the synovial fluid after intra-articular ankle fracture. Foot Ankle Int. 2015;36(11):1264–71. LOE: This level V study examined inflammatory cytokines in synovial fluid of 21 patients with an intra-articular ankle fracture. The contralateral ankle was used as matched control. The synovial fluid exhibits a largely pro-inflammatory and extra-cellular matrix degrading environment similar to that described in idiopathic osteoarthritis.
16. Stauffer RN, Chao EYS, Brewster RC. Force and motion analysis of the normal, diseased, and prosthetic ankle joint. Clin Orthop Relat Res. 1977;127:189–96.
17. Lindsjo U. Operative treatment of ankle fracture-dislocations. A follow-up study of 306/321 consecutive cases. Clin Orthop Relat Res. 1985;199:28–38.
18. Lomax A, Singh A, et al. Complications and early results after operative fixation of 68 pilon fractures of the distal tibia. Scott Med J. 2015;60(2):79–84. This level IV study reviewed 68 closed pilon fractures retrospectively with mean follow up of 7.7 months and found 1.6% deep infection rate, 6.3% wound breakdown, 7.8% nonunion and malunion, and 26.6% posttraumatic arthritis.
19. Daniels TR, Smith JW. Talar neck fractures. Foot Ankle. 1993;14(4):225–34.

20. Mei-Dan O, Kish B, Shabat S, et al. Treatment of osteoarthritis of the ankle by intra-articular injections of hyaluronic acid: a prospective study. J Am Podiatr Med Assoc. 2010;100(2):93–100.
21. Witteveen AG, Hofstad CJ, Kerkhoffs GM. Hyaluronic acid and other conservative treatment options for osteoarthritis of the ankle. Cochrane Database Syst Rev. 2015;(10):Cd010643. This level IV study reviewed six randomized controlled trials including 240 patients with ankle osteoarthritis comparing hyaluronic acid to placebo and found insufficient data to conclude whether there is benefit or harm for HA as treatment for ankle OA compared to placebo.
22. Angthong C, Khadsongkram A, Angthong W. Outcomes and quality of life after platelet-rich plasma therapy in patients with recalcitrant hindfoot and ankle diseases: a preliminary report of 12 patients. J Foot Ankle Surg. 2013;52(4):475–80. This study reviewed 12 patients with hindfoot and ankle osteoarthritis treated with platelet-rich plasma and 16 month follow up. Mean visual analog score was significantly greater than the pretreatment score and 33% of the patients had unsatisfactory results.
23. Mei-Dan O, Carmont MR, Laver L, Mann G, Maffulli N, Nyska M. Platelet-rich plasma or hyaluronate in the management of osteochondral lesions of the talus. Am J Sports Med. 2012;40(3):534–41. This level II randomized controlled trial had 32 patients aged 18 to 60 years were allocated to intra-articular injections of HA or PRP for OCLs of the talus and followed for 28 weeks. The pain scores and functional scores for both groups improved for 6 months and PRP had significantly better outcome than HA.
24. Chahla J, Cinque ME, Shon JM, et al. Bone marrow aspirate concentrate for the treatment of osteochondral lesions of the talus: a systematic review of outcomes. J Exp Orthop. 2016;3(1):33. This systematic review identified 47 studies on the outcomes of BMAC for the treatment of chondral defect and osteoarthritis of the talus. There is paucity of long-term data and high-level evidence supporting BMAC.
25. Mann RA, Rongstad KM. Arthrodesis of the ankle: a critical analysis. Foot Ankle Int. 1998;19(1):3–9.
26. Mann RA. Arthrodesis of the foot and ankle. In: Mann RA, Coughlin MJ, editors. Surgery of the foot and ankle. St. Louis: CV Mosby; 1999. p. 651–69.
27. Buchner M, Sabo D. Ankle fusion attributable to posttraumatic arthrosis: a long-term followup of 48 patients. Clin Orthop. 2003;406:155–64.
28. Coester LM, Saltzman CL, Leupold J, Pontarelli W. Long-term results following ankle arthrodesis for post-traumatic arthritis. J Bone Joint Surg Am. 2001;83(2):219–28.
29. O'Brien TS, Hart TS, Shereff MJ, Stone J, Johnson J. Open versus arthroscopic ankle arthrodesis: a comparative study. Foot Ankle Int. 1999;20(6):368–74.
30. Winson IG, Robinson DE, Allen PE. Arthroscopic ankle arthrodesis. J Bone Joint Surg. 2005;87(3):343–7.
31. Kitaoka HB, Patzer GL. Clinical results of the Mayo total ankle arthroplasty. J Bone Joint Surg Am. 1996;78(11):1658–64.
32. Easley ME, Vertullo CJ, Urban WC, Nunley JA. Total ankle arthroplasty. J Am Acad Orthop Surg. 2002;10(3):157–67.
33. Pyevich MT, Saltzman CL, Callaghan JJ, Alvine FG. Total ankle arthroplasty: a unique design. Two to twelve-year follow-up. J Bone Joint Surg Am. 1998;80(10):1410–20.
34. Haddad SL, Coetzee JC, Estok R, Fahrbach K, Banel D, Nalysnyk L. Intermediate and long-term outcomes of total ankle arthroplasty and ankle arthrodesis. A systematic review of the literature. J Bone Joint Surg. 2007;89(9):1899–905. LOE: 4.
35. Saltzman CL, Mann RA, Ahrens JE, et al. Prospective controlled trial of STAR total ankle replacement versus ankle fusion: initial results. Foot Ankle Int. 2009;30(7):579–96.
36. Daniels TR, ASE Y, Penner M, et al. Intermediate-term results of total ankle replacement and ankle arthrodesis: a COFAS multicenter study. J Bone Joint Surg Am. 2014;96(2):135–42. This level IV study reviewed 321 patients in the Canadian Orthopaedic Foot and Ankle Society Prospective Ankle Reconstruction Database treated with total ankle replacement or ankle arthrodesis at a mean follow-up of 5.5 years. The major complication rate was 7% for arthrod-

esis and 19% for ankle replacement. There were minimal differences in AOS and SF-36 scores between the two groups at follow up.

37. Tan EW, Maccario C, Talusan PG, Schon LC. Early complications and secondary procedures in transfibular total ankle replacement. Foot Ankle Int. 2016;37(8):835–41. This level IV study reviewed 20 total ankle replacements aged 41 to 80 years with a mean follow-up of 18 months. There was no fibular nonunion, delayed union, or implant failure.
38. Arnold H. Posttraumatic impingement syndrome of the ankle–indication and results of arthroscopic therapy. Foot Ankle Surg. 2011;17(2):85–8. This level IV study reviewed 32 patients aged 16 to 65 years who underwent arthroscopic debridement for posttraumatic ankle impingement. 26 patients had good or excellent results according to the West Point Ankle Score, 5 patients rated fair result and 1 bad.
39. Rasmussen S, Hjorth JC. Arthroscopic treatment of impingement of the ankle reduces pain and enhances function. Scand J Med Sci Sports. 2002;12(2):69–72.
40. Hahn DB, Aanstoos ME, Wilkins RM. Osteochondral lesions of the talus treated with fresh talar allografts. Foot Ankle Int. 2010;31(4):277–82.
41. Giannini S, Buda R, Pagliazzi G, et al. Survivorship of bipolar fresh total osteochondral ankle allograft. Foot Ankle Int. 2014;35(3):243–51. This level IV case series reviewed 26 patients who underwent BFTOA with a mean follow-up of 40.9 months. AOFAS score improved significantly from 26.6 to 77.8 and 6 failures occurred.
42. Bugbee WD, Khanna G, Cavallo M, McCauley JC, Gortz S, Brage ME. Bipolar fresh osteochondral allografting of the tibiotalar joint. J Bone Joint Surg. 2013;95(5):426–32. This level IV study reviewed 86 ankles that underwent BFTOA with a mean follow-up of 5.3 years in young, active patients with tibiotalar arthritis. 29% of the ankle underwent graft-related reoperations. Graft surgical was 76% at 5 years and 44% at 10 years.
43. Hintermann B, Knupp M, Barg A. Supramalleolar osteotomies for the treatment of ankle arthritis. J Am Acad Orthop Surg. 2016;24(7):424–32. This review article discussed supramalleolar osteotomy in patients with asymmetric valgus or varus ankle arthritis.
44. Takakura Y, Takaoka T, Tanaka Y, Yajima H, Tamai S. Results of opening-wedge osteotomy for the treatment of a post-traumatic varus deformity of the ankle. J Bone Joint Surg Am. 1998;80(2):213–8.
45. Pagenstert G, Knupp M, Valderrabano V, Hintermann B. Realignment surgery for valgus ankle osteoarthritis. Oper Orthop Traumatol. 2009;21(1):77–87.
46. Knupp M, Stufkens SA, Bolliger L, Barg A, Hintermann B. Classification and treatment of supramalleolar deformities. Foot Ankle Int. 2011;32(11):1023–31. This level IV study reviewed 92 patients who underwent supramalleolar osteotomy for asymmetric arthritis of the ankle joint with a mean follow-up of 43 months and found significant improvement of clinical scores with 10.6% converted to total ankle replacement or arthrodesis.
47. Paley D, Lamm BM, Purohit RM, Specht SC. Distraction arthroplasty of the ankle–how far can you stretch the indications? Foot Ankle Clin. 2008;13(3):471–84, ix.
48. Tellisi N, Fragomen AT, Kleinman D, O'Malley MJ, Rozbruch SR. Joint preservation of the osteoarthritic ankle using distraction arthroplasty. Foot Ankle Int. 2009;30(4):318–25.
49. Nguyen MP, Pedersen DR, Gao Y, Saltzman CL, Amendola A. Intermediate-term follow-up after ankle distraction for treatment of end-stage osteoarthritis. J Bone Joint Surg Am. 2015;97(7):590–6. This level IV study reviewed 36 patients who underwent ankle distraction surgery with a mean follow-up of 8.3 years. 45% had undergone either ankle arthrodesis or total ankle arthroplasty. Positive predictors of ankle survival included a better AOS score at 2 years, older age at surgery and fixed distraction.

Chapter 13
Post-traumatic Arthritis of the Foot

Ram K. Alluri and Eric W. Tan

> **Key Points**
> - The most common traumatic orthopaedic injuries of the hindfoot and midfoot are calcaneus fractures and tarsometatarsal (TMT) fracture-dislocations (Lisfranc injury), respectively.
> - The hindfoot is structurally composed of the talus and calcaneus, and its functionality is primarily dependent on motion through the talonavicular and subtalar (talocalcaneal) joints.
> - The Lisfranc complex is a major stabilizer of the midfoot and is composed of the five metatarsal base articulations with the cuboid and cuneiforms.
> - The mainstay for surgical treatment involves selective arthrodesis with the goal of a creating a stable, functional, and painless plantigrade foot.

Introduction

Traumatic injuries of the foot are common after high-energy trauma, and second only to hip, thigh, and knee injuries [1]. Although these injuries of the foot are typically not life threatening, they can result in significant long-term functional disability, and in patients with multiple injuries, those with foot injuries have significantly worse outcomes than matched patients without foot injuries [2]. Much of the disability sustained after traumatic injuries to the foot is due to acute and chronic post-traumatic degenerative changes of the articular surfaces.

R. K. Alluri · E. W. Tan (✉)
Department of Orthopaedic Surgery, Keck School of Medicine of USC,
Los Angeles, CA, USA
e-mail: Ram.Alluri@med.usc.edu; erictan@usc.edu

© Springer Nature Switzerland AG 2021
S. C. Thakkar, E. A. Hasenboehler (eds.), *Post-Traumatic Arthritis*,
https://doi.org/10.1007/978-3-030-50413-7_13

The most common traumatic orthopaedic injuries of the hindfoot and midfoot are calcaneus fractures and tarsometatarsal (TMT) fracture-dislocations (Lisfranc injury), respectively. Calcaneus fractures account for approximately 2% of all fractures, and it is the most frequently fractured bone of the foot [3]. Fracture-dislocations of the TMT joint are relatively uncommon, only accounting for 0.2% of all fractures; [4] however, up to 20% of these TMT injuries are initially missed or misdiagnosed [5]. In both injuries, patients can develop symptomatic posttraumatic osteoarthritis due to intraarticular fracture fragments, altered biomechanics resulting in pathologic force distribution, and direct articular surface damage. Previous studies have demonstrated that chondrocyte injury and death can immediately occur due to forceful impaction during the traumatic event [6].

In this chapter, we will discuss the relevant anatomy, evaluation, and management of patients who sustain a calcaneus fracture or TMT fracture-dislocation and, subsequently, develop posttraumatic osteoarthritis of the hindfoot or midfoot.

Anatomy and Biomechanics

Anatomy

The hindfoot is structurally composed of the talus and calcaneus, and its functionality is primarily dependent on motion through the talonavicular and subtalar (talocalcaneal) joints. The majority of hindfoot motion occurs through the talonavicular joint with fusion of this joint resulting in 90% loss of subtalar motion. Conversely, subtalar fusion only results in 26% loss of talonavicular motion [7]. The subtalar joint is composed of two articulations. Anteriorly, the lip and sustentaculum of the calcaneus rotate about the talar head; posteriorly, the posterior facet of the calcaneus provides a surface for which the talus can glide upon. The spring ligament and the proximal articular surface of the navicular bone augment the calcaneus to form a complete socket stabilizing the talar head. Overall, the axis of the subtalar joint is oblique due to the more medial anterior talocalcaneal articulation relative to the posterior articulation.

The midfoot is composed of navicular, cuboid, and three cuneiform bones and articulates proximally with the hindfoot and distally with the forefoot. Functionally, the midfoot is often described in terms of medial, middle, and lateral columns. The rigid medial and middle columns are composed of articulations between the first metatarsal base and medial cuneiform, second metatarsal base and intermediate cuneiform, and third metatarsal base and lateral cuneiform. The mobile lateral column consists of the cuboid and fourth and fifth metatarsal bases. There are 5–10 degrees of motion at the first TMT joint and minimal motion occurs at the second and third TMT joints. The fourth and fifth TMT joints are most mobile, with 10–20 degrees of movement. The osseous stability of the midfoot is partly because of the wedge shape of the metatarsal bases and cuneiforms resulting in a transverse arch, or "Roman arch," of the foot in the coronal plane. A second osseous stabilizer is provided by recession of the second metatarsal base relative to the first and third tarsometatarsal joints.

The Lisfranc complex is a major stabilizer of the midfoot and is composed of the five metatarsal base articulations with the cuboid and cuneiforms. This complex is stabilized by a combination of ligamentous attachments and a unique bony configuration at the second metatarsal base. The dorsal ligaments are the weakest while the interosseous and plantar ligaments are the strongest [8]. The specific Lisfranc ligament stabilizes 1–2 intermetatarsal bases, attaching the second metatarsal base to the medial cuneiform. While intermetatarsal ligaments are present between the second, third, fourth, and fifth metatarsal bases, there is no intermetatarsal ligament stabilizing the 1–2 metatarsal bases directly. Therefore, the integrity of the Lisfranc ligament is critical for stability.

Altered Biomechanics

Fractures of the calcaneus can result in significant articular damage and progressive hindfoot deformity resulting in a heel that is wide, flattened, and in varus (Figs. 13.1 and 13.2). Widening of the hindfoot may cause significant difficulty with shoe wear. The varus deformity can cause lateral deviation of the peroneal tendons and sural nerve compression [9]; severe varus deformity can cause symptomatic subfibular impingement between the lateral wall of the calcaneus and distal fibula [9]. When

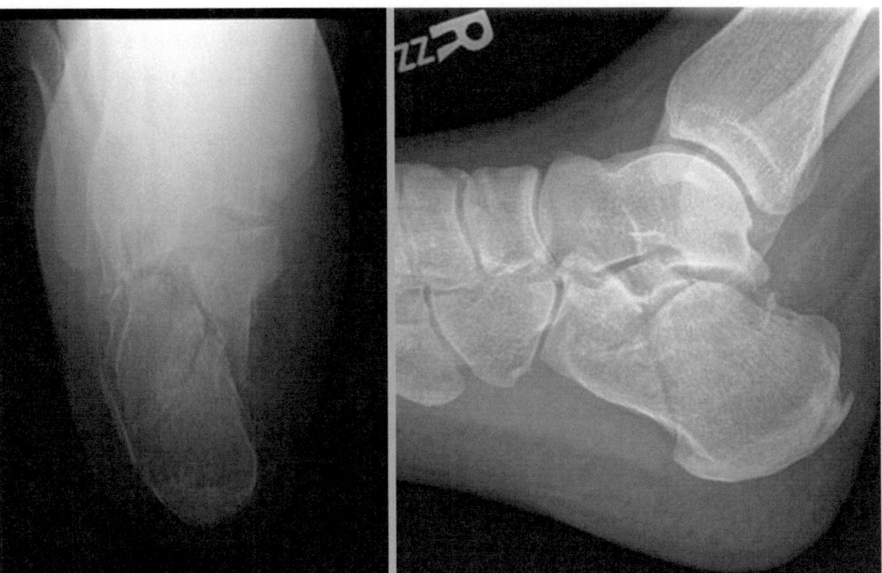

Fig. 13.1 Axial heel view and lateral radiographs of a simple, intraarticular calcaneal fracture

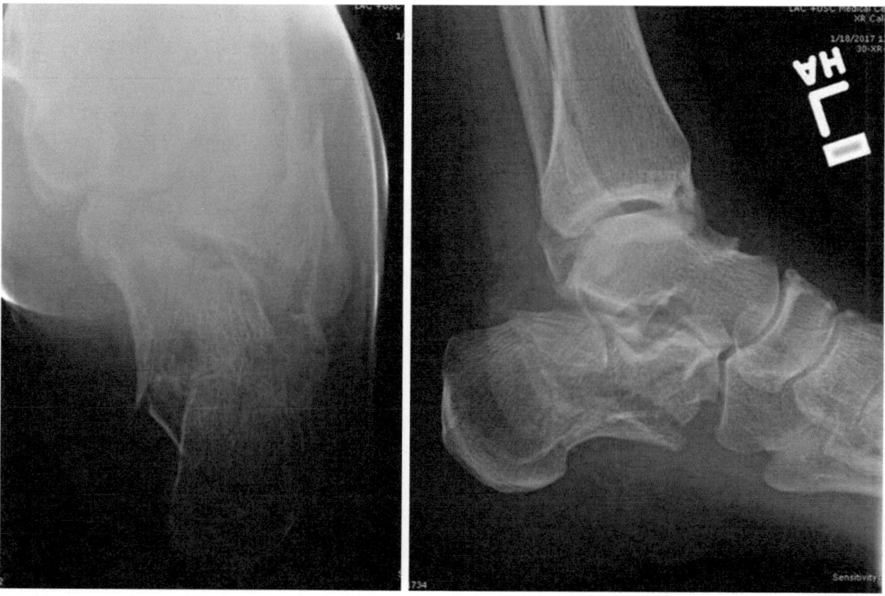

Fig. 13.2 Axial heel view and lateral radiographs of a complex, intraarticular calceanal fracture with significant intraarticular comminution and joint depression

the hindfoot assumes a pathological varus alignment, the transverse tarsal joint remains locked, resulting in subsequent degeneration of the adjacent midfoot joints due to persistently increased loads during gait [9]. Hindfoot varus deformity can also cause lateral column overloading of the midfoot. In addition to varus deformity, loss of hindfoot height from depression of the posterior calcaneal facet can also occur after calcaneal fractures [9]. This causes the talus to adopt a more dorsiflexed position, which may result in anterior impingement of the talus on the anterior tibial plafond [9]. Additionally, the lever arm of the Achilles tendon is reduced, which can significantly alter normal gait patterns [9].

Traumatic injuries to the Lisfranc complex occur during torsion of the forefoot and axial load transmission to the midfoot (Figs. 13.3 and 13.4). These injuries result in direct articular damage and altered midfoot biomechanics due to instability and resultant collapse of the longitudinal arch. The normal intact midfoot arch functions as a lever, efficiently transmitting force from the forefoot to hindfoot, and loss of this arch results in decreased mechanical efficiency [10]. This leads to abnormal loading of the midfoot and adjacent joints, resulting in arthritic degeneration. Commonly, patients develop a valgus deformity of the hindfoot, midfoot flattening from the loss of the longitudinal arch, and forefoot abduction and dorsiflexion because of pathologic changes in the peroneus brevis and posterior tibialis tendons, respectively.

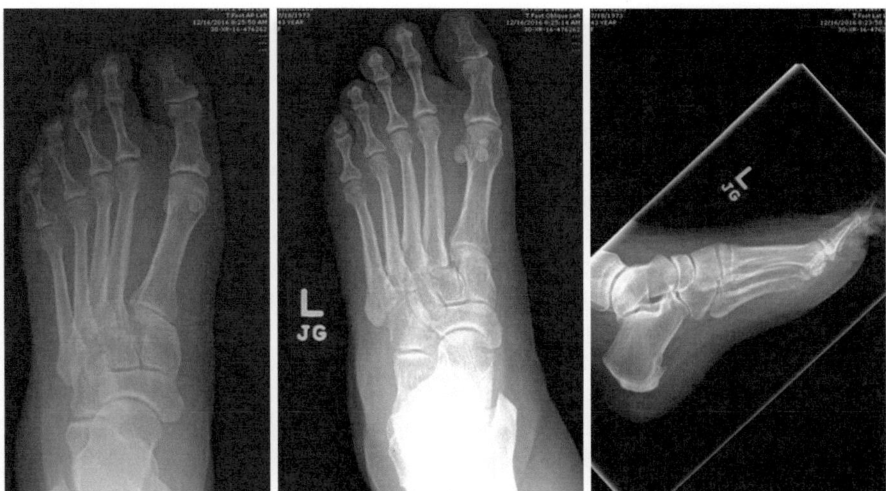

Fig. 13.3 Anteroposterior (AP), oblique, and lateral radiographs of a subtle Lisfranc injury with mild diastasis between the medial cuneiform and the base of the second metatarsal that could be missed during initial presentation

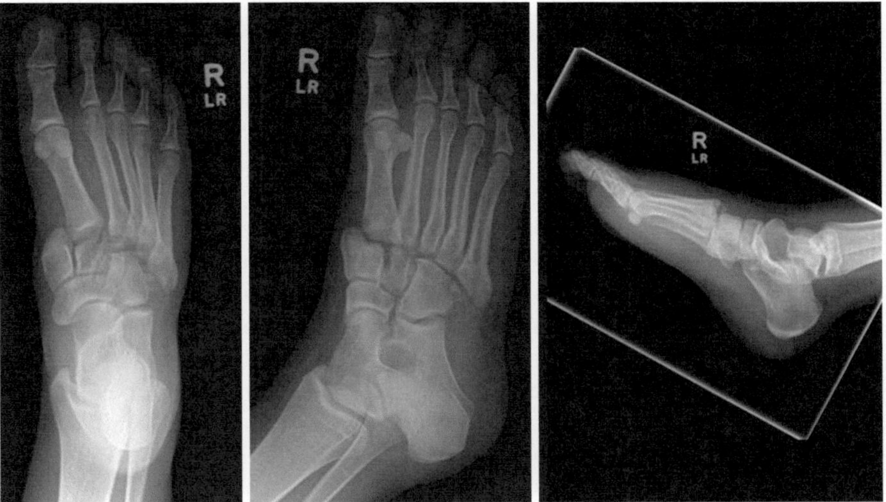

Fig. 13.4 Anteroposterior (AP), oblique, and lateral radiographs of a severe Lisfranc injury with homolateral shift of the first through fifth tarsometatarsal joints

Natural History of Initial Hindfoot and Midfoot Fracture Healing

During the acute injury, a calcaneus fracture can be treated operatively or nonoperatively; however, no definite consensus exists with regard to ideal treatment. Current relative indications for operative management include large extraarticular fractures, fractures with greater than 2 mm of intraarticular displacement, flattening of Bohler's angle and the angle of Gissane, varus malalignment of the tuberosity, impending skin necrosis from displaced tongue-type fractures, and open fractures. Relative nonoperative indications include anterior process fractures involving <25% of the calcaneocuboid joint, fractures with preserved calcaneal height, nondisplaced fractures, fractures with less than 2 mm of intraarticular displacement, or patients with comorbidities (smoking, diabetes, vascular disease) placing them at increased risk for postoperative complications [11].

Prior studies have stressed the importance of achieving an anatomic reduction to prevent accelerated wear of the subtalar joint. Minimal displacement of 1–2 mm has been shown to alter contact pressures of the subtalar joint and posterior facet, resulting in significant gait disturbance [12, 13]. Whether achieved through open or closed reduction, anatomic reduction of calcaneal fractures attempts to recreate a congruent subtalar joint, reduce the lateral wall, and take the hindfoot out of varus while restoring calcaneal height. Therefore, most surgeons advocate initial operative management to achieve an anatomic reduction of the joint surface to potentially decrease the incidence of subtalar osteoarthritis requiring secondary arthrodesis [14, 15].

Several prior studies have attempted to delineate the ideal management of displaced intraarticular calcaneal fractures. In a study by Agren et al., surgical treatment was associated with higher complications and similar functional outcomes at 1 year compared to nonoperative management [16]. Buckley et al. also found little difference in SF-36 or VAS outcome scores between operatively and nonoperatively treated calcaneus fractures [15]. However, the authors did note higher rates of eventual arthrodesis in patients who received initial nonoperative management [15]. Csizy et al. noted similar findings with a six times higher subtalar arthrodesis rate in patients receiving initial nonoperative management [14].

Regardless of initial operative or nonoperative management, a high number of patients who sustain calcaneal fractures with significant intraarticular involvement will develop posttraumatic osteoarthritis [17]. The initial injury results in the displacement of intraarticular fracture fragments and irreversible cartilage damage. In a study by Radnay et al., 69 patients who sustained a calcaneal fracture requiring eventual arthrodesis were reviewed [18]. Thirty-four (49%) underwent initial operative management, and 35 (51%) were treated initially nonoperatively [18]. Worse functional outcomes after subtalar arthrodesis were noted in patients who were initially treated with nonoperative management [18]. Patients with initial nonoperative management also had greater postoperative wound complications, potentially due to greater restoration of calcaneal height resulting in postoperative tension along the surgical wound [18].

The initial management of Lisfranc injuries also remains without consensus, partly because the term "Lisfranc injury" reflects a wide and poorly defined injury spectrum. Initial management includes nonoperative interventions versus open reduction and internal fixation (ORIF) or primary partial arthrodesis of the midfoot. Nonoperative management is generally reserved for patients who are minimally ambulatory, have an insensate foot, or inflammatory osteoarthritis [19]. In patients without these preexisting comorbidities, nonoperative management is generally only recommended in patients with a stable injury (no diastasis of the Lisfranc complex).

Any measurable incongruity greater than 2 mm at the Lisfranc joint is generally an indication for surgical treatment, ideally within the first two weeks after injury to optimize outcomes [19]. The most accurate predictor of postoperative outcome is achieving a stable anatomic reduction after which good to excellent postoperative outcomes can be expected in 85% of patients whereas nonanatomic alignment results in similar outcomes in only 17% of patients [20]. Even after adequate reduction, the incidence of posttraumatic osteoarthritis can be as high as 25–72% [21, 22]. However, up to 100% of patients with an inadequate initial reduction will develop posttraumatic osteoarthritis [21], and initial radiographic findings are generally not predictive of which patients will develop this complication [23]. Some authors have stated that developing osteoarthritis after a Lisfranc injury is almost inevitable given the damage to the articular surface at the time of initial injury [24]. Given these findings, some surgeons recommend primary partial fusion in Lisfranc injuries at high risk for developing posttraumatic osteoarthritis such as injuries with ligamentous disruption and multidirectional instability, significant comminution, or crush injuries [25]. Although partial midfoot arthrodesis may limit or eliminate the eventual development of posttraumatic midfoot osteoarthritis, the stiffness and limited function of the foot following the arthrodesis may not be well tolerated in young, active patients.

Patient Evaluation

History

The preoperative examination of all patients with posttraumatic osteoarthritis secondary to a hindfoot or midfoot injury should begin with a thorough history. The history should focus on the initial mechanism of injury and soft tissue damage, previous nonoperative or operative treatment received, degree of current disability and pain, and a discussion of current expectations in terms of functional outcome. An assessment of current medical comorbidities, work status, and tobacco use can allow for perioperative risk stratification and assessment of nonunion risk.

Physical Exam

The physical exam should consist of a gait assessment, range of motion measurement, and careful inspection of ankle and foot alignment. Alignment should be assessed with the patient standing as this best allows for examination of hindfoot varus or valgus, medial arch height, and forefoot abduction. Patients should also be asked to walk to assess for dynamic flatfoot deformity or subfibular impingement. Abnormal alignment should be assessed for passive correctability, and in a patient with unilateral injury, the contralateral, uninjured side can serve as a reliable control. In cases of severe deformity, the quality of the soft tissue and presence of ulcers or impending skin breakdown should be assessed. Previous surgical scars should be examined as they can dictate choice of surgical exposure. The dorsalis pedis and posterior tibial pulses should be assessed; nonpalpable pulses may require a preoperative vascular consult. Lastly, the strength and sensation of the foot should also be formally assessed and documented.

In patients with posttraumatic hindfoot deformity and osteoarthritis, the hindfoot is often in varus and collapsed, and therefore evaluation for contractures of the gastrocnemius-soleus complex and anterior ankle impingement is important. Additionally, patients with posttraumatic hindfoot osteoarthritis may have a widened calcaneus that can cause skin breakdown over the lateral malleolus from contact friction.

In patients with posttraumatic midfoot deformity and osteoarthritis, excessive pronation and midfoot collapse may be noted secondary to loss of the longitudinal arch and acquired forefoot abduction. These patients may have pain with palpation over the midfoot; however, the degree of arthrosis visualized on radiographs may not correlate with symptoms found on physical examination. In most cases, patients endorse greatest pain at the second TMT joint as this is the least mobile joint of the midfoot and undergoes the greatest posttraumatic arthritic change. To a lesser extent, they may endorse pain at the first and third TMT joints. Patients with arthrosis of the lateral column may not endorse significant pain because of the inherent mobility of this column. Stress testing of individual metatarsocuneiform joints (the "piano key" test) may also help elicit pain across the affected midfoot TMT joints as it places compression along the medial and lateral midfoot [26]. A positive test will produce localized pain at the involved tarsometatarsal joint. Additionally, the examiner may be able to aggravate posttraumatic midfoot osteoarthritis symptoms by having the patient perform a single heel rise or stair ascent as these activities require significant load transmission across the midfoot. Lastly, dorsal osteophytes may cause difficulty with shoe wear, neuritis, or tendonitis.

Imaging

Weight-bearing anteroposterior, lateral, and oblique plain radiographs of the foot are necessary to diagnose and characterize the degree of arthrosis in the hindfoot or midfoot based on the presence of joint space narrowing, subchondral sclerosis, and osteophyte formation. The lateral view is particularly useful to assess talar declination, hindfoot collapse, and the presence of anterior impingement of the talar neck on the tibial plafond. Measurement of Bohler's angle or the angle of Gissane can help quantify the loss of calcaneal height due to posterior facet collapse (Fig. 13.5). Additionally on the lateral view, Meary's angle can be calculated in patients with loss of the medial longitudinal arch and subsequent pes planus deformity (Fig. 13.5). An axial heel view, or Harris view, can be useful to assess hindfoot alignment and heel widening. Some surgeons may elect to obtain plain radiographs of the uninjured foot for comparative purposes.

The role of computed tomography (CT) in evaluating posttraumatic arthrosis of the hindfoot and midfoot is unclear. Many surgeons recommend routinely obtaining CT imaging as it can assist in preoperative planning, particularly in cases of complex deformity. CT imaging allows for more accurate characterization of the degree

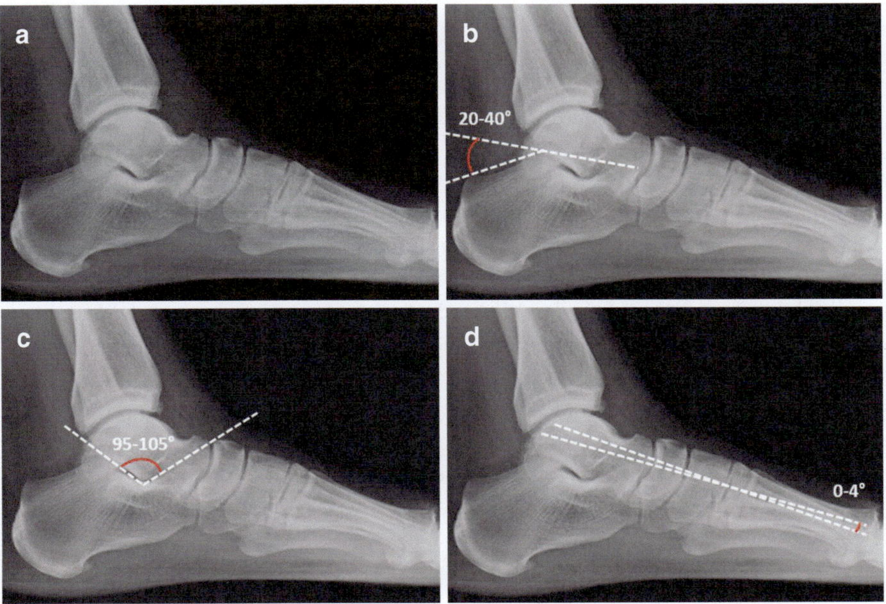

Fig. 13.5 (**a**) Normal lateral radiograph of the foot. (**b**) Bohler's angle. (**c**) Angle of Gissane. (**d**) Meary's angle. Normal values for the respective angles are listed within the image. The curved red line demonstrates where the angle should be measured

and location of hindfoot and midfoot arthrosis. Specifically, in hindfoot posttraumatic arthrosis, CT may allow for the determination of whether there is subfibular impingement of the calcaneus and distal tip of the fibula. With regards to midfoot posttraumatic arthrosis, CT images in three planes can allow for determining which specific midfoot joint is undergoing posttraumatic degeneration, potentially allowing for limited fusion, thus preserving greater function.

Magnetic resonance imaging (MRI) is not routinely utilized. In rare cases, a technetium Tc- 99 m bone scan can be ordered in patients with normal plain radiographs to identify early-onset arthritic changes in patients with persistent posttraumatic hindfoot or midfoot pain.

Nonoperative Management

The central treatment modalities of nonoperative management for posttraumatic osteoarthritis of the hindfoot and midfoot center on physical therapy, nonsteroidal antiinflammatory medications (NSAIDs), injections, and bracing. Activity modification, physical therapy, and NSAIDs are generally firstline treatments in this patient population. Selective injection of corticosteroids or hyaluronic acid in the hindfoot or midfoot is also an option, but scientific evidence proving their efficacy is lacking.

Braces and orthotics provide pain relief and increased function for patients with hindfoot and midfoot osteoarthritis by decreasing force transmission and motion across the arthritic joint. The selection of the appropriate brace or orthotic depends on the degree of osteoarthritis present as well as the flexible or rigid nature of the deformity. In addition, the provider should be cognizant about the materials used and pressure applied by the brace or orthotic, as this may result in skin breakdown or ulceration. In early stages of hindfoot or midfoot osteoarthritis with flexible or minimal deformity, a semirigid ankle brace or custom orthotic may provide enough stability to support and realign the foot and ankle. As the severity of the osteoarthritis and deformity increases, a more rigid brace, such as a double-upright brace or custom Arizona brace, or rigid orthotic may be necessary to reduce motion at the affected hindfoot or midfoot joints, respectively. However, many patients find these braces cumbersome and difficult to use. Shoe wear modification, particularly rocker-bottom shoes or customized shoes, may also be effective nonoperative treatment options.

Operative Management

Patients that have failed nonoperative management of posttraumatic hindfoot and midfoot osteoarthritis with continued debilitating symptoms may be candidates for surgical intervention. Patient factors such as age, medical comorbidities, smoking history, profession, and workers' compensation status should be considered as these can significantly affect postoperative outcomes. The mainstay for surgical treatment involves selective arthrodesis with the goal of a creating a stable, functional, and painless plantigrade foot.

Hindfoot

Fractures of the calcaneus that develop posttraumatic osteoarthritis can be surgically treated with in situ subtalar arthrodesis or distraction bone-block arthrodesis with or without additional corrective osteotomies, lateral wall decompression, or soft tissue procedures.

In situ arthrodesis can provide significant pain relief with satisfactory functional outcomes (Fig. 13.6). It is indicated for patients with minimal deformity, significant subtalar osteoarthritis, and gross preservation of calcaneal height such that there is no evidence of anterior talar impingement on the tibial plafond. Patient selection is key for this in situ procedure as patients with deformity that is not addressed will inevitably have poorer long-term outcomes [27]. The choice of surgical approach for in situ arthrodesis must be given careful consideration. If previous hardware is present, but asymptomatic, it can be left in place [9, 28]. If the hardware is symptomatic, some surgeons elect to use the previous surgical incision, which is commonly an extensile lateral approach or, more recently, a sinus tarsi approach [9, 28]. After adequate exposure of the subtalar joint has been achieved, cartilage and nonviable bone are completely removed from the subtalar joint with care taken to

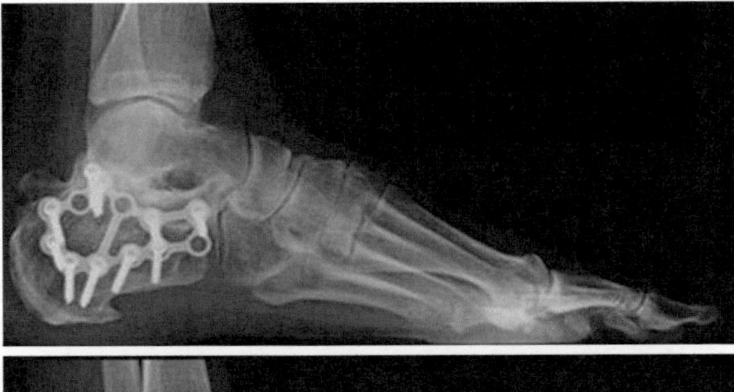
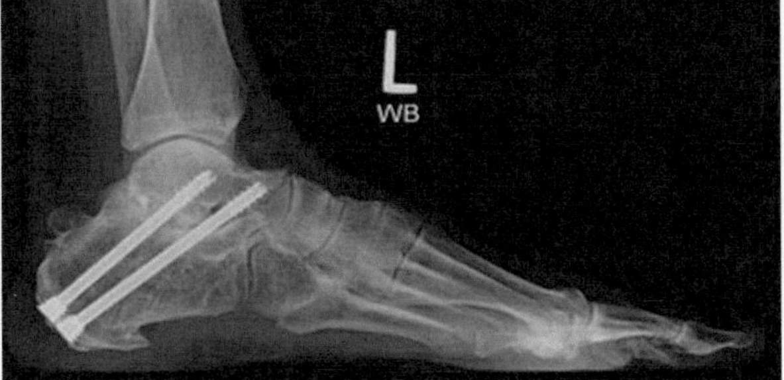

Fig. 13.6 Lateral radiograph of an intraarticular calcaneus fracture that was initially treated with open reduction and internal fixation (upper image). The patient eventually developed significant subtalar posttraumatic osteoarthritis. Postoperative lateral radiograph after removal of hardware and in situ subtalar arthrodesis (lower image). (Images courtesy of Dr. David E. Oji, MD)

preserve the normal bone contour and subchondral bone. The exposed subchondral bone is then meticulously prepared and perforated to improve blood flow. The subtalar joint is then aligned in approximately 0–5 degrees of valgus and fixed using partially threaded 6.5 mm screws. It is important to obtain correct hindfoot positioning prior to arthrodesis to maximize functional outcomes. Residual bony deficits can be filled with autologous bone graft, bone allograft, synthetic bone, or cancellous chips.

Previous studies have demonstrated union rates ranging from 84% to 98% after in situ arthrodesis on average 12 weeks after surgery [29, 30] and improvement in functional outcomes after arthrodesis: [18, 31] the AOFAS hindfoot score can be as high as 89 at final follow-up [32], and 93% of patients have good to fair outcomes using the Angus and Cowell rating system [31]. Overall patient satisfaction can range from 70% to 90% [33, 34]. The most common complication after this procedure is wound infection, which has recently been shown to be as high as 18%, especially in patients with an original open fracture or infection after the index operation [30]. Other complications include neuromas and chronic regional pain syndrome. Patients at higher risk for poorer functional outcomes include those initially treated nonoperatively, smokers, diabetics, and patients of advanced age [18, 35, 36].

In patients with loss of hindfoot height and symptomatic anterior tibial impingement, distraction bone-block subtalar arthrodesis is indicated (Fig. 13.7). An in situ arthrodesis in these patients, even with lateral wall decompression, will not optimize posttraumatic hindfoot function. The added distraction with a structural bone graft and arthrodesis will reestablish the calcaneal height as well as the inclination of the talus and normalize the gastrocnemius-soleus lever arm. Most commonly, the subtalar joint is approached with a posterior or posterolateral incision for this procedure. Alternatively, a sinus tarsi incision may also be utilized. However, an extensile lateral approach, commonly used for initial operative fixation of calcaneal fractures, should be avoided due to concerns about wound healing after distraction, particularly along the horizontal limb. After initial dissection through the soft tissues, a lateral wall exostectomy may be performed; the bone can be used as bone graft. The subtalar joint is then distracted using a large distractor or laminar spreader to correct the calcaneal height and varus malalignment. The joint surfaces are then prepared in a similar fashion to in situ subtalar arthrodesis. Next, the structural bone graft is inserted into the distraction gap and the hindfoot is placed into 0–5 degrees of valgus. Once aligned, the fusion may be secured using partially threaded 6.5 mm screws placed from the posteroinferior aspect of the calcaneus into the talar dome.

Tricortical iliac crest bone autograft is the main choice for structural grafting. However, structural allografts such as the femoral neck allograft and tricortical iliac crest allograft are alternative options. Initial reports comparing structural allograft to autograft demonstrated significantly lower union rates with allograft [37]; however, more recent studies report 92% union rates with allograft and favorable outcomes [38]. Augmentation of structural graft with synthetic bone graft substitutes or cancellous chips can be utilized at the surgeon's discretion.

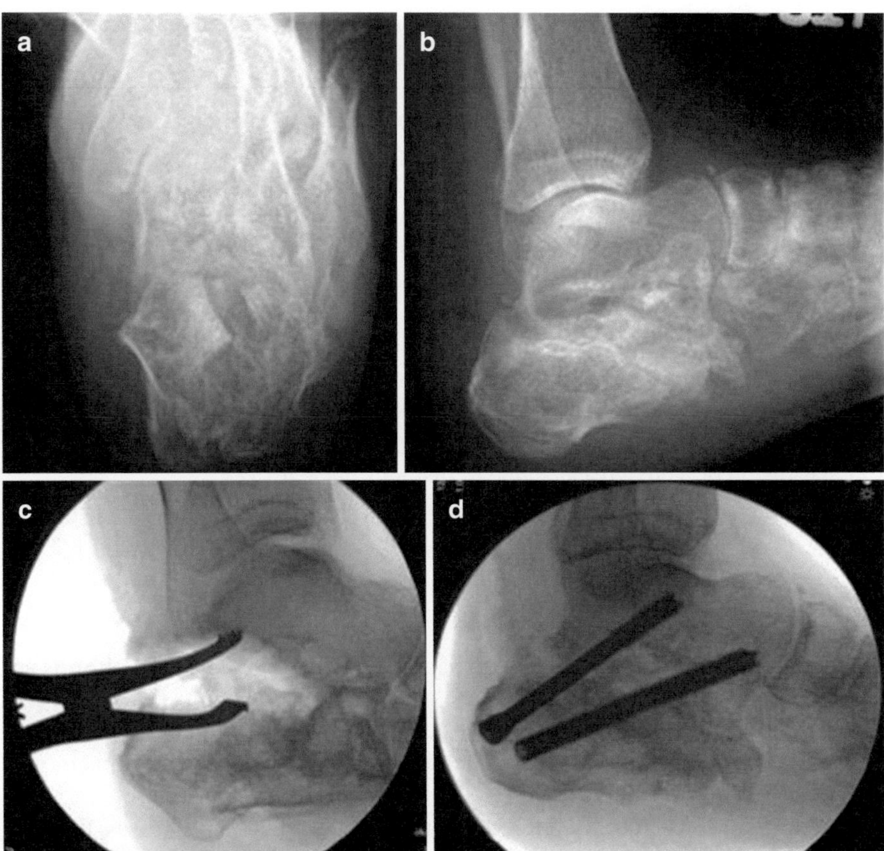

Fig. 13.7 (**a**, **b**) Axial heel view and lateral radiographs of an intraarticular calcaneus fracture initially treated nonoperatively. The patient developed significant subtalar posttraumatic osteoarthritis with varus hindfoot alignment and anterior talar impingement due to loss of calcaneal height. (**c**). Intraoperative fluoroscopic image demonstrating distraction of the subtalar joint using a laminar spreader (**d**). Intraoperative fluoroscopic image after distraction bone-block arthrodesis of the subtalar joint

Outcomes after distraction bone-block subtalar arthrodesis are generally favorable. Although the procedure is technically more challenging, as two osseous surfaces need to be united, union rates are similar to that for in situ subtalar arthrodesis, ranging from 87% to 95% [35, 37]. In a prospective study by Rammelt et al., AOFAS hindfoot scores increased from 23.5 to 73.2 at 33 months after distraction arthrodesis [39]. Other studies have demonstrated similar results, all with AOFAS hindfoot scores ranging from 70 to 76 at final follow-up [40–42], and over 90% of patients report satisfaction with the procedure [37, 39]. Although distraction bone-block subtalar arthrodesis is generally a successful procedure, complications can occur in up to 13% of patients [39]. The most common complications include infection, plantar exostosis, and nerve injury. Patients at risk for complications and poorer postoperative outcomes include diabetics, smokers, and workers' compensation patients [35, 41].

Occasionally with both subtalar arthrodesis techniques, additional soft tissue procedures may be needed. In the setting of peroneal subluxation or tendonitis, the peroneal tendons may need to be debrided, repaired, or reconstructed. Furthermore, percutaneous lengthening of the Achilles tendon or a Strayer gastrocnemius recession may be indicated in the setting of equinus deformity.

Importantly, fusion of the hindfoot for symptomatic posttraumatic osteoarthritis can result in increased stress across adjacent joints. Subtalar joint arthrodesis can result in greater force transmission across the adjacent transverse tarsal joint and tibiotalar joint. However, the clinical significance of adjacent joint degenerative changes remains unclear. Previous studies have demonstrated adjacent joint degenerative changes in the tibiotalar and transverse tarsal joints in 10–40% of patients [32, 33, 36, 37]. Whether these adjacent degenerative changes were present prior to subtalar fusion or were advanced due to fusion is unclear [32].

Midfoot

Fracture-dislocations of the TMT joint that develop posttraumatic osteoarthritis are commonly treated with arthrodesis of the medial three TMT joints (Fig. 13.8) [10, 28]. Similar to posttraumatic hindfoot osteoarthritis, the main indication for midfoot arthrodesis is patients who continue to have symptomatic pain refractory to nonoperative management.

The midfoot can be accessed through multiple incisions. In most cases, the incision used for arthrodesis is similar to that used for primary open reduction of acute Lisfranc injuries. A longitudinal incision made along the dorsal first intermetatarsal space allows access to the first and second tarsometatarsal joints. A second incision can be made over the dorsal fourth metatarsal with care to maintain an adequate skin bridge to access the third, fourth, and fifth TMT joints, if necessary. Alternatively, fusion of the first, second, and third TMT joints can be performed through a medial incision in conjunction with a central dorsal incision just lateral to the second metatarsal. Regardless of the approach, care should be taken to avoid and protect the dorsal pedis artery, first dorsal metatarsal artery, and the superficial and deep peroneal nerves.

The decision of which midfoot joints to fuse is critical and selective fusion is advocated to avoid making the midfoot overly rigid. Most commonly, the first, second, and third TMT joints are included in the arthrodesis. Additional fusion or interpositional tendon arthroplasty of the fourth and fifth TMT joints is rarely indicated but may be needed in cases of significant midfoot osteoarthritis. The selected joints of the midfoot arthrodesis construct should be denuded of residual cartilage and fibrous tissue. The subchondral bone is then debrided and perforated to improve blood flow to the fusion site. After adequate preparation of the bony surfaces, the mechanical alignment of the midfoot must be restored. A Hintermann distractor or

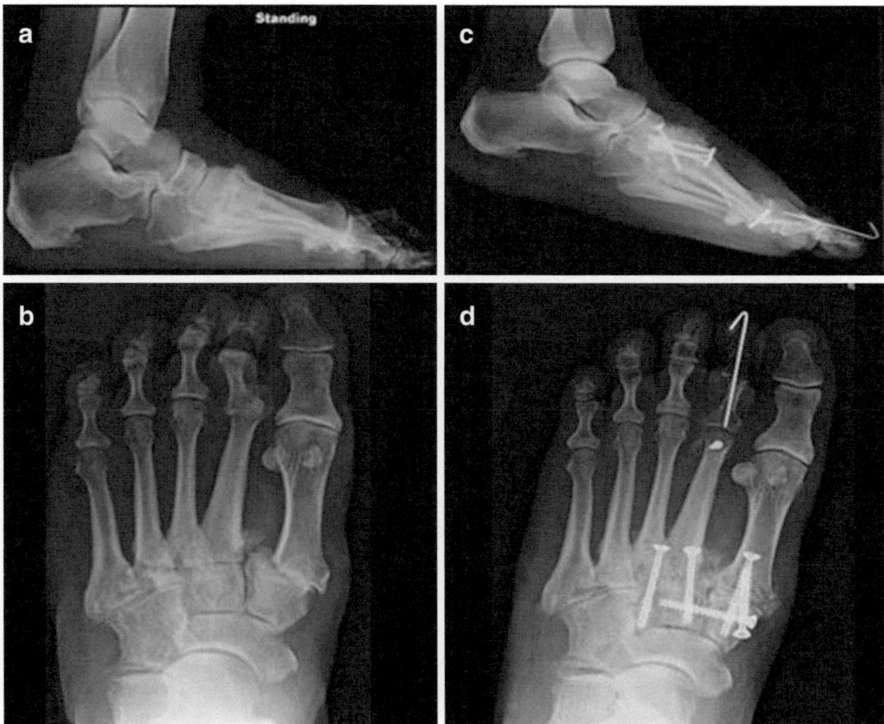

Fig. 13.8 (**a, b**) Anteroposterior (AP) and lateral radiographs of a patient with a prior Lisfranc injury who developed significant midfoot posttraumatic osteoarthritis. (**c, d**) Postoperative radiographs after arthrodesis of the first, second, and third tarsometatarsal joints of the midfoot. (Images courtesy of Dr. David E. Oji, MD)

lamina spreader can aid in restoring alignment and, occasionally, in more severe deformities, a wedge resection across the midfoot may be necessary [28].

In addition, soft tissue procedures may be needed to fully correct the deformity. In the presence of severe abduction deformity, lengthening or complete release of the peroneus brevis tendon may be needed. The tendon can also be transferred to the peroneus longus to help stabilize the medial column of the midfoot. Furthermore, in the presence of equinus deformity, percutaneous lengthening of the Achilles tendon or a Strayer gastrocnemius recession may be necessary.

After reestablishing alignment of the midfoot, residual bony deficits should be filled with autologous bone graft, bone allograft, synthetic bone graft substitutes, or cancellous chips. To stabilize the arthrodesis, multiple techniques are available including use of Kirschner wires, staples, compression screws as well as dorsal, medial, and plantar plates. There is no clear evidence indicating which construct leads to the best clinical outcomes [10]. However, Marks et al. demonstrated that midfoot fusions fixed with a plantarly applied plate result in superior biomechanical stability compared to midfoot fusion constructs with screw fixation [43]. In most cases, adequate stability can be achieved with partially threaded cancellous screws or cortical lag screws placed across each joint of the arthrodesis construct. In cases of severe deformity, the addition of compression plates or plantar plate fixation will add additional stability and should be considered.

The results of midfoot fusion for posttraumatic osteoarthritis after a TMT joint fracture-dislocation are generally favorable. Union is achieved in greater than 90% of patients with some studies demonstrating 98% union rates [44, 45]. Sangeorzan et al. reported good to excellent results in 11 of 16 patients (69%), and 15 of 16 (94%) were satisfied with the procedure [46]. Mann et al. reported 93% patient satisfaction following selective arthrodesis [44], and Johnson and Johnson reported 84% patient satisfaction [47]. AOFAS-midfoot scores can improve by up to 34 points with final scores ranging from 71 to 78 [48, 49]. Several studies have shown that the quality of the initial reduction during the acute TMT fracture-dislocation correlates with better outcomes after secondary midfoot arthrodesis [20, 46] while workplace injuries and delay to treatment can negatively affect outcomes [46]. The most common complications after midfoot fusion include superficial infections, neuritis, and neuromas [44, 47, 48]. Nerve injuries are common in midfoot fusion due to the anatomic location of the cutaneous nerves, particularly the deep peroneal nerve, and the soft tissue retraction needed for adequate exposure and preparation of the joint surfaces.

Similar to subtalar fusion of the hindfoot, concerns exist for adjacent joint degenerative changes after select midfoot fusion; however, no clinical studies exist that have objectively evaluated this potential complication.

Conclusions

Calcaneus fractures and TMT fracture-dislocations of the hindfoot and midfoot, respectively, can result in significant long-term morbidity primarily due to the development of posttraumatic osteoarthritis secondary to acute articular damage at the time of initial injury and chronic malalignment and abnormal force distribution across the foot resulting in progressive degeneration. Restoration of the articular surface and a stable reduction during initial treatment can decrease the risk of developing posttraumatic osteoarthritis, but, regardless of initial treatment, a certain subset will inevitably develop posttraumatic osteoarthritis. In symptomatic patients with posttraumatic osteoarthritis refractory to nonoperative management, select fusion of the subtalar joint with or without bone block distraction or medial and middle columns of the midfoot can result in good to excellent postoperative functional outcomes and high rates of patient satisfaction.

References

1. Chong M, Sochor M, Ipaktchi K, Brede C, Poster C, Wang S. The interaction of "occupant factors" on the lower extremity fractures in frontal collision of motor vehicle crashes based on a level I trauma center. J Trauma. 2007;62(3):720–9.
2. Turchin DC, Schemitsch EH, McKee MD, Waddell JP. Do foot injuries significantly affect the functional outcome of multiply injured patients? J Orthop Trauma. 1999;13(1):1–4.
3. O'Connell F, Mital MA, Rowe CR. Evaluation of modern management of fractures of the os calcis. Clin Orthop Relat Res. 1972;83:214–23.
4. English TA. Dislocation of the metatarsal bone and adjacent toe. J Bone Joint Surg Br. 1964;46:700–4.
5. Goossens M, De Stoop N. Lisfranc's fracture-dislocations: etiology, radiology, and results of treatment. A review of 20 cases. Clin Orthop Relat Res. 1983;176:154–62.
6. Borrelli J Jr, Silva MJ, Zaegel MA, Franz C, Sandell LJ. Single high-energy impact load causes posttraumatic OA in young rabbits via a decrease in cellular metabolism. J Orthop Res. 2009;27(3):347–52.
7. Astion DJ, Deland JT, Otis JC, Kenneally S. Motion of the hindfoot after simulated arthrodesis. J Bone Joint Surg Am. 1997;79(2):241–6.
8. Desmond EA, Chou LB. Current concepts review: Lisfranc injuries. Foot Ankle Int. 2006;27(8):653–60.
9. Banerjee R, Saltzman C, Anderson RB, Nickisch F. Management of calcaneal malunion. J Orthop Trauma Rehabil. 2011;19(1):27–36. A review article on the management of calcaneus malunion which specifically addresses the management of post-traumatic osteoarthritis of the subtalar joint. Multiple calcaneal malunion classification systems are discussed that can help guide management. Level of Evidence: N/A.
10. Patel A, Rao S, Nawoczenski D, Flemister AS, Digiovanni B, Baumhauer JF. Midfoot arthritis. J Am Acad Orthop Surg. 2010;18(7):417–25.
11. Sharr PJ, Mangupli MM, Winson IG, Buckley RE. Current management options for displaced intra-articular calcaneal fractures: non-operative, ORIF, minimally invasive reduction and fixation or primary ORIF and subtalar arthrodesis. Foot Ankle Surg. 2016;22(1):1–8. A systematic review article analyzing the operative and nonoperative management options for intra-articular calcaneal fractures. The review demonstrates a progressive trend towards increased operative fixation and reviews evidence to guide management decisions. Level of Evidence: III.
12. Sangeorzan BJ, Wagner UA, Harrington RM, Tencer AF. Contact characteristics of the subtalar joint: the effect of talar neck misalignment. J Orthop Res. 1992;10(4):544–51.
13. Catani F, Benedetti MG, Simoncini L, Leardini A, Giannini S. Analysis of function after intra-articular fracture of the os calcis. Foot Ankle Int. 1999;20(7):417–21.
14. Csizy M, Buckley R, Tough S, Leighton R, Smith J, McCormack R, et al. Displaced intra-articular calcaneal fractures: variables predicting late subtalar fusion. J Orthop Trauma. 2003;17(2):106–12.
15. Buckley R, Tough S, McCormack R, Pate G, Leighton R, Petrie D, et al. Operative compared with nonoperative treatment of displaced intra-articular calcaneal fractures: a prospective, randomized, controlled multicenter trial. J Bone Joint Surg Am. 2002;84(10):1733–44.
16. Agren PH, Wretenberg P, Sayed-Noor AS. Operative versus nonoperative treatment of displaced intra-articular calcaneal fractures: A prospective, randomized, controlled multicenter trial. J Bone Joint Surg Am. 2013;95(15):1351–7. Eighty-two patients with an intra-articular calcaneus fracture were randomized to operative or nonoperative management. At 8–12 years post-operatively there was a trend towards better functional outcomes in the operatively treated group. Post-traumatic osteoarthritis was lower in the operatively treated group. Level of Evidence: II.

17. Flemister AS Jr, Infante AF, Sanders RW, Walling AK. Subtalar arthrodesis for complications of intra-articular calcaneal fractures. Foot Ankle Int. 2000;21(5):392–9.
18. Radnay CS, Clare MP, Sanders RW. Subtalar fusion after displaced intra-articular calcaneal fractures: does initial operative treatment matter? J Bone Joint Surg Am. 2009;91(3):541–6.
19. Watson TS, Shurnas PS, Denker J. Treatment of Lisfranc joint injury: current concepts. J Am Acad Orthop Surg. 2010;18(12):718–28.
20. Myerson MS, Fisher RT, Burgess AR, Kenzora JE. Fracture dislocations of the tarsometatarsal joints: end results correlated with pathology and treatment. Foot Ankle. 1986;6(5):225–42.
21. Dubois-Ferrière V, Lübbeke A, Chowdhary A, Stern R, Dominguez D, Assal M. Clinical outcomes and development of symptomatic osteoarthritis 2 to 24 years after surgical treatment of tarsometatarsal joint complex injuries. J Bone Joint Surg Am. 2016;98(9):713–20. A retrospective study of 61 patients who underwent operative management for TMT joint complex injuries. 72.1% of patients had radiographic evidence of arthrosis but only 54.1% were symptomatic. Risk factors for osteoarthritis included nonanatomic reduction and a history of smoking. Level of Evidence: IV.
22. Kuo RS, Tejwani NC, Digiovanni CW, Holt SK, Benirschke SK, Hansen ST Jr, et al. Outcome after open reduction and internal fixation of Lisfranc joint injuries. J Bone Joint Surg Am. 2000;82(11):1609–18.
23. Philbin T, Rosenberg G, Sferra JJ. Complications of missed or untreated Lisfranc injuries. Foot Ankle Clin. 2003;8(1):61–71.
24. Jeffreys TE. Lisfranc's fracture-dislocation: a clinical and experimental study of tarsometatarsal dislocations and fracture-dislocations. J Bone Joint Surg Br. 1963;45:546–51.
25. Coetzee JC. Making sense of Lisfranc injuries. Foot Ankle Clin. 2008;13(4):695–704.
26. Keiserman LS, Cassandra J, Amis JA. The piano key test: a clinical sign for the identification of subtle tarsometatarsal pathology. Foot Ankle Int. 2003;24(5):437–8.
27. Ågren PH, Tullberg T, Mukka S, Wretenberg P, Sayed-Noor AS. Post-traumatic in situ fusion after calcaneal fractures: a retrospective study with 7-28 years follow-up. Foot Ankle Surg. 2015;21(1):56–9. A retrospective review of 29 patients who underwent in situ arthrodesis for calcaneal malunion and subtalar arthritis. Patients with significant deformity who underwent in situ arthrodesis without restoring hindfoot alignment generally had poor outcomes. Level of Evidence: IV.
28. Thordarson DB. Fusion in posttraumatic foot and ankle reconstruction. J Am Acad Orthop Surg. 2004;12(5):322–33.
29. Haskell A, Pfeiff C, Mann R. Subtalar joint arthrodesis using a single lag screw. Foot Ankle Int. 2004;25(11):774–7.
30. Dingemans SA, Backes M, Goslings JC, de Jong VM, Luitse JS, Schepers T. Predictors of nonunion and infectious complications in patients with posttraumatic subtalar arthrodesis. J Orthop Trauma. 2016;30(10):e331–5. A retrospective study of 93 patients who underwent subtalar arthrodesis. Patients at risk for complications included those who had an initial open fracture or infection. Alcohol, nicotine, and drug abuse were not associated with a higher risk for complications. Level of Evidence: IV.
31. Davies MB, Rosenfeld PF, Stavrou P, Saxby TS. A comprehensive review of subtalar arthrodesis. Foot Ankle Int. 2007;28(3):295–7.
32. Mann R, Beaman D, Horton GA. Isolated subtalar arthrodesis. Foot Ankle Int. 1998;19(8):511–9.
33. Dahm D, Kitaoka HB. Subtalar arthrodesis with internal compression for posttraumatic arthritis. J Bone Joint Surg Br. 1998;80(1):134–8.
34. Sammarco GJ, Tablante EB. Subtalar arthrodesis. Clin Orthop Relat Res. 1998;349:73–80.
35. Chahal J, Stephen DJ, Bulmer B, Daniels T, Kreder HJ. Factors associated with outcome after subtalar arthrodesis. J Orthop Trauma. 2006;20(8):555–61.
36. Easley ME, Trnka HJ, Schon LC, Myerson MS. Isolated subtalar arthrodesis. J Bone Joint Surg Am. 2000;82(5):613–24.

37. Trnka HJ, Easley ME, Lam PW, Anderson CD, Schon LC, Myerson MS. Subtalar distraction bone block arthrodesis. J Bone Joint Surg Br. 2001;83(6):849–54.
38. Myerson MS, Neufeld SK, Uribe J. Fresh-frozen structural allografts in the foot and ankle. J Bone Joint Surg Am. 2005;87(1):113–20.
39. Rammelt S, Grass R, Zawadski T, Biewener A, Zwipp H. Foot function after subtalar distraction bone-block arthrodesis. A prospective study. J Bone Joint Surg Br. 2004;86(5):659–68.
40. Garras DN, Santangelo JR, Wang DW, Easley ME. Subtalar distraction arthrodesis using interpositional frozen structural allograft. Foot Ankle Int. 2008;29(6):561–7.
41. Bednarz PA, Beals TC, Manoli A 2nd. Subtalar distraction bone block fusion: an assessment of outcome. Foot Ankle Int. 1997;18(12):785–91.
42. Burton DC, Olney BW, Horton GA. Late results of subtalar distraction fusion. Foot Ankle Int. 1998;19(4):197–202.
43. Marks RM, Parks BG, Schon LC. Midfoot fusion technique for neuroarthropathic feet: biomechanical analysis and rationale. Foot Ankle Int. 1998;19(8):507–10.
44. Mann RA, Prieskorn D, Sobel M. Midtarsal and tarsometatarsal arthrodesis for primary degenerative osteoarthrosis or osteoarthrosis after trauma. J Bone Joint Surg Am. 1996;78(9):1376–85.
45. Suh JS, Amendola A, Lee KB, Wasserman L, Saltzman CL. Dorsal modified calcaneal plate for extensive midfoot arthrodesis. Foot Ankle Int. 2005;26(7):503–9.
46. Sangeorzan BJ, Veith RG, Hansen ST Jr. Salvage of Lisfranc's tarsometatarsal joint by arthrodesis. Foot Ankle Int. 1990;10(4):193–200.
47. Johnson JE, Johnson KA. Dowel arthrodesis for degenerative arthritis of the tarsometatarsal (Lisfranc) joints. Foot Ankle. 1986;6(5):243–53.
48. Komenda GA, Myerson MS, Biddinger KR. Results of arthrodesis of the tarsometatarsal joints after traumatic injury. J Bone Joint Surg Am. 1996;78(11):1665–76.
49. Richter M, Wippermann B, Krettek C, Schratt HE, Hufner T, Therman H. Fractures and fracture dislocations of the midfoot: occurrence, causes and longterm results. Foot Ankle Int. 2001;22(5):392–8.

Index

A

Acetabular fractures, 31
   antero-lateral approach, 124, 131
   bimodal distribution, 112
   cement-less acetabular components,
      128, 129
   complications, 131
   Harris hip score, 124, 128, 129
   heterotopic ossification, 130
   hypotensive anesthesia, 114
   implant loosening, 130
   implant selection, 114
   incidence, 112
   internal fixation, 112, 114
   intra-operative fluoroscopy, 114
   Kaplan–Meier survivorship, 131
   open reduction, 112
   open reduction internal fixation, 115, 130
   postero-lateral approach, 114, 124,
      130, 131
   post-operative care, 115
   revision surgery, 128
   surgical planning, 113, 114
   total hip arthroplasty, 112, 115, 128–132
Affordable Care Act (ACA), 38
Ankle osteoarthritis
   allograft transplantation, 191
   anatomy, 186
   ankle arthrodesis, 188
   bipolar fresh total osteochondral
      allograft, 191
   conservative treatment, 187, 188
   epidemiology, 186, 187
   fibular osteotomy, 190
   operative treatment, 188–191
   patient evaluation, 187
   prevalence, 185
   Scadanavian Total Ankle Replacement, 189
   supramalleolar osteotomy, 191
   total ankle arthroplasty, 188
Anterior cruciate ligament (ACL), 27
Arthroplasty
   hemiarthroplasty, 50, 51
   humeral resurfacing, 51
   reverse shoulder arthroplasty, 51, 52
   total shoulder arthroplasty, 49, 50
Articular cartilage
   functional unit, 5
   homeostasis, 10
   osteoarthritic, 7–9

B

Bipolar fresh total osteochondral allograft
      (BFTOA), 191
Bone marrow aspirate concentrate (BMAC)
      injection, 188
Bone marrow edema, 21, 22
Bone remodeling, 5

C

Calcaneus fracture, 200, 201
Capsulorrhaphy arthropathy, 47
Carpal instability adaptive (CIA), 78
Carpal instability dissociative (CID), 75
Carpometacarpal (CMC) arthritis, 105, 106
Carpus and intercarpal joints, 74, 76
Cartilage degeneration, 7
Cartilage homeostasis, 5

© Springer Nature Switzerland AG 2021
S. C. Thakkar, E. A. Hasenboehler (eds.), *Post-Traumatic Arthritis*,
https://doi.org/10.1007/978-3-030-50413-7

Conventional radiography (CR)
    arthroscopy confirmed grade II femoro-
        tibial chondromalacia, 18
    disadvantages, 18
    5-point K-L scoring system, 16
    joint space narrowing, 16, 19
    K-L method, 18
    malleolar fracture, 18
    Takakura method, 18
    talar tilt angle, 18
    Van Dick method, 18

D
Darrach procedure, 91
Distal femur fractures
    epidemiology, 153, 154
    intra-articular correction of deformity,
        162, 164
    natural history, 154, 155
    nonoperative management of post-
        traumatic arthritis, 155
    operative management of post-traumatic
        arthritis, 155, 156
    patient evaluation, 155
    primary arthroplasty, 156, 157
    staged osteotomy, 158, 159
    total knee arthroplasty, 158
Distal humerus hemiarthroplasty, 67
Distal interphalangeal (DIP) arthritis
    arthroplasty, 100
    bony mallet finger injuries, 98
    carpometacarpal arthritis, 105, 106
    complications, 98
    compression screw, 98
    conservative treatment, 98
    flexor digitorum profundus avulsion
        injuries, 98
    Herbert compression screws, 99
    K-wire, 98
    metacarpophalangeal joint arthritis,
        103, 104
    proximal interphalangeal joint
        injuries, 100–103
    steroid injections, 98
Distal radioulnar joint (DRUJ), 76

E
Elbow arthrodesis, 69
Elbow fracture
    bimodal age distribution, 60
    classification, 60
    distal humerus hemiarthroplasty, 67
    elbow arthrodesis, 69
    interpositional arthroplasty, 66, 67
    intra-articular distal humerus fractures, 60
    nonsurgical treatment, 62
    osteocapsular debridement
        arthroplasty, 63–66
    post-traumatic elbow stiffness, 61
    radiocapitellar arthroplasty, 67
    surgical planning, 61, 62
    surgical treatment, 62
    total elbow arthroplasty, 68, 69
Extensor pollicis longus (EPL), 88

F
Finite element simulation study, 5
Foot injuries
    anatomy, 200, 201
    arthritic degeneration, 202
    calcaneus fracture, 200, 201
    hondrocyte injury, 200
    hindfoot and midfoot fracture healing,
        204, 205
    hindfoot varus deformity, 202
    imaging, 207, 208
    long-term functional disability, 199
    nonoperative management, 208
    operative management
        hindfoot, 209, 210, 212
        midfoot, 212–214
    physical examination, 206
    preoperative examination, 205
    symptomatic subfibular impingement, 201
    TMT injuries, 200
5-point K-L scoring system, 16

G
Garden III or IV fractures, 139

H
Hand arthritis
    artificial joint replacement, 97
    distal interphalangeal arthritis, 98–100
    prevalence, 97
Hemiarthroplasty, 50, 51
Hip
    management
        primary prevention, 33
        secondary prevention, 34
        tertiary prevention, 34

post-traumatic osteoarthritis
   acetabular fractures, 31
   hip dislocations, 33
   osteonecrosis, 33
   total direct cost, 35, 36
   total indirect cost, 36, 37
Humeral resurfacing, 51
Hyaline cartilage, 21

I
ICD-10 coding system, 37, 38
Intercarpal and radiocarpal arthritis
   management, 81–83
   S4CF vs. *PRC*, 83, 85
   scaphoid nonunion advanced collapse, 79
   scapholunate advanced collapse, 78, 79
   surgical technique, 88
   total wrist arthrodesis, 86, 87
   total wrist arthroplasty, 86
   wrist denervation, 85, 86
International osteoarthritis research society
   (IOARS), 172
Interpositional arthroplasty, 66, 67
Intra-articular distal humerus fractures, 60
Intra-articular fractures, 28, 32
Isolated intercarpal arthritis
   lunotriquetral arthritis, 89, 90
   pisotriquetral arthritis, 90, 91
   scaphotrapeziotrapezoidal arthritis, 89

J
Joint space narrowing (JSN), 16, 19

K
Knee
   management
      primary prevention, 28
      secondary prevention, 29
      tertiary prevention, 29, 30
   post-traumatic osteoarthritis
      anterior cruciate ligament injury, 27
      intra-articular fractures, 28, 32
      meniscal injuries, 27, 28
      total direct cost, 35, 36
      total indirect cost, 36, 37

L
Latency-associated peptide (LAP), 6
Lunotriquetral arthritis, 89, 90
Lunotriquetral interosseous ligament (LTIL), 75

M
Malleolar fracture, 18
Mayo Elbow Performance Index
   (MEPI), 66
Medial opening wedge
   osteotomy, 191
Medicare Severity Diagnosis-Related Groups
   (MS-DRGs), 38
Meniscal injuries, 27, 28
Mesenchymal stem cells (MSCs), 7
Metacarpophalangeal (MCP) joint arthritis,
   103, 104

N
Non-inflammatory arthritis, 9

O
Osteoarthritic synovial system, 9
Osteoarthritis (OA)
   atypical locations, 16, 17
   pain and imaging findings, 21, 22
   posttraumatic vs. idiopathic, 16
Osteocapsular debridement
   arthroplasty, 63–66
Osteochondral allografts (OCA), 173
Osteonecrosis, 33

P
Parathyroid hormone (PTH), 10
Patient-specific finite element stress
   analysis, 4
Pauwel III fractures, 139
Pipkin I fractures, 138
Pipkin III fractures, 138
Pipkin IV fractures, 136, 139
Pisotriquetral arthritis, 90, 91
Posttraumatic arthritis (PTOA)
   arthroplasty, 143, 145, 146
   core decompression, 145
   epidemiology, 135, 136
   femoral head fracture, 138, 139
   femoral neck fracture, 139
   hip arthrodesis, 146
   hip arthroscopy, 143, 144
   hip dislocation, 138
   hip preservation, 144
   intertrochanteric fractures, 141, 142
   non-operative management, 143
   pathophysiology, 136, 137
   trochanteric fractures, 142
   varus malunion, 145

Post-traumatic glenohumeral arthritis
    arthroplasty
        hemiarthroplasty, 50, 51
        humeral resurfacing, 51
        reverse shoulder arthroplasty, 51, 52
        total shoulder arthroplasty, 49, 50
    causes
        fractures, 46, 47
        instability, 47
        isolated chondral lesions/
            osteochaondral injury, 48
    complications, 53
    non-arthroplasty surgery, 52, 53
    nonoperative management, 48, 49
    preoperative evaluation, 49
Proximal humerus fractures, 46
Proximal interphalangeal (PIP) joint
        injuries, 100–103
PTH type-I receptor (PTH1R), 11

R
Radial head and neck fractures, 60
Radiocapitellar arthroplasty, 67
Reverse shoulder arthroplasty, 51, 52

S
Scaphoid nonunion advanced collapse
        (SNAC), 79, 81
Scapholunate advanced collapse
        (SLAC), 78, 79
Scaphotrapeziotrapezoidal arthritis, 89
Subchondral bone
    functional unit, 5
    osteoarthritic, 6, 7, 10
Supramalleolar osteotomy, 191

T
Tibial plateau fractures, 32
    bicondylar fracture, 168
    classifications systems, 168
    CT imaging, 168
    genetic and environmental factors, 169
    incidence, 167
    ligamentous injuries, 168
    medial unicondylar fracture, 168
    meniscal injuries, 168
    posttraumatic osteoarthritis (OA)
        conservative treatment, 172
        ligamentous instability treatment, 168

        long-term outcomes, 168
        osteochondral allografts, 173
        osteotomies, 173, 175
        risk factors, 169
        total knee arthroplasty, 174, 177, 178
        unicompartmental knee
            arthroplasty, 174
    reconstructive surgery, 169
    soft-tissue injuries, 168
Total elbow arthroplasty (TEA), 68, 69
Total knee arthroplasty (TKA), 29
Total shoulder arthroplasty, 49, 50
Total wrist arthrodesis, 86, 87
Total wrist arthroplasty, 86
Transforming growth factor-beta (TGF-β)
    activation mechanism, 6
    articular cartilage
        functional unit, 5
        homeostasis, 10
        osteoarthritic, 7–9
    bisphosphonates, 10
    clinical effects, 10
    disease-modifying efficacy, 10
    function and behavior, 10
    isoforms, 5
    latency-associated peptide, 6
    osteoarthritic synovial system, 9
    parathyroid hormone, 10
    patient-specific finite element stress
        analysis, 4
    potential therapy, 10
    PTH upregulates BMP and Wnt
        signaling, 11
    Smad-dependent canonical pathway, 6
    subchondral bone
        functional unit, 5
        osteoarthritic, 6, 7, 10
    temporal-spatial regulation, 6
    type-I and type-II receptors, 6
Triangular fibrocartilage complex (TFCC), 77
Tricortical iliac crest bone autograft, 210

U
Ulnohumeral arthritis, 60

W
Wrist
    anatomy
        carpus and intercarpal joints, 74, 76
        distal radioulnar joint, 76

arthritis
    distal radioulnar joint and ulnocarpal
       arthritis, 91, 92
    evaluation, 77, 78
    intercarpal and radiocarpal arthritis (*see*
       Intercarpal and radiocarpal arthritis)
    isolated radiocarpal arthritis, 88
    lunotriquetral arthritis, 89, 90
    pisotriquetral arthritis, 90, 91
    scaphotrapeziotrapezoidal
       arthritis, 89
  denervation, 85, 86

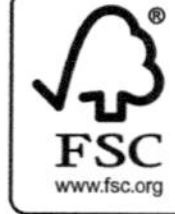

MIX
Papier aus verantwortungsvollen Quellen
Paper from responsible sources
FSC® C105338

If you have any concerns about our products,
you can contact us on
ProductSafety@springernature.com

In case Publisher is established outside the EU,
the EU authorized representative is:
**Springer Nature Customer Service Center GmbH
Europaplatz 3, 69115 Heidelberg, Germany**

Printed by Libri Plureos GmbH
in Hamburg, Germany